Blueprints Notes & Cases
Pathophysiology:
Renal, Hematology, and Oncology

Blueprints Notes & Cases
Series Editor: Aaron B. Caughey MD, MPP, MPH

Blueprints *Notes & Cases—Microbiology and Immunology*
Monica Gandhi, Paul Baum, C. Bradley Hare, Aaron B. Caughey

Blueprints *Notes & Cases—Biochemistry, Genetics, and Embryology*
Juan E. Vargas, Aaron B. Caughey, Annie Tan, Jonathan Z. Li

Blueprints *Notes & Cases—Pharmacology*
Katherine Y. Yang, Larissa R. Graff, Aaron B. Caughey

Blueprints *Notes & Cases—Pathophysiology: Cardiovascular, Endocrine, and Reproduction*
Gordon Leung, Susan H. Tran, Tina O. Tan, Aaron B. Caughey

Blueprints *Notes & Cases—Pathophysiology: Pulmonary, Gastrointestinal, and Rheumatology*
Michael Filbin, Lisa M. Lee, Brian L. Shaffer, Aaron B. Caughey

Blueprints *Notes & Cases—Pathophysiology: Renal, Hematology, and Oncology*
Aaron B. Caughey, Christie del Castillo, Nancy Palmer, Karen Spizer, Dana N. Tuttle

Blueprints *Notes & Cases—Neuroscience*
Robert T. Wechsler, Alexander M. Morss, Courtney J. Wusthoff, Aaron B. Caughey

Blueprints *Notes & Cases—Behavioral Science and Epidemiology*
Judith Neugroschl, Jennifer Hoblyn, Christie del Castillo, Aaron B. Caughey

Blueprints **Notes & Cases**
Pathophysiology:
Renal, Hematology, and Oncology

Aaron B. Caughey, MD, MPP, MPH
Clinical Instructor, Division of Maternal-Fetal Medicine
Department of Obstetrics & Gynecology
University of California, San Francisco
Division of Health Services and Policy Analysis
University of California, Berkeley
Berkeley & San Francisco, California

Christie del Castillo, MD
Class of 2003
University of California, San Francisco, School of Medicine
San Francisco, CA

Nancy Palmer, MD
Class of 2003
University of California, San Francisco, School of Medicine
San Francisco, California

Karen Spizer, MD
Chief Resident
California Pacific Medical Center
San Francisco, California

Dana N. Tuttle, MD
Class of 2003
University of California, San Francisco, School of Medicine
San Francisco, California

Series Editor: Aaron B. Caughey, MD, MPP, MPH

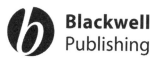

Blackwell
Publishing

© 2004 by Blackwell Publishing

Blackwell Publishing, Inc., 350 Main Street, Malden, Massachusetts 02148-5018, USA
Blackwell Publishing Ltd, 9600 Garsington Road, Oxford OX4 2DQ, UK
Blackwell Science Asia Pty Ltd, 550 Swanston Street, Carlton, Victoria 3053, Australia

04 05 06 07 5 4 3 2 1

ISBN: 1–4051-0352–3

Library of Congress Cataloging-in-Publication Data

Pathophysiology. Renal, hematology, and oncology / Aaron B. Caughey . . . [et al.]. ? 1st ed.
    p. ; cm.— (Blueprints notes & cases)
  Includes index.
  ISBN 1-4051-0352-3 (pbk.)
  1. Cancer—Pathophysiology—Case studies. 2. Kidneys—Pathophysiology—Case studies. 3. Blood—Pathophysiology—
Case studies. I. Caughey, Aaron B. II. Title: Renal, hematology, and oncology. III. Series.
  [DNLM: 1. Kidney Diseases—physiopathology—Problems and Exercises. 2. Hematologic Diseases—physiopathology—
Problems and Exercises. 3. Neoplasms—physiopathology—Problems and Exercises. WJ 18.2 P297 2003]
  RC254.6.P38 2003
  616.6'107—dc21
                                                  2003007430

A catalogue record for this title is available from the British Library

Acquisitions: Beverly Copland
Development: Selene Steneck
Production: Jennifer Kowalewski
Cover design: Hannus Design Associates
Interior design: Janet Bollow Associates
Typesetter: Peirce Graphic Services, in Stuart, FL
Printed and bound by Courier Companies, in Westford, MA

For further information on Blackwell Publishing, visit our website: www.blackwellpublishing.com

Notice: The indications and dosages of all drugs in this book have been recommended in the
medical literature and conform to the practices of the general community. The medications
described do not necessarily have specific approval by the Food and Drug Administration for
use in the diseases and dosages for which they are recommended. The package insert for each
drug should be consulted for use and dosage as approved by the FDA. Because standards for
usage change, it is advisable to keep abreast of revised recommendations, particularly those
concerning new drugs.

Contents

I. RENAL

II. HEMATOLOGY

III. ONCOLOGY

Acknowledgments

We would like to thank the staff at Blackwell Publishing for all of their work on our book, particularly Selene and Jen who coordinated our efforts. I would like to acknowledge the support I receive from my colleagues, mentors, residents, and students at UCSF and UC Berkeley. And most importantly to my dearest friends, Jim and Wendy, whose strength and courage during difficult times is inspiring, and my wife, Susan, whose faith in me keeps me hopeful.
—Aaron Caughey

To God, for all the life and the lessons She has given me. To Tante and Beth, my parents, whose never-ending love and support have been with me throughout both my darkest and most triumphant hours. To Roehl, Carlo, Arnel, and Dennis, my brothers, for teaching me to read, multiply, and stick up for myself. To Jovie, Michelle, and Len, my new sisters. To Dana, Mac Mac, and Ronin, my beautiful niece and nephews. And to Kevin, whose love keeps me grounded while setting me free.
—Christie del Castillo

To my loving and supportive family, especially Dave and Amanda who keep me smiling, and to UCSF for an education that has allowed me to spread my wings and fly.
—Nancy Palmer

To Mom, Dad, Susan, and Miklane my very loving, supportive, and tolerant family. To my friends who have shown me how to live life to its fullest. To California Pacific Medical Center for providing me with a great education.
—Karen Spizer

To my parents, Thomas and Cheryl, for all their hard work and encouragement from the beginning; I would not be here without you. To my amazing husband and best friend, Ted, for his love and support—my gratitude is endless.
—Dana Tuttle

Contributors

Holbrook E. Kohrt
Class of 2004
Stanford University School of Medicine
Stanford, California

Elaine Yu
Class of 2004
University of California, San Francisco, School of Medicine
San Francisco, California

Reviewers

Simon M. Adanin
Class of 2004
Chicago College of Osteopathic Medicine/MWU
Downers Grove, Illinois

Heather Simpkins
Class of 2004
Temple University School of Medicine
Philadelphia, Pennsylvania

Michael Tomblyn
Class of 2004
Rush Medical College
Chicago, Illinois

Angela Turalba
Class of 2004
Brown Medical School
Providence, Rhode Island

Syam Vasireddy
Class of 2005
University of Illinois at Chicago
Chicago, Illinois

Thomas Wong
Class of 2004
SUNY Downstate
Brooklyn, New York

Warren Yunker
MD/PhD Program
University of Alberta
Edmonton, Alberta

Preface

The first two years of medical school are a demanding time for medical students. Whether the school follows a traditional curriculum or one that is case-based, every student is expected to learn and be able to apply basic science information in a clinical situation.

Medical schools are increasingly using clinical presentations as the background to teach the basic sciences. Case-based learning has become more common at many medical schools as it offers a way to catalogue the multitude of symptoms, syndromes and diseases in medicine.

Blueprints Notes & Cases is a new series by Blackwell Publishing designed to provide students a textbook to study the basic science topics combined with clinical data. This method of learning is also the way to prepare for the clinical case format of USMLE questions. The eight books in this series will make the basic science topics not only more interesting, but also more meaningful and memorable. Students will be learning not only the why of a principle, but also how it might commonly be seen in practice.

The books in the *Blueprints* Notes & Cases series feature a comprehensive collection of cases which are designed to introduce one or more basic science topics. Through these cases, students gain an understanding of the coursework as they learn to:

- Think through the cases
- Look for classic presentations of most common diseases and syndromes
- Integrate the basic science content with clinical application
- Prepare for course exams and Step 1 USMLE
- Be prepared for clinical rotations

This series covers all the essential material needed in the basic science courses. Where possible, the books are organized in an organ-based system.

Clinical cases lead off and are the basis for discussion of the basic science content. A list of **"thought questions"** follows the case presentation. These questions are designed to challenge the reader to begin to think about how basic science topics apply to real-life clinical situations. The **answers to these questions** are integrated within the **basic science review and discussion** that follows. This offers a clinical framework from which to understand the basic content.

The discussion section is followed by a high-yield **Thumbnail table and Key Points box** which highlight and summarize the essential information presented in the discussion.

The cases also include two to four **multiple-choice questions** that allow readers to check their knowledge of that topic. Many of the answer explanations provide an opportunity for further discussion by delving into more depth in related areas. An **answer key** for these questions is at the end of the section for easy reference, and **full answer explanations** can be found at the end of the book.

This new series was designed to provide comprehensive content in a concise and templated format for ease in learning. A dedicated attempt was made to include sufficient art, tables, and clinical treatment, all while keeping the books from becoming too lengthy. We know you have much to read and that what you want is high-yield, vital facts.

The authors and series editor for these eight books, as well as everyone in editorial, production, sales and marketing at Blackwell Publishing, have worked long and hard to provide new textbooks to help you learn and be able to apply what you've learned. We engaged in multiple student email surveys and many focus groups to "hear what you needed" in new basic science level textbooks to meet the current curriculums, tests, and coursework. We know that you value this "student to student" approach, and sincerely hope you like what we have put together **just for you.**

Blackwell Publishing and the authors wish you success in your studies and your future medical career. Please feel free to offer us any comments or suggestions on these new books at blue@bos.blackwellpublishing.com.

Abbreviations

α-IFN	alpha interferon		ASA	acetylsalicylic acid
2°	"due to" or "secondary to"		ASO	antistreptolysin O (streptococcal antigen)
5HT	serotonin		AST	aspartate aminotransferase
°C	degrees Celsius		ATL	adult T-cell leukemia/lymphoma
°F	degrees Fahrenheit		ATM	ataxia-telangiectasia
A	adenine		ATN	acute tubular necrosis
Ab	antibody		ATP	adenosine triphosphate
Abd	abdomen		ATPase	enzyme that uses adenosine triphosphate
ABO	blood types with surface antigens A, B, and O		AZT	zidovudine
ACD	anemia of chronic disease		B19	parvovirus B19
ACE	angiotensin-converting enzyme		BC	Bowman's capsule
ACEI	angiotensin-converting enzyme inhibitor		BCC	basal cell carcinoma
ACTH	adrenocorticotropic hormone		bFGF	basic fibroblast growth factor
AD	autosomal dominant		BM	basement membrane
ADH	antidiuretic hormone		BM	bone marrow
ADP	adenosine diphosphate		BP	blood pressure
ADPKD	autosomal-dominant polycystic kidney disease		BPH	benign prostatic hypertrophy
Ag-Ab	antigen-antibody		B-PLL	B-cell prolymphocytic leukemia
AIHA	autoimmune hemolytic anemia		BRCA	breast cancer
AII	angiotensin II		BS	bowel sounds
AIN	acute interstitial nephritis		BS	breath sounds
AJCC	American Joint Committee on Classification (of colorectal cancer)		BUN	blood urea nitrogen
			C1–4	complement 1–4
ALL	acute lymphocytic leukemia		C	cytosine
ALT	alanine aminotransferase		Ca²⁺	serum calcium
AML	acute myelogenous leukemia		CABG	coronary artery bypass graft
ANA	anti-nuclear antibody		cAMP	cyclic adenosine monophosphate
ANC	absolute neutrophil count		CBC	complete blood count
ANCA	antineutrophil cytoplasmic autoantibodies		CD	cluster of differentiation (leukocyte surface markers)
Anti-dsDNA	anti–double-stranded DNA		CD	collecting duct
aPC	activated Protein C		CDK	cyclin-dependent kinase
APC	adenomatous polyposis coli		CEA	carcinoembryonic antigen
APC	antigen-presenting cell		CFU	colony-forming unit
APSAC	acylated plasminogen streptokinase activator complex		Cl, Cl⁻	chloride
AR	autosomal recessive		CLL	chronic lymphocytic leukemia
ARF	acute renal failure			

CML	chronic myeloid (myelogenous) leukemia	ESRD	end-stage renal disease
CMV	cytomegalovirus	ET	essential thrombocytopenia
CN	cranial nerves	EtOH	ethanol, alcohol
CNS	central nervous system	Ext	extremities
CO_2	carbon dioxide	F	factor
Cr	creatinine	FamHx	family history
CRF	chronic renal failure	FAP	familial adenomatous polyposis
CRH	corticotropin-releasing hormone	Fc	constant fragment of immunoglobulin
CSF	cerebral spinal fluid	$Fca\gamma R$	receptor recognizing the constant fragment of immunoglobulin G
CT	computed tomography	$Fc\epsilon R$	receptor recognizing the constant fragment of immunoglobulin E
CV	cardiovascular		
CVA	cerebrovascular accident	Fe	iron
CVA	costovertebral angle	FE_{Na+}	fractional excretion of sodium
CVD	collagen vascular disease	FGF	fibroblast growth factor
DCIS	ductal carcinoma in situ	FH	family history
DCT	distal convoluted tubule	fL	fluid liters
DDAVP	deamino-8-D-arginine vasopressin	FNA	fine needle aspiration
DI	diabetes insipidus	FNHTR	febrile nonhemolytic transfusion reaction
DIC	disseminated intravascular coagulation	FOBT	fecal occult blood test
dL	deciliter	FS	flexible sigmoidoscopy
DNA	deoxyribonucleic acid	FSGS	focal segmental glomerulosclerosis
DRE	digital rectal exam	FT_4	free thyroxine (T_4)
dsDNA	double-stranded DNA	g	grams
DTR	deep tendon reflex	G	guanine
DVT	deep vein thrombosis	G^- or $^+$	Gram stain − or +
EBV	Epstein-Barr virus	G6PD	glucose-6-phosphate dehydrogenase
ECF	extracellular fluid compartment	GBM	glioblastoma multiforme
ECF-A	eosinophil chemotactic factor of anaphylaxis	GBM	glomerular basement membrane
ECM	extracellular matrix	G-CSF	granulocyte–colony-stimulating factor
ED	emergency department	Gen	general
EDGF	epidermal-derived growth factor	GERD	gastroesophageal reflux
EGFR	epidermal growth factor receptor	GFR	glomerular filtration rate
EM	electron microscopy	GI	gastrointestinal
EMB	eosin methylene blue agar	GM-CSF	granulocyte monocyte–colony-stimulating factor
EOMI	extraocular movements intact	GN	glomerulonephritis
Epo	erythropoietin	GnRH	gonadotropin-releasing hormone
ERPF	effective renal plasma flow		

GU	genitourinary	Ig	immunoglobulin
GVHD	graft-versus-host disease	IgA	immunoglobulin A
G# P#	gravida (pregnancies) and para (deliveries)	IgD	immunoglobulin D
H^+	proton/hydrogen ion	IgE	immunoglobulin E
H_2CO_3	carbonic acid	IGF	insulin-like growth factor
H_2O	water	IgG	immunoglobulin G
H4 folate	tetrahydrofolate	IgM	immunoglobulin M
Hb S	hemoglobin S	IL	interleukin
HBV	hepatitis B virus	INR	international normalized ratio
HCC	hepatocellular carcinoma	ITP	idiopathic thrombocytopenic purpura
HCL	hairy cell leukemia	IV	intravenous
HCO3, HCO_3^-	bicarbonate	IVDU	intravenous drug use
Hct	hematocrit	IVP	intravenous pyelogram
HCV	hepatitis C virus	JVD	jugular venous distension
HD	Hodgkin's disease	K, K^+	potassium
HEENT	head, eyes, ears, nose, throat	KOH	potassium hydroxide
Hgb	hemoglobin	L	left
HIT	heparin-induced thrombocytopenia	L + H cells	lymphohistiocytic cells ("popcorn cells")
HIV	human immunodeficiency virus	LAD	leukocyte adhesion deficiencies
HLA	human lymphocytic antigen	LAD	lymphadenopathy
HNPCC	hereditary nonpolyposis colon cancer	LCIS	lobular carcinoma in situ
hpf	high power field	LDH	lactate dehydrogenase
HPI	history of present illness	LFT	liver function test
HPV	human papilloma virus	LGL	large granular lymphocytic leukemia
HR	heart rate	LH	loop of Henle
HS	hereditary spherocytosis	LLQ	left lower quadrant
HSM	hepatosplenomegaly	LM	light microscopy
HTLV-1	human T-cell leukemia virus	LMW	low molecular weight
HTN	hypertension	LPS	lipopolysaccharide (component of endotoxin of gram-negative bacteria)
HUS	hemolytic-uremic syndrome		
IBD	inflammatory bowel disease	LUQ	left upper quadrant
IBS	irritable bowel syndrome	LV	left ventricle
ICF	intracellular fluid compartment	MAHA	microangiopathic hemolytic anemia
ICU	intensive care unit	MCHC	mean corpuscular hemoglobin concentration
IF	immunofluorescence	MCV	mean corpuscular volume
IF	intrinsic factor	MDS	myelodysplastic syndromes
IFN	interferon	Meds	medications

MEN	multiple endocrine neoplasia	PE	physical exam
MF	myelofibrosis	PE	pulmonary embolism
MHC	major histocompatibility complex	PERRLA	pupils equally round and reactive to light and accommodation
MI	myocardial infarction		
mL	milliliter	pg	picogram
MM	multiple myeloma	PG	prostaglandin
MMM	myelofibrosis with myeloid metaplasia	PID	pelvic inflammatory disease
MPO	myeloperoxidase	*PKD1*	polycystic kidney disease 1 gene
MRG	murmurs, rubs, gallops	*PKD2*	polycystic kidney disease 2 gene
MRI	magnetic resonance imaging	Plt	platelets
M/S	musculoskeletal	PMD	primary medical doctor
MW	molecular weight	PMH, PMHx	past medical history
Na, Na$^+$	sodium	PMN	polymorphonuclear cell (neutrophil)
NaCl	sodium chloride	PNH	paroxysmal nocturnal hemoglobinuria
NADPH	reduced nicotinamide adenine dinucleotide phosphate	PO$_4^{2-}$	phosphate
		PPD	purified protein derivative (tuberculin antigen)
Neuro	neurologic	PSA	prostate serum antigen
ng	nanogram	PSH, PSHx	past surgical history
NHL	non-Hodgkin's lymphoma	PT	prothrombin time
NK	natural killer	PTH	parathyroid hormone
NI	normal	PTHrP	parathyroid hormone related peptide
NSAIDs	nonsteroidal anti-inflammatory drugs	PTT	partial thromboplastin time
NSE	nonspecific esterase	PUD	peptic ulcer disease
NST	no special type	PV	polycythemia vera
O$_2$Sat	hemoglobin oxygen saturation	R	right
OR	operating room	RA	rheumatoid arthritis
ORF	open reading frame	RA	room air
P	plasma concentration	RBC	red blood cell
P	pulse	RBF	renal blood flow
P#	para (deliveries)	RFLP	restriction fragment length polymorphism
PAH	para-aminohippuric acid	RH	rhesus factor
PAMP	pathogen-associated molecular patterns	RLQ	right lower quadrant
PBS	peripheral blood smear	ROS	review of systems
PCR	polymerase chain reaction	RR	respiratory rate
PCRV	polycythemia rubra vera	RRR	regular rate and rhythm
PCT	proximal convoluted tubule	RS cells	Reed-Sternberg cells
PDGF	platelet-derived growth factor	RTA	renal tubular acidosis

RUQ	right upper quadrant	TLR	toll-like receptor
s_1	first heart sound	TNF	tumor necrosis factor
s_2	second heart sound	TNM	tumor, node, metastasis (classification system)
s_3	abnormal heart sound heard right after s_2; sound of ventricle filling	tPA	tissue plasminogen activator
s_4	abnormal heart sound heard right before s_1; atrial kick	T-PLL	T-cell prolymphocytic leukemia
		TRUS	transrectal ultrasound
SaO_2	oxygen saturation	TSH	thyroid-stimulating hormone
SCC	squamous cell carcinoma	TT	thrombin time
SCD	sickle cell disease	TTP	thrombotic thrombocytopenic purpura
SCU-PA	single-chain urokinase type plasminogen activator	TURP	transurethral radical prostatectomy
SH	social history	U	urine concentration
SIADH	syndrome of inappropriate antidiuretic hormone	UA	urine analysis
		UG	urogenital
SLE	systemic lupus erythematosus	UPEP	urine protein electrophoresis
SPEP	serum protein electrophoresis	US	ultrasound
SRS-A	slow-reacting substance of anaphylaxis	UTI	urinary tract infection
S/Sx	signs and symptoms	UV	ultraviolet
T	temperature	VA	Veterans Administration
T	thymine	VEGF	vascular endothelial growth factor
$t(x,y)$	translocation between chromosome x and chromosome y	VHL	von Hippel–Lindau
		VIP	vasoactive intestinal polypeptide
T_3	triiodothyronine (active form of thyroid hormone)	VS	vital signs
TB	tuberculosis	vWD	von Willebrand's disease
TBW	total body water	vWF	von Willebrand's factor
TdT	terminal deoxynucleotidyl transferase	WAGR	*W*ilms' tumor, *a*niridia, *g*enital anomalies, mental *r*etardation syndrome
TF	tubular fluid		
TFPI	tissue factor pathway inhibitor	WBC	white blood cell
TFT	thyroid function test	WHO	World Health Organization
TGF-α	transforming growth factor-alpha	*WT-1*	Wilms' tumor 1 gene (11p13)
TGF-β	transforming growth factor-beta	*WT-2*	Wilms' tumor 2 gene
T_h-cell	T-helper cell (type 1 or 2)		
T*is*	Tumor in situ		

Normal Ranges of Laboratory Values

BLOOD, PLASMA, SERUM

Alanine aminotransferase (ALT, GPT at 30 C)	8–20 U/L
Amylase, serum	25–125 U/L
Asparatate aminotransferase (AST, GOT at 30 C)	8–20 U/L
Bilirubin, serum (adult) Total // Direct	0.1–1.0 mg/dL // 0.0–0.3 mg/dL
Calcium, serum (Ca^{2+})	8.4–10.2 mg/dL
Cholesterol, serum	Rec: < 200 mg/dL
Cortisol, serum	0800 h: 5–23 μg/dL // 1600 h: 3–15 μg/dL
	2000 h: ≤ 50% of 0800 h
Creatine kinase, serum	Male: 25–90 U/L
	Female: 10–70 U/L
Creatinine, serum	0.6–1.2 mg/dL
Electrolytes, serum	
Sodium (Na^+)	136–145 mEq/L
Chloride (Cl^-)	95–105 mEq/L
Potassium (K^+)	3.5–5.0 mEq/L
Bicarbonate (HCO_3^-)	22–28 mEq/L
Magnesium (Mg^{2+})	1.5–2.0 mEq/L
Ferritin, serum	Male: 15–200 ng/mL
	Female: 12–150 ng/mL
Follicle-stimulating hormone, serum/plasma	Male: 4–25 mIU/mL
	Female: premenopause 4–30 mIU/mL
	midcycle peak 10–90 mIU/mL
	postmenopause 40–250 mIU/mL
Gases, arterial blood (room air)	
pH	7.35–7.45
P_{CO_2}	33–45 mm Hg
P_{O_2}	75–105 mm Hg
Glucose, serum	Fasting: 70–110 mg/dL
	2-h postprandial: < 120 mg/dL
Growth hormone—arginine stimulation	Fasting: < 5 ng/mL
	provocative stimuli: > 7 ng/mL
Iron	50–70 μg/dL
Lactate dehydrogenase, serum	45–90 U/L
Luteinizing hormone, serum/plasma	Male: 6–23 mIU/mL
	Female: follicular phase 5–30 mIU/mL
	midcycle 75–150 mIU/mL
	postmenopause 30–200 mIU/mL
Osmolality, serum	275–295 mOsmol/kg
Parathyroid hormone, serum, N-terminal	230–630 pg/mL
Phosphate (alkaline), serum (p-NPP at 30 C)	20–70 U/L
Phosphorus (inorganic), serum	3.0–4.5 mg/dL
Prolactin, serum (hPRL)	< 20 ng/mL
Proteins, serum	
Total (recumbent)	6.0–7.8 g/dL
Albumin	3.5–5.5 g/dL
Globulin	2.3–3.5 g/dL
Thyroid-stimulating hormone, serum or plasma	0.5–5.0 μU/mL
Thyroidal iodine (^{123}I) uptake	8–30% of administered dose/24 h
Thyroxine (T_4), serum	5–12 μg/dL
Triglycerides, serum	35–160 mg/dL
Triiodothyronine (T_3), serum (RIA)	115–190 ng/dL
Triiodothyronine (T_3), resin uptake	25–35%
Urea nitrogen, serum (BUN)	7–18 mg/dL
Uric acid, serum	3.0–8.2 mg/dL

CEREBROSPINAL FLUID

Cell count	0–5 cells/mm^3
Chloride	118–132 mEq/L
Gamma globulin	3–12% total proteins
Glucose	40–70 mg/dL
Pressure	70–180 mm H$_2$O
Proteins, total	< 40 mg/dL

HEMATOLOGIC

Bleeding time (template)	2–7 minutes
Erythrocyte count	Male: 4.3–5.9 million/mm^3
	Female: 3.5–5.5 million/mm^3
Erythrocyte sedimentation rate (Westergren)	Male: 0–15 mm/h
	Female: 0–20 mm/h
Hematocrit	Male: 41–53%
	Female: 36–46%
Hemoglobin A$_{1C}$	≤ 6%
Hemoglobin, blood	Male: 13.5–17.5 g/dL
	Female: 12.0–16.0 g/dL
Leukocyte count and differential	
Leukocyte count	4500–11,000/mm^3
Segmented neutrophils	54–62%
Bands	3–5%
Eosinophils	1–3%
Basophils	0–0.75%
Lymphocytes	25–33%
Monocytes	3–7%
Mean corpuscular hemoglobin	25.4–34.6 pg/cell
Mean corpuscular hemoglobin concentration	31–36% Hb/cell
Mean corpuscular volume	80–100 μm^3
Partial thromboplastin time (activated)	25–40 seconds
Platelet count	150,000–400,000/mm^3
Prothrombin time	11–15 seconds
Reticulocyte count	0.5–1.5% of red cells
Thrombin time	< 2 seconds deviation from control
Volume	
Plasma	Male: 25–43 mL/kg
	Female: 28–45 mL/kg
Red cell	Male: 20–36 mL/kg
	Female: 19–31 mL/kg

SWEAT

Chloride	0–35 mmol/L

URINE

Calcium	100–300 mg/24 h
Chloride	Varies with intake
Creatine clearance	Male: 97–137 mL/min
	Female: 88–128 mL/min
Osmolality	50–1400 mOsmol/kg
Oxalate	8–40 μg/mL
Potassium	Varies with diet
Proteins, total	< 150 mg/24 h
Sodium	Varies with diet
Uric acid	Varies with diet

Part I

Renal

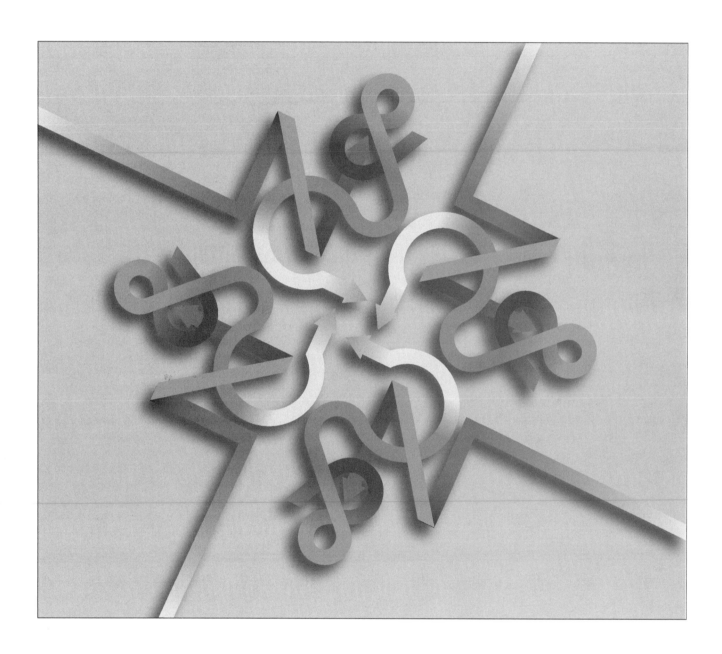

HPI: DD is a 22-year-old Caucasian female brought to the emergency department (ED) by ambulance following several stab wounds to the flank inflicted by her estranged husband.

PE: A congenitally absent right kidney is incidentally discovered during her ED evaluation.

Thought Questions

- What is normal kidney anatomy?

- What are the functional divisions of the nephron?

- What is the normal histology of the nephron?

Basic Science Review and Discussion

The Kidneys The kidneys are paired **retroperitoneal** organs, lying at the level of the first lumbar vertebrae. The right kidney lies slightly lower than the left due to displacement by the large right lobe of the liver. They are approximately the size of a fist and weigh about 150 g each. The left renal vein lies anterior to the abdominal aorta and posterior to the superior mesenteric artery. The kidney is covered by a fibrous capsule, perirenal fat, renal fascia continuous with the transversalis fascia, and extensive pararenal fat that anchors and protects the kidney. The adrenal glands lie on the upper poles of each kidney.

The kidney is composed of two major components: the functional renal parenchyma made up of the cortex and medulla, and the collecting system composed of the minor and major calyces, renal pelvis, and ureters (Figure 1-1). The renal cortex contains the glomeruli, and the medullary pyramids contain the long tubules and vasculature responsible for concentrating the urine.

The kidney is a highly vascularized organ and receives 20% of cardiac output with each heartbeat, filtering 1700 L of blood per day, producing 1 L of urine per day. The resulting glomerular filtration rate (GFR) is 120 mL/min.

The Nephron The nephron is composed of distinct parts with distinct roles. The **proximal convoluted tubule** (PCT) is responsible for absorbing 75% of the glomerular filtrate including all glucose and amino acids, and most of the sodium, bicarbonate, and water. As fluid flows down the PCT, solutes are reabsorbed by transporters (many Na$^+$ dependent), and water follows via osmotic forces. Inulin is used experimentally to measure water reabsorption along the PCT. Although it is neither reabsorbed nor secreted, its concentration in the tubular fluid (TF) increases to three times that of its plasma concentration (P) because so much water is reabsorbed along the length of the PCT. Solutes that

are primarily secreted (para-aminohippuric acid, PAH) have steeply increasing TF/P ratios and solutes that are primarily reabsorbed have sharply decreasing TF/P ratios (Figure 1-2).

Most solutes are reabsorbed by secondary active cotransport with Na$^+$. The necessary electrochemical gradient is maintained by a Na$^+$/K$^+$ adenosine triphosphatase (ATPase) in the PCT cell membrane. K$^+$ and Cl$^-$ are absorbed paracellularly (between cells). The PCT cells are also critically involved in acid-base homeostasis. They have a **brush border,** which provides ample surface area for absorption and which contains **carbonic anhydrase**, an enzyme responsible for both steps in the reaction $H^+ + HCO_3^- \leftrightarrow H_2CO_3 \leftrightarrow H_2O + CO_2$. The end result is essentially secretion of H$^+$ ions and regeneration of HCO$_3^-$ (Figure 1-3). The PCT secretes bases like ammonia, which buffer luminal H$^+$.

The loop of Henle is responsible for establishing the medullary gradient via the **countercurrent multiplier**

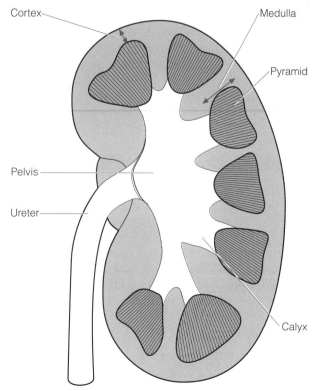

Figure 1-1 The kidney.

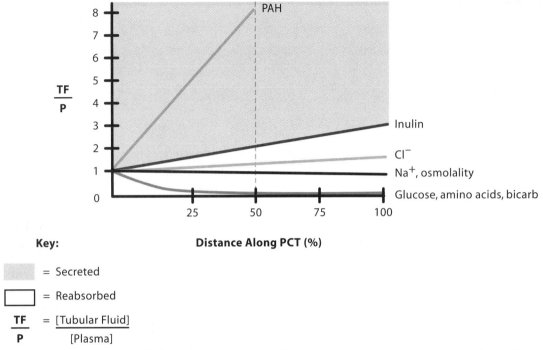

Figure 1-2 Proximal convoluted tubule. The concentrations of various substances change as they are reabsorbed or secreted and as water is reabsorbed along the length of the PCT.

mechanism (discussed in a later case), which then enables the concentration of urine in the collecting tubules. The **thin descending limb** is permeable to water but impermeable to sodium. The **thick ascending limb** is impermeable to water but Na^+, K^+, and $2Cl^-$ are absorbed via a secondary active transporter. As these osmotically active substances cross into the interstitium, the osmotic gradient in the medulla increases. The osmolarity of the deep medulla can reach 1200 to 1400 mOsm. Highly diffusible urea also plays an important role in creating the medullary osmotic gradient.

The **distal convoluted tubule** (DCT) is mainly involved in reabsorbing Na^+ and Ca^{2+}. The luminal side of the distal convoluted tubule cell has a Na^+/Cl^- symport and a Ca^{2+} channel under the control of parathyroid hormone (PTH). (See Figure 1-3.) A specialized portion of the DCT, the **macula densa**, abuts the afferent arteriole of the glomerulus. The macula densa detects decreased delivery of NaCl, indicative of decreased fluid flow (and thus decreased GFR), and causes increased **renin** release from juxtaglomerular granular cells, specialized smooth muscle cells of the afferent arteriole. Renin has multiple downstream effects that increase renal sodium and fluid reabsorption.

Several collecting tubules converge into a **collecting duct** (CD) made up of two types of cells, the principal cell and the intercalated cell. The **principal cell** contains Na^+ channels under the influence of **aldosterone**, K^+ secretion

channels, and H_2O channels inserted by the actions of **antidiuretic hormone (ADH)** on the cell. Aldosterone also increases the activity of the Na^+/K^+ ATPase on the interstitial border, thereby increasing the total amount of sodium reabsorbed and potassium secreted. As water follows sodium, aldosterone increases the amount of water reabsorbed and thus the concentration of urine. The water channels (aquaporins) inserted in response to ADH allow for maximal concentration of urine. ADH (vasopressin) is secreted from the posterior pituitary in response to low osmolality or blood pressure. The **intercalated cells** contain an ATP driven H^+ pump and a HCO_3^-/Cl^- antiport and are thus critical in influencing acid-base homeostasis.

Vasculature   The **vasa recta** are the blood vessels that run the length of the renal medulla, perfusing the renal parenchyma itself. They are not significantly involved in the solute reabsorption function of the kidney and do not affect the medullary gradient (in truth, the ascending and descending limbs both affect the gradient, cancelling each other out). The **peritubular capillaries** run directly along the PCT surface in the renal cortex and receive the solutes absorbed by the tubular cells.

The **afferent** and **efferent arterioles** control the amount of blood flow through the kidney, and thus, the GFR. This mechanism ensures that in times of low flow, renal perfusion is preserved both to protect this important organ and to ensure proper electrolyte and fluid homeostasis.

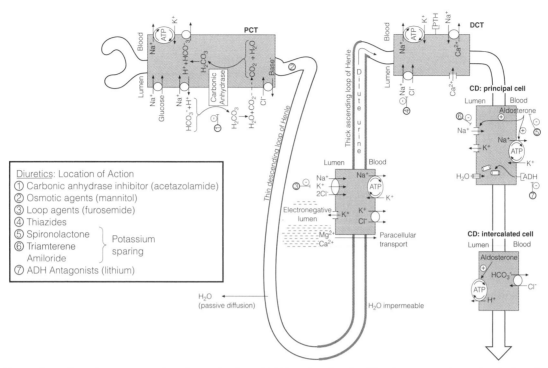

Figure 1-3 The nephron. (Drawing courtesy of Tracie Harris, Class of 2003, University of California, San Francisco, School of Medicine.)

Diuretics: Location of Action
① Carbonic anhydrase inhibitor (acetazolamide)
② Osmotic agents (mannitol)
③ Loop agents (furosemide)
④ Thiazides
⑤ Spironolactone ⎫
⑥ Triamterene   ⎬ Potassium
   Amiloride   ⎭ sparing
⑦ ADH Antagonists (lithium)

Case Conclusion Domestic violence is encountered often in ERs, women's health clinics, and all primary care clinics. It should always be on the differential diagnosis. This patient had had several visits to the ER previously, but the domestic violence was not picked up. The congenitally absent kidney is a relatively common finding with significance only when the functional reserve of a second kidney is indispensable (trauma, renal damage or disease). Fortunately for DD, the stab wounds narrowly missed the artery supplying her only functional kidney. Since domestic violence tends to escalate, next time she might not be so lucky.

Thumbnail: Nephron Histology

	Proximal convoluted tubule (PCT)	Loop of Henle: thin descending	Loop of Henle: thick ascending	Distal convoluted tubule (DCT)	Collecting duct (CD)
Main role	Reabsorption of 75% of the glomerular filtrate	Establish medullary concentration gradient via countercurrent multiplication		Reabsorption of Na^+, secretion of H^+ and K^+	Reabsorption of water, Na^+, with ADH and aldosterone
Location	Cortex	Medulla	Medulla	Renal cortex	Medullary rays
Epithelium	Cuboidal	Simple squamous	Cuboidal	Cuboidal	Columnar
Appearance under light microscope	• Prominent **brush border** of microvilli + artifactual microvilli debris in lumen • Indistinct boundaries between cells • **Intensely staining** due to mitochondria, which give rise to **basal striations** (microvilli at basal surface)	• No brush border + clear, well-defined lumen without debris		• No brush border + clear, well-defined lumen without debris • Less intensely stained due to less organelles	• Principal cells are poorly stained w/**clear boundaries** between cells

Key Points

▶ The kidneys are retroperitoneal.

▶ The PCT is responsible for absorption of 75% of filtered solutes.

▶ The loop of Henle establishes the medullary interstitial concentration gradient.

▶ The DCT is responsible for calcium reabsorption under the influence of PTH.

▶ The collecting duct allows for the secretion of acid and the concentration of urine under the influence of aldosterone and ADH.

Questions

1. A 58-year-old man reports to his primary care clinic every 6 months to be monitored for his chronic hypertension. He takes spironolactone, a potassium-sparing diuretic that competitively inhibits the actions of aldosterone on the kidney. Aldosterone's actions include which of the following:

   A. Blocking the $Na^+/K^+/2Cl^-$ channel in the thick ascending loop of Henle.

   B. Inserting aquaporins (water channels) into the principal cells of the cortical collecting duct.

   C. Increasing Ca^{2+} reabsorption in the distal convoluted tubule.

   D. Increasing the activity of the Na^+/K^+ ATPase and the sodium channels in the collecting tubules.

   E. Increasing the activity of carbonic anhydrase in the proximal convoluted tubule.

2. A 33-year-old Hispanic woman presents to her Ob/Gyn office for prenatal care. She is found to have 3+ glucose in her urine. If her nephron was examined under the light microscope, what would be the appearance of the segment responsible for absorbing all filtered glucose?

   A. Pale staining with distinct borders between cells.

   B. Dark staining with basal striations and debris in the lumen.

   C. Thin squamous epithelium lining a clear lumen.

   D. Pale-staining with debris in the lumen.

   E. Dark staining with distinct borders between cells.

3. A 28-year-old woman with bipolar disorder is diagnosed with nephrogenic diabetes insipidus caused by lithium. Her kidneys are unable to concentrate urine in response to ADH. As a result, she urinates huge volumes of dilute urine even though her serum sodium is elevated. Prolonged diuresis from any cause leads to washout of the medullary osmotic gradient established by which of the following:

   A. The vasa recta

   B. The peritubular capillaries

   C. The principal cells

   D. The loop of Henle

   E. The intercalated cells

HPI: RL is a 16-year-old boy who is brought to the ER by paramedics following a motor vehicle accident 3 days after receiving his driver's license. His past medical history includes asthma as a child and allergic rhinitis. He uses albuterol rarely. He is a high school student and lives with his single mother. He does not smoke, drink, or use any drugs.

PE: T 37.8 HR 90 BP 112/70
Abdominal exam reveals some guarding and a firm mass in the left pelvic region. Abdominal and pelvic plain films (x-rays) are ordered to rule out pelvic fractures. A pelvic kidney, lying close to the left common iliac artery, is incidentally discovered on the plain film. There are no pelvic or other fractures.

Thought Questions

- What are the embryologic origins of adult genitourinary structures?

- How does knowledge of kidney embryology help to explain the existence of a pelvic kidney or a horseshoe kidney?

- What are the other significant congenital kidney anomalies?

Basic Science Review and Discussion

The kidneys are formed from **intermediate mesoderm** (Figure 2-1). Kidney development begins in the fourth week with the formation of the first of three kidney scaffolds that arise and regress sequentially before the permanent kidney develops (Figure 2-2). This first scaffold is the **pronephros**, which is nonfunctional. In the following week, the **mesonephros** develops and functions briefly, creating the **mesonephric duct (wolffian duct).** The **ureteric bud** is an offshoot of the mesonephric duct that dilates and subdivides to form the **urinary collecting system** (collecting tubules, calyces, renal pelvis, and ureter) in both males and females. In males, in the presence of testosterone, the mesonephric duct also forms the **vas deferens, epididymis, ejaculatory duct, and seminal vesicles.** In females, it degen-

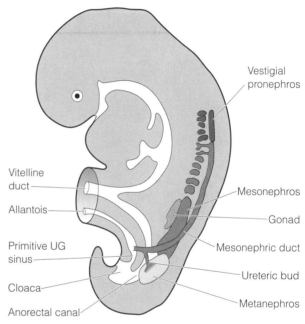

Figure 2-2 Embryonic renal development.

erates entirely except for the vestigial Gartner's duct that can form a benign cyst along the broad ligament. The **para-mesonephric duct (müllerian duct)** runs alongside the mesonephric duct. It is involved in genital tract embryology but not in urinary tract or renal embryology and is thus not discussed in detail here. The third scaffold, the **meta-nephros** appears in the 5th week of gestation and becomes the functioning kidney by the 9th week of gestation. The ureteric bud from the mesonephric duct contacts the meta-nephros and induces it to form nephrons. If this contact does not occur, **renal agenesis** results. The adjacent dorsal aorta also sends out collaterals into the metanephros that ultimately develop into glomerular tufts.

Before the seventh week, the **cloaca** (the proximal portion of the allantois, distally connected to the yolk sac) is divided into the **urogenital (UG) sinus** and the anorectal canal. During this process, the caudal-most portion of the mesonephric duct is absorbed. Thus, the ureteric bud no longer buds off of the mesonephric duct but enters the UG

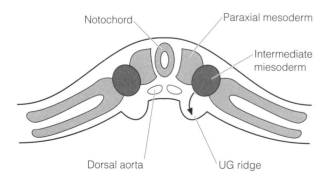

Figure 2-1 Cross-section of 4-week embryo.

sinus directly. As such, the UG sinus forms the bladder and the ureteric buds form the ureters. As the kidneys ascend, the ureteric buds (ureters in the adult) are pulled cranially, and the mesonephric ducts (the ejaculatory ducts in the adult) move caudally until coming to rest in the prostatic urethra. The resulting relationship is that of *"water (urine) flowing under the bridge (ejaculatory duct)"* (Figure 2-3). In the male, buds from the urethra form the **prostate** gland. The UG sinus forms the bladder and is in continuity with the urethra caudally and the allantois cranially. The **urachus** is the fibrotic cord that remains when the allantois is obliterated and becomes the **median umbilical ligament** in the adult.

Congenital Anomalies   The kidney, a retroperitoneal organ, is initially located in the pelvic region and ascends with fetal growth in the lumbar and sacral regions. During its ascent, it is vascularized by arteries that originate from the aorta at continuously higher levels while the lower vessels degenerate. If they do not degenerate, **accessory renal arteries** remain. During their ascent, the kidneys pass through a fork formed by the umbilical arteries. If a kidney gets stuck, as it does in one in 20,000 people, a **pelvic kidney** results. Alternately, the kidneys can pass so closely that they fuse, forming a **horseshoe kidney.** The horseshoe gets stuck on the inferior mesenteric artery during the ascent, forcing the kidney to remain in the lower lumbar area. This is a common abnormality found in 1/600 people and has no functional significance. Clinically *significant* congenital renal malformations are rare. Most abnormalities are likely due to acquired developmental defects that arise in utero. Because of their similar embryologic origins, patients with renal anomalies are at higher risk of other GU tract anomalies such as uterine, cervical, and vaginal defects.

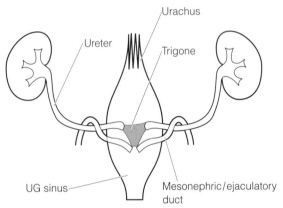

Figure 2-3 Ureters and mesonephric duct.

Case Conclusion: The patient's parents are very concerned about this "pelvic mass." The third year medical student on her trauma surgery rotation is asked to explain that this is a benign condition that is unlikely to cause any problems. However, the patient should tell future medical providers about his left pelvic kidney to avoid unnecessary work-ups and to alert them to the possibility of kidney injury in the event of pelvic trauma.

Thumbnail: Renal Embryology

Embryonic origin	Male	Female
Mesonephric (wolffian) duct	Epididymis Vas deferens Ejaculatory duct Seminal vesicle Urinary collecting system	Gartner's duct Urinary collecting system
Paramesonephric (müllerian) duct	No major structures	Fallopian tubes Uterus
Urogenital sinus	Prostate Bulbourethral (Cowper's) glands Urinary bladder Urethra	Vagina Urethral and paraurethral glands Greater vestibular (Bartholin's) glands Urinary bladder Urethra
Allantois	Urachus → median umbilical ligament	Urachus → median umbilical ligament

Thumbnail: Congenital Renal Anomalies

Bilateral renal agenesis (Potter's syndrome)	Agenesis of the ureteric bud → agenesis of the kidney Causes **oligohydramnios** → pulmonary hypoplasia → limb and facial deformities Not compatible with life ex utero (**stillbirth**)
Accessory renal arteries	End arteries that arise from the aorta and supply a particular area of a kidney
Congenital polycystic kidney disease	Bilateral multiple small cysts → renal insufficiency Present at birth → death in infancy or childhood
Horseshoe kidney	Fusion of inferior poles of kidney → trapped in pelvis by the inferior mesenteric artery
Pelvic kidney	One kidney does not make the ascent

Key Points

▶ The mesonephric (wolffian) duct forms predominantly male sex organs.

▶ The paramesonephric (müllerian) duct forms the female sex organs.

▶ The development of the urinary and genital systems are inextricably linked.

▶ Knowledge of renal embryology helps us understand how congenital anomalies occur.

Questions

1. A nurse in the well-baby nursery comes to you concerned that urine is draining out of a neonate's umbilicus. You suspect an **urachal fistula.** This is the abnormal patency of what structure?

   A. Median umbilical ligament
   B. Vitelline duct
   C. Paramesonephric duct
   D. Wolffian duct
   E. Medial umbilical ligament

2. A 22-year-old G1 P0 woman at 36 weeks' gestation presents to her obstetrician with signs and symptoms of preterm labor. She has received no prenatal care. A stillborn infant is delivered by vaginal delivery. An autopsy reveals lung hypoplasia, limb deformities, and several other abnormalities. What could have caused this syndrome?

   A. Unilateral renal agenesis
   B. Tracheoesophageal atresia
   C. Duodenal atresia
   D. Bilateral agenesis of the ureteric buds
   E. Congenital polycystic kidneys

HPI: AB, a 55-year-old man, is referred to you, the nephrologist, by his primary care physician for a rising serum creatinine. The patient has long-standing, poorly controlled hypertension. He has difficulty remembering to take his hypertension medications. He has no other medical problems but does smoke a pack a day. His primary care physician reports that his serum creatinine 1 year ago was 1.0 mg/dL and has now risen to 1.7 mg/dL. He has a family history of hypertension, stroke, and heart disease.

PE: BP 178/100

Aside from the elevated blood pressure, his vital signs are otherwise normal. He is mildly obese, has a normal lung exam, and on cardiac exam has a regular rate and rhythm with a notable S_4. The rest of his exam is normal.

Labs: Na^+ 140 mEq/L, K^+ 4.2 mEq/L, HCO_3^- 24 mEq/L, Cl^- 101 mEq/L, BUN 20 mg/dL, creatinine 2.0 mg/dL, WBC 10,000/mL, hematocrit 40%, platelets 230,000/mL. Urine dipstick: 1+ protein. 24-hour urine collection: volume 720 mL, creatinine 200 mg/dL, protein 1.1 g.

Thought Questions

- How do we estimate kidney function?
- What are autoregulation and tubuloglomerular feedback?
- What is the GFR and what factors determine it?
- What is creatinine clearance?

Basic Science Discussion and Review

The kidney receives 25% of the cardiac output and maintains consistent perfusion over a wide range of blood pressures. Between systolic blood pressures of 80 to 220 mm Hg, the kidneys maintain blood flow, being neither over- nor underperfused, by **autoregulation** of blood flow. Two theories seek to explain the localized response of the kidney to changes in systemic blood pressure. If the systemic blood pressure rises, the renal arterioles constrict, limiting the amount of renal blood flow. If the systemic pressure drops, the arterioles dilate to maintain blood flow. This response of the renal arterioles is an intrinsic response of smooth muscle to stretch and is termed **myogenic.**

Tubuloglomerular feedback also aids in maintaining consistent renal perfusion and is mediated by the juxtaglomerular apparatus. A drop in renal perfusion transiently decreases the amount of fluid delivered to the cells of the macula densa, which senses this drop and initiates a dilation of the afferent arteriole maintaining blood flow. Conversely, an elevation in blood pressure and thus in delivery of filtrate to the macula densa results in constriction of the afferent arteriole. Autoregulation of the kidneys is an important mechanism by which glomerular filtration rate (GFR) is maintained.

Control of the Glomerular Filtration Rate The renal afferent (carrying blood toward the glomerulus) and efferent (carrying blood away from the glomerulus) arterioles are under the influence of a number of vasoactive substances (Figure 3-1). Renal blood vessel tone is regulated by local mecha-

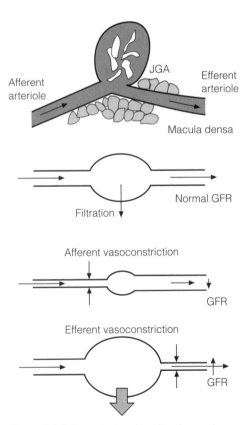

Figure 3-1 Schematic drawing of a glomerulus, depicting the afferent and efferent arterioles and their relationships to the macula densa.

nisms but also by sympathetic tone. Both the afferent and efferent arterioles constrict in response to catecholamines, which decrease renal blood flow (RBF) and thus GFR. The powerful vasoconstrictor angiotensin II preferentially constricts the efferent arteriole, preserving GFR. This effect may be abolished by angiotensin I converting enzyme inhibitors and angiotensin II receptor blockers. Renally produced prostaglandins have vasodilatory effects on the afferent and efferent arterioles (afferent greater than efferent), protecting the kidney against drastic decreases in RBF. Nonsteroidal anti-inflammatory drugs (NSAIDs) decrease production of prostaglandins, blunting their vasodilatory effect, potentially damaging renal function.

Measuring GFR Renal plasma flow can be measured by the clearance from the blood of PAH, an organic anion not normally found in the body. Clearance (C), in general terms, is the volume of a substance removed from the plasma per unit time.

$$C = UV/P$$

U = concentration of substance in urine = mg/mL

V = urine volume/flow = mL/min

P = concentration of substance in the plasma = mg/mL

$$\text{mL/min} = \frac{\text{mg/mL} * \text{mL/min}}{\text{mg/mL}}$$

Infused PAH is readily filtered by and almost completely secreted by tubular cells and is thus a good estimate of renal plasma flow. Only 90% of PAH is secreted, because a portion of the blood flowing through the kidney is not in contact with the renal tubules; thus the clearance of PAH from the plasma actually underestimates the renal plasma flow by 10%. We use the term *effective* **renal plasma flow (ERPF)** to indicate this estimate.

$$ERPF = C_{PAH} = U_{PAH} * V/P_{PAH} = \text{mL/min}$$

The **RBF** can be extrapolated from the above information:

$$RBF = ERPF/(1 - \text{hematocrit}) = \text{mL/min}$$

The **GFR** is the volume of plasma filtered into Bowman's capsule per unit time. The GFR is determined by the net ultrafiltration pressure (Starling forces) across the glomerular capillaries, the net oncotic pressure, and the permeability and surface area of the filtering membrane.

$$GFR = K_f(P_{gc} - P_t) - (\Pi_{pc} - \Pi_t) = \text{mL/min}$$

K_f is the filtration coefficient and takes into consideration the permeability of the glomerular basement membrane and the surface area available to filter the plasma. In general, small, neutral particles are most easily filtered. The glomerular basement membrane is negatively charged and thus does not readily permit the passage of negatively

charged particles such as albumin. $P_{gc} - P_t$ is the difference between the hydrostatic pressure of the glomerular capillary and the renal tubule. The hydrostatic pressure of the glomerular capillary is usually greater than the hydrostatic pressure of the tubule, thus favoring filtration. Opposing filtration is the oncotic pressure of the plasma in the capillary as plasma proteins attempt to hold onto fluid (Π_{pc}). The oncotic pressure of the tubule (Π_t) is negligible, as there is usually no protein in the filtrate. Over the course of the glomerular capillary loop the direction of filtration, i.e., the formation of urine, is favored. These forces equilibrate toward the end of the capillary as fluid from the plasma has been removed, decreasing the net hydrostatic pressure, and increasing the oncotic pressure of the capillary. By the end of the capillary, forces are balanced, no longer favoring filtration.

Glomerular filtration can be estimated by the clearance of **inulin,** a synthetic polymer of fructose, which is filtered and neither reabsorbed nor secreted by the renal tubules. The clearance of inulin can be represented by the equation below:

$$C_{inulin} = (U_{inulin} * V)/P_{inulin} = GFR$$

GFR can also be estimated by creatinine (Cr) clearance. Creatinine is an endogenous substance formed from the metabolism of creatine in the muscles. Because it is derived from muscles, muscle mass influences the serum creatinine concentration. Creatinine is a small molecule, freely filtered, only minimally secreted, and not reabsorbed, and its rate of formation is fairly constant; thus its clearance from the blood can be used as an estimate of GFR.

$$C_{Cr} = (U_{Cr} * V)/P_{Cr} = \text{mL/min}$$

Normal GFR is approximately 125 mL/min. The **Cockcroft-Gault equation** is an estimate of creatinine clearance that takes into account the age-related decrease in creatinine clearance, body weight, and sex.

$$C_{Cr} = \text{mL/min} = (140 - \text{age}) * \frac{\text{weight (in kg)}}{P_{Cr} \text{(mg/dL)} * 72}$$

multiply by 0.85 for women

Because creatinine is minimally secreted, creatinine clearance is a slight overestimation of the glomerular filtration rate.

The **filtration fraction** is the ratio of GFR to RPF and ranges between 0.16 and 0.20.

$$\text{Filtration fraction} = GFR/RPF = 0.20$$

Due to autoregulation and tubuloglomerular feedback, the RBF, RPF, and GFR remain relatively constant with approximately 20% of the fluid that reaches the glomerulus being filtered into Bowman's capsule.

Case Conclusion The benefits of blood pressure control are explained to the patient: decreased risk of further renal damage, stroke, and heart attack. His rising creatinine and loss of 1 g of protein in his urine are ominous signs and herald a continuing decline in his renal function. An angiotensin I converting enzyme inhibitor (ACEI) is added to his blood pressure treatment, as it has been shown to decrease proteinuria and the rate of functional decline in those with renal disease. At present the patient is taking his medications and eating a low-salt diet, and his proteinuria has improved.

Thumbnail: Renal Pathophysiology — Key Formulas

$C = UV/P$

$ERPF = C_{PAH} = U_{PAH} \, V/P_{PAH}$

$RBF = ERPF/ \, 1 - hematocrit$

$GFR = K_f \, (P_{gc} - P_t) - (\Pi_{pc} - \Pi_t)$

$C_{Cr} = mL/min = ((140 - age) * weight \, (in \, kg)/(P_{Cr} \, (mg/dL) * 72))$
$* (0.85 \, for \, women)$

Filtration fraction = GFR/RPF = GFR/ERPF = 0.20

Key Points

▶ Renal function is essentially determined by the GFR.

▶ Control of GFR depends primarily on control of RPF by dilation or constriction of the afferent and efferent arterioles.

▶ Catecholamines lead to constriction of both arterioles, decreasing GFR. Angiotensin II leads to preferential constriction of the efferent arteriole, preserving GFR.

▶ Prostaglandins dilate the arterioles, especially the afferent arteriole, preserving GFR. Thus, prostaglandin inhibitors (e.g., NSAIDs) can lead to a dangerous unopposed drop in GFR when RPF is compromised for any reason.

Questions

1. Referring again to our patient, if our patient's clearance of PAH is 600 mL/min what is his renal blood flow? (Reminder: His hematocrit is 40%.)

   A. 500 mL/min
   B. 1000 mL/min
   C. 1250 mL/min
   D. 1000 mL/min
   E. 2000 mL/min

2. What is our patient's creatinine clearance? (Reminder: The 24-hour urine collection had 720 mL and a Cr of 200 mg/dL.)

   A. 10 mL/min
   B. 50 mL/min
   C. 125 mL/min
   D. 150 mL/min
   E. 200 mL/min

3. A 29-year-old female diabetic comes to see you for dysuria, hematuria, and urinary frequency. Upon urine dipstick you note the presence of 2+ white blood cells, 2+ red blood cells, and 2+ protein. Which of the following is freely filtered at the glomerulus?

   A. Dextran
   B. Albumin
   C. Glucose
   D. Protein
   E. Red blood cells

4. A 60-year-old man with type II diabetes, weighing 72 kg, is found to have a serum creatinine concentration of 2.0 mg/dL. What is his estimated creatinine clearance?

   A. 115 mL/min
   B. 90 mL/min
   C. 40 mL/min
   D. 25 mL/min
   E. Unable to calculate

HPI: KR is a 70-year-old man who is seen in the doctor's office at a resort in Mexico. He has just returned from a long hike in the noonday sun exploring some Mayan ruins. He didn't drink water during the hike and did not wear a hat. He has no medical problems but is usually sedentary.

PE: Pulse 110 BP 100/60
The patient appears fatigued and flushed. His heart is tachycardic and his lungs are clear.

Labs: His chemistry panel is significant for sodium 150 mEq/L, BUN 52 mg/dL, and creatinine 1.3 mEq/L.

Thought Questions

- What is the distribution of water and electrolytes among the body fluid compartments?

- What are osmolality and tonicity?

- How does the kidney maintain salt and water balance?

- What is the role of thirst in maintaining fluid balance?

Basic Science Review and Discussion

Our bodies are approximately 60% water by weight. The percentage of total body water differs between men and women. Men have a higher percent total body water, 60%, due to a greater amount of lean muscle mass. Women have a larger amount of anhydrous adipose tissue, and their total body water comprises approximately 50% of their weight. As we age, lean muscle mass decreases, adipose tissue increases, and our percent total body water decreases. Total body water can be broken down into two compartments: the extracellular fluid compartment (ECF) and the intracellular fluid compartment (ICF). The ECF is composed of the plasma and interstitial fluid (fluid between cells, not in the vasculature).

The ECF is one third of the total body water (TBW) or 20% of the body weight. The ICF is two thirds of the TBW or 40% of the body weight. The ECF can be further broken down into plasma, which is one fourth of the ECF, and interstitial fluid, which makes up three fourths of the ECF.

To measure the **TBW** one needs a measurable substance, such as tritiated water, that will equilibrate across semipermeable membranes. The formula below allows us to calculate the volume of a fluid compartment if we first know the concentration (C) and the volume (V) we have instilled.

$$C_1V_1 = C_2V_2$$
$$mg/L * L = mg/L * x$$
$$x = mg/L * L/mg * L$$

The **ICF** cannot be directly measured as there is no substance that will stay isolated to the intracellular compartment. Mannitol, inulin, and sucrose, all large molecules, will stay distributed in the **ECF** and are good markers of ECF. Evans blue dye is a substance that is largely bound to plasma proteins and is used to measure the **plasma volume.**

The distribution of electrolytes between the intracellular compartment and the extracellular compartment is not the same. The differences in electrolyte composition among the plasma, interstitial fluid, and intracellular compartments are maintained by the electrical potential difference across cell membranes, the semipermeable phospholipid bilayer of cells, which hinders the diffusion of certain ions, and the presence of nondiffusable, negatively charged proteins in the plasma and the ICF. **Potassium is a primarily intracellular ion and is the ion most responsible for the resting potential of cell membranes.** There is a high concentration of protein in both the plasma and ICF but none in interstitial fluid. These nondiffusable proteins create oncotic pressure preventing fluid from "leaking" into the interstitium. The concentration of **sodium is much higher in the ECF** than the ICF and is the main determinant of the ECF osmolality and thus ECF and intravascular (plasma) volume.

Osmolality, Osmolarity, and Tonicity **Plasma osmolality** is the total solute concentration of plasma measured as the number of osmoles per kg of plasma and ranges from 285 to 295 mOsm/kg. It can be estimated with the formula below:

Osmolality =

$$2(Na^+ \text{ mEq/L}) + \frac{\text{glucose mg/dL}}{18} + \frac{\text{BUN mg/dL}}{2.8} = \text{mOsm/kg}$$

The contribution of BUN and glucose to plasma osmolality is usually small but may become larger if diabetes or renal failure is present. The term **osmolarity** has units of number of milliosmoles per liter and may also be used when referring to body fluids.

Tonicity is a unitless term that allows us to make comparisons of concentrations between fluids. It describes the hydrostatic force created by osmotically active particles across a semipermeable membrane. A hypertonic fluid has a higher effective osmolar concentration than plasma. A 0.9% saline solution ("normal saline") is used as plasma replace-

Table 4-1 Changes that occur with water loss

Disorder	Osmolality of lost fluid	ECF volume	ICF volume	Serum Na+
Diarrhea	Iso-osmotic	↓	↔	↔
Sweating	Hypo-osmotic	↓	↓	↑
Diabetes insipidus	Hypo-osmotic	↓	↓	↑
Adrenal insufficiency	Hypo-osmotic	↓	↑	↓

ment fluid because it is approximately isotonic to plasma having 154 mEq/L of sodium chloride (2 × 154 mEq = 308 mOsm/L). A 0.45% saline solution ("half normal saline") is hypotonic to plasma with only 154 mOsm/L of sodium chloride.

Serum osmolality is tightly controlled by ADH, also known as vasopressin for its vasoconstrictive properties. **ADH** is a nonapeptide synthesized in the supraoptic nucleus of the hypothalamus and released from the posterior pituitary. It is released when osmoreceptors in the anterolateral hypothalamus are stimulated by increases in serum osmolarity as small as 1%. ADH acts on V_2 luminal receptors in the collecting ducts via the cyclic adenosine monophosphate (cAMP) messenger system. Upon binding ADH, there is an up-regulation of transmembrane water channels, **aquaporins,** which results in an increased reabsorption of water. In the absence of ADH, the distal tubule and collecting ducts are almost impermeable to water but with ADH, the kidney is able to reabsorb large amounts of water.

Fluid Shifts   Water equilibrates freely across cell membranes to establish an osmotic equilibrium between the ECF and the ICF. Thus, ICF volume varies inversely with the plasma concentration of sodium. The volume of ECF in the intravascular space (i.e., plasma) is a central determinant of blood pressure. Several disorders causing water loss can disrupt plasma volume, leading to dangerously low blood pressures. The effect of fluid loss on ECF volume, ICF volume, and plasma sodium concentration can be determined if we know the osmolarity of the fluid being lost. Table 4-1 catalogues changes that occur with pathologic gastrointestinal, renal, and insensible water losses. The

average daily loss of water in the urine is approximately 1.5 to 2.0 L and from the feces 0.1 to 0.2 L. Insensible losses include loss of water from the skin and lungs and account for approximately 0.5 L per day.

The effects of ECF volume contraction, decreased cardiac output, tachycardia, and hypotension result in a cascade of events aimed at maintaining blood pressure and perfusion to vital organs. Hypotension is sensed by the cardiac and carotid baroreceptors, which stimulate the sympathetic nervous system and angiotensin-renin-aldosterone hormonal axis. Systemic vasoconstriction due to sympathetic nervous system activation and increased reabsorption of salt and water by the kidney under the influence of aldosterone act to restore normal blood pressure. Under circumstances of hypovolemia ADH is also secreted in an attempt to increase intravascular volume.

Extracellular fluid volume can be expanded by the addition of hypertonic or isotonic saline. Hypertonic, 3% saline, contains 513 mEq/L of sodium chloride and will draw water from the ICF, thereby expanding plasma volume but dehydrating individual cells. Isotonic saline expands the intravascular volume without causing fluid to shift from the cells because the osmolarity of 0.9% saline is similar to the ICF and ECF osmolarity (Table 4-2).

Thirst   What about the role of thirst in preserving intravascular volume? In states of dehydration, a rise of plasma osmolarity of only 2% will stimulate our thirst center located anterolaterally to the preoptic nucleus of the hypothalamus (near the area that controls the release of ADH). Other stimulants of thirst include decreased blood pressure and a dry mouth.

Table 4-2 Changes that occur with fluid gained

Situation	Osmolarity of fluid gained	ECF volume	ICF volume	Serum Na+
3% saline infusion	Hypertonic	↑	↓	↑
0.9% saline infusion	Isotonic	↑	↔	↔
5% dextrose	Hypotonic	↑	↑	↓

Case Conclusion Our weekend warrior went out hiking unprepared. Sweating leads to a loss of hypotonic fluid and volume contraction. As a result, the patient's serum sodium concentration is increased, blood pressure is decreased, and he is tachycardic. Keep in mind that the blood urea nitrogen (BUN) concentration can also be a useful indication of volume status. Dehydration causes increased reabsorption of urea resulting in an elevation of the normal BUN-creatinine ratio of 10:1. **A ratio of BUN:creatinine of 20:1 or greater is not unusual in dehydrated patients.**

Thumbnail: Renal Physiology—Body Fluids

Compartment	% TB weight	% TB water	Marker	Volume for a 70-kg person (L)
TBW	60 ♂ 50 ♀	100	Tritiated water, deuterium oxide (D$_2$O)	42
ICF	40	67	TBW − ECF	28
ECF	20	33	Mannitol, inulin, sucrose	14
Plasma	5	8 (1/4 of ECF)	Evans blue dye, Radioiodinated serum albumin	3.5
Interstitial	15	25 (3/4 of ECF)	ECF − plasma	10.5

Key Points

▶ Serum sodium concentration is the main determinant of extracellular fluid volume.

▶ Osmolality is the number of particles per kg of water and osmolarity is the number of particles per liter of water.

▶ Tonicity is a measure of the osmotic activity or hydrostatic force exerted by particles in a solution across a semipermeable membrane.

▶ Antidiuretic hormone, the main regulator of serum osmolality, is stimulated with small increases in serum osmolality.

Questions

1. A 100-kg man is injected with 250 mL of Evans blue dye with a concentration of 500 mg/mL. After 10 minutes his blood is drawn and the concentration of Evans blue dye is 25 mg/mL. What is his plasma volume?

   A. 1000 mL
   B. 2500 mL
   C. 4000 mL
   D. 5000 mL
   E. 10,000 mL

2. A 24-year-old man presents to your clinic with a history of episodes of diarrhea and crampy abdominal pain for the last 6 years. He comes to your office today after 3 days of severe diarrhea and because he has noticed blood in his stool. Measurement of his blood pressure in the supine position is 100/60 and his heart rate is 90 beats per minute. His upright blood pressure drops to 80/50 and his heart rate increases to 110 beats per minute and he complains of feeling dizzy and nauseous. His serum sodium is 140 mEq/L. What is the most appropriate replacement fluid?

   A. Intravenous 0.9% saline
   B. Intravenous 0.45% saline
   C. Intravenous 5% dextrose
   D. Intravenous 3% saline
   E. Chicken soup

HPI: BB is a 67-year-old woman brought to the ED by her son because of confusion. Her son states that over the past 2 days his mother became increasingly lethargic. When he arrived home from work today his mother was sleeping on the couch and he could not wake her. The son notes that his mother recently started a new medication for hypertension.

PE: BP 130/90 mm Hg Pulse 80 T 36.6°C SaO$_2$ 97% at room air
The patient's heart rate is within normal limits and regular. Her lungs are clear. She is somnolent, responds to voice but quickly returns to sleep, and cannot follow commands. There is no facial droop, she resists eye opening, and her pupils are equal and reactive to light. She moves all extremities when stimulated to do so and her reflexes are intact.
Medication: Hydrochlorothiazide

Labs: Na$^+$ 120 mEq/L, K$^+$ 3.0 mEq/L, Cl$^-$ 90 mEq/L, HCO$_3^-$ 26 mEq/L, BUN 32 mg/dL, Cr 1.0 mg/dL.

Thought Questions

- What is the renal regulation of sodium?
- What are the causes of hypernatremia and hyponatremia?
- Why is this patient so lethargic?

Basic Science Review and Discussion

Sodium is the major cation of the ECF. Normal serum levels range between 135 and 145 mEq/L. The high sodium concentration in the ECF and low concentration intracellularly is an important determinant of the potential difference across cell membranes. The abundance of sodium in the ECF also determines the osmolality of the extracellular fluid. The serum osmolality is normally regulated by ADH acting to regulate water reabsorption in the distal nephron. The osmolality may be deranged in disease states as we shall see below.

Sodium Homeostasis Approximately 99% of filtered sodium is reabsorbed by the end of the nephron (see Figure 1-3). The action of the Na$^+$/K$^+$ ATPase at the basolateral membrane of the tubular cells facilitates sodium movement from lumen to tubular cell to peritubular capillary. The reabsorption of water and chloride (and most other filtered solutes) is closely coupled to the sodium reabsorption throughout the nephron.

Two thirds of the filtered sodium and water is reabsorbed in the proximal convoluted tubule (PCT). When sodium is reabsorbed it creates an osmotic gradient, which facilitates the passive absorption of water, and a negative potential in the tubular lumen, which facilitates the absorption of chloride down its electrical and chemical gradient. Fluid entering the loop of Henle is iso-osmolar with respect to plasma.

Countercurrent Multiplication and Countercurrent Exchange
The primary role of the loop of Henle is to establish a hyperosmolar medullary interstitium that can be used by the collecting tubules to concentrate urine. The loop of Henle establishes this gradient by the mechanism of **countercurrent multiplication.** The flow of urine through the limbs of the loop run counter to one another. The descending loop of Henle is permeable to water and impermeable to ions. As fluid flows down the descending loop, it becomes increasingly concentrated as water is reabsorbed into the peritubular capillaries. The ascending loop is impermeable to water and actively transports, via an ATPase pump, Na$^+$, 2Cl$^-$, and K$^+$ from the tubular lumen to the medullary interstitium. As the filtrate flows up the ascending loop it becomes more dilute. The active transport of ions into the medulla creates an osmotic gradient that ranges from 300 mOsm/L at the outer medulla to up to 1400 mOsm/L at the tips of the loops of Henle. The gradient is maintained by vasa recta, capillaries that course parallel to the loops of Henle. Because of their ability to perpetuate the high osmotic pressure of the medulla, the vasa recta are termed **countercurrent exchangers.** During their course through the kidney, the plasma within the vasa recta becomes more concentrated as it descends and more dilute as it ascends. The net effect is that the vasa recta are able to perfuse the kidney interstitium without disrupting the steep medullary gradient essential for the production of concentrated urine.

The Concentration of Urine The collecting tubule becomes permeable to water only under the influence of ADH, which acts on V$_2$ luminal receptors in the collecting ducts. Upon binding ADH, transmembrane water channels, aquaporins, are inserted into the luminal cell surface. Water passively flows through these channels down the osmotic gradient created by countercurrent multiplication and is reabsorbed, resulting in concentration of urine. The concentration of urine varies directly with the plasma concentration of ADH, with urine osmolarity ranging from 50 to 1400 mOsm/L.

Urea is a product of protein metabolism. Approximately 50% of filtered urea is reabsorbed at the PCT. Most nephron segments are relatively impermeable to urea except for the medullary collecting ducts, which, under the influence of ADH, allow urea to diffuse into the medullary interstitium. In this manner, urea contributes to the hyperosmolarity of the medulla and maximal urine concentration.

Hypernatremia   Hypernatremia is defined as a serum sodium concentration above 150 mEq/L. There are only two ways to become hypernatremic, either to ingest too much salt or to lose too much water. The latter is far more common. Hypernatremia occurs most commonly in patients with inadequate water intake due to an altered state of consciousness or in elderly patients who are less sensitive to thirst. Insensible water loss via the skin or respiratory tract without replenishment leads to hypernatremia. Diarrhea leads to water loss greater than salt loss causing hypernatremia. Renal water losses include osmotic diuresis due to diabetes insipidus or hyperglycemia.

Diabetes Insipidus   Diabetes insipidus (DI) is the renal wasting of water due to a lack of or resistance to ADH. Patients with DI present with polyuria, intense thirst, and signs of volume depletion such as hypotension and tachycardia. Patients with DI urinate large volumes of dilute urine, greater than 2 to 3 L/day, that may disrupt sleep or result in enuresis (bedwetting).

Central DI occurs with damage to the hypothalamus or posterior pituitary, leading to impaired ADH secretion. Central DI may be caused by central nervous system (CNS) tumors, surgery, intracranial hemorrhage, anoxic injury, infection, or infiltrating disease such as sarcoidosis. Central DI can be primary or idiopathic if no proximate cause is found. Renal insensitivity to ADH leads to the same clinical picture with normal or elevated ADH secretion and is referred to as **nephrogenic DI.** Nephrogenic diabetes insipidus is caused by chronic renal insufficiency, drugs such as **lithium** and **alcohol, hypercalcemia,** and long-standing **hypokalemia.**

The clinical presentation of hypernatremia depends on the rapidity of onset. Acute hypernatremia results in alterations of consciousness, from lethargy to coma, due to cerebral intracellular dehydration. Other neurologic symptoms include weakness, tremor, muscle rigidity, ataxia, and seizures. Hypernatremia that develops over time allows the body, especially the neurons, to produce osmolytes, solutes that allow the cells of the CNS to maintain intracellular volume. This moderates damage to the brain and may not produce any specific pattern of symptoms.

Treatment of hypernatremia includes restoring body water, ADH replacement when indicated, and removing the offending drug. The TBW deficit may be estimated by the following equation:

Water deficit = ((measured serum Na$^+$/normal serum Na$^+$) * TBW) − TBW

where TBW = 0.60 * normal body weight in kg.

The rate of water repletion is determined by how acutely the hypernatremia developed. Chronic onset (greater than 36 hours) allows for the compensatory response by neurons, and care must be taken to correct the hypernatremia slowly. If hypernatremia has occurred over time, rapid correction may result in cerebral edema.

Hyponatremia   Hyponatremia is a serum sodium of less than 135 mEq/L with a resulting parallel decrease in the osmolality of the serum. This distinguishes true hyponatremia from **pseudohyponatremia,** which is a factitious lowering of the serum sodium concentration due to hyperlipidemia, hyperproteinemia, or hyperglycemia, in which there is increased serum osmolality.

Like hypernatremia, the clinical picture in hyponatremia depends on the rapidity of onset. Mild hyponatremia is usually asymptomatic but the rapid onset of severe hyponatremia (less than 120 mEq/L) can result in serious morbidity and death due to cerebral edema. Patients commonly present with lethargy, seizures, anorexia, headaches, and muscle cramps.

Patients with hyponatremia can be hypovolemic, euvolemic, or hypervolemic. The serum sodium concentration does not give any information about the patient's volume status. For volume status, we look for clinical signs of dehydration (dry mucous membranes, tachycardia, etc.) or fluid overload (edema).

Disorders that present with hyponatremia and **hypovolemia** include water losses due to diarrhea, excessive sweating with solute-free water replacement, and renal losses due to diuretics, osmotic diuresis, salt-losing nephropathy, and adrenal insufficiency.

Several disorders present with **euvolemia** and hyponatremia. The syndrome of inappropriate antidiuretic hormone (SIADH), deficiencies of glucocorticoid and thyroid hormones, primary polydipsia, and medications that potentiate the effect of ADH all cause euvolemic hyponatremia. The list of drugs that cause an SIADH-like syndrome include nicotine, chlorpropamide, morphine, and carbamazepine. Primary polydipsia or compulsive water drinking usually occurs in psychiatric patients taking psychotropic medications that cause a dry mouth.

SIADH is a diagnosis of exclusion and is often secondary to ectopic ADH production by tumors (especially non–small cell lung cancer), pulmonary disorders, CNS disorders, or pain. Patients maintain euvolemia in the presence of excess ADH because any increase in TBW leads to sodium excretion to rid the body of the excess water. In addition to elevation of urine sodium concentration, the urine osmolarity will be inappropriately concentrated, i.e., greater than 100 mOsm/L. The hallmarks of SIADH are euvolemia and inappropriately concentrated urine in the presence of hyponatremia.

Disorders that present with **hypervolemia** and hyponatremia include nephrotic syndrome, cirrhosis, and congestive heart failure. In all of these disorders TBW is increased, but water is not retained in the circulation and intravascular hypovolemia is present. Inadequate filling of the arterial circulation leads to inadequate sodium delivery to the renal tubules and increased ADH secretion, culminating in hyponatremia. In addition, diuretics used in the treatment of these disorders also perpetuate hyponatremia.

The treatment of hyponatremia depends on the underlying cause, the volume status of the patient, and the severity of symptoms. Hormonal causes of hyponatremia are treated with hormone replacement. If hyponatremia is drug induced, the offending drug should be discontinued. SIADH, regardless of the cause, usually responds to water restriction.

Emergent treatment of hyponatremia is required if patients have an alteration of consciousness or seizures. The emergent treatment is administration of hypertonic saline (3% NaCl = 513 mEq/L) to replace the sodium deficit to at least 120 mEq/L at a rate not more than 0.5 mEq/L/h. The sodium deficit to be replaced can be calculated as follows:

$$Na^+ \text{ deficit} = TBW * (Na^+ \text{ desired} - Na^+ \text{ measured}) = 0.60 * \text{wt in kg} * (120 \text{ mEq/L} - Na^+ \text{ measured mEq/L}) = \text{mEq } Na^+ \text{ deficit}$$

Too rapid correction of hyponatremia may result in **central pontine myelinosis,** a selective demyelination of the pons that can result in quadriparesis and death.

Case Conclusion   The patient has a symptomatic hyponatremia most likely due to diuretic use. She also has hypokalemia. Treatment includes discontinuation of hydrochlorothiazide, restriction of water, repletion of potassium, and infusion of normal saline.

Thumbnail: Renal Physiology—Sodium Regulation

	Hypernatremia	Hyponatremia
Etiology	Decreased water intake Increased salt intake Diabetes insipidus Diarrhea Insensible losses	Pseudohyponatremia **Hypovolemic** Renal losses (diuretics) Gastrointestinal losses (diarrhea) Insensible losses Addison's disease (adrenal insufficiency) **Euvolemic** SIADH Hypothyroidism Glucocorticoid deficiency Primary polydipsia Medications **Hypervolemic** Nephrotic syndrome Congestive heart failure Cirrhosis
Symptoms	Impaired consciousness, weakness, tremor, hyperreflexia	Anorexia, headaches, muscle cramps, impaired consciousness, seizure, coma

Key Points

▸ The reabsorption of sodium occurs throughout the nephron and is coupled to the reabsorption of chloride, amino acids, and glucose.

▸ The ascending loop of Henle is the site of active transport of Na^+, K^+, and $2Cl^-$ into the medulla of the kidney.

▸ The collecting ducts are permeable to water only under the influence of ADH and are responsible for the final concentration of urine.

▸ ADH is the hormone primarily responsible for maintaining serum osmolality but is elevated in states of hypovolemia even when the patient is hyponatremic.

▸ SIADH results in euvolemic hyponatremia and inappropriate renal sodium wasting.

▸ Diabetes insipidus is caused by a lack of ADH or a resistance to ADH resulting in large volumes of dilute urine.

Questions

1. A 33-year-old, 70-kg woman remains lethargic after surgery for removal of an ovarian cyst. She has no other health problems. She was given 2.5 L of 0.45% saline during her operation and recovery. Her serum sodium is 122 mEq/L. How many milliequivalents of sodium are needed to raise her sodium to 130 mEq/L and how fast should it be replaced?

   A. 200 mEq, 10 hours
   B. 336 mEq, 16 hours
   C. 448 mEq, 40 hours
   D. 513 mEq, 20 hours
   E. No replacement is needed

2. A 70-year-old man is admitted to the intensive care unit (ICU) for a subarachnoid hemorrhage. After 12 hours of observation, the astute ICU nurse informs you that the patient's urine output has increased to 400 cc/h. What is his most likely diagnosis?

   A. SIADH
   B. Diuresis after urinary obstruction
   C. Diabetes mellitus
   D. Diabetes insipidus
   E. Administration of diuretics

3. A 35-year-old woman comes to see you for a checkup required by her new place of employment. She feels well and takes no medication. She complains of a weight gain of 5 pounds over the last year. Her blood pressure is mildly elevated at 130/80. Her serum chemistry profile reveals hyponatremia. Laboratory examination is as follows: Na^+ 125 mEq/L, Cl^- 100 mEq/L, K^+ 4.2 mEq/L, HCO_3^- 24 mEq/L, BUN 9 mEq/L, Cr 0.9 mg/dL, glucose 90 mg/dL. Which of the following is the most likely diagnosis?

   A. Hyperthyroidism
   B. Diabetes mellitus
   C. Hypercholesterolemia
   D. Diuretic abuse
   E. SIADH

HPI: DK, an 81-year-old man, is brought to the ED by his wife for increasing lethargy over the last week. She also reports that he has complained of feeling ill and has had little to eat or drink over the past week.
His past medical history includes hypertension, myocardial infarction, and congestive heart failure. His medical regimen includes metoprolol, furosemide, and lisinopril.

PE: BP 100/60 Pulse 62 T 37°C SaO$_2$ 97% at room air
The patient is a thin, frail-appearing man. His oral mucosa is dry. His cardiac rhythm is regular and his lungs are clear to auscultation. He is lethargic but easily aroused and answers questions appropriately.

Labs/Studies: Na$^+$ 148 mEq/L, K$^+$ 6.1 mEq/L, Cl$^-$ 102 mEq/L, HCO$_3^-$ 20 mEq/L, BUN 60 mg/dL, creatinine 3.4 mg/dL. ECG (Figure 6-1).

Thought Questions

- What regulates the serum concentration of potassium?

- What is the renal handling of potassium?

- How does the acid-base balance affect the serum potassium concentration?

- What are the physiologic affects of hyper- and hypokalemia?

- What is the cause of hyperkalemia in this patient?

Basic Science Discussion and Review

Most of the potassium within the body is **intracellular.** The ratio of intracellular to extracellular concentrations deter-mines the resting membrane potential of cell membranes, and alterations in this ratio have profound effects on membrane excitability. Normal serum potassium levels are 3.5 to 5.0 mEq/L. The serum concentration of potassium is regulated by renal excretion and by changes in the distribution of potassium between extracellular and intracellular fluid compartments. **Aldosterone,** via its action on the kidney, is the main determinant of serum potassium concentration.

Renal Handling of Potassium   Approximately 60% to 80% of filtered potassium is passively reabsorbed in the PCT. An additional 25% is actively reabsorbed at the thick ascending loop of Henle by cotransport of Na$^+$, K$^+$ and Cl$^-$. Only 10% to 15% of filtered potassium reaches the distal nephron. Aldosterone determines the final concentration of potassium in the urine. An increased serum concentration of potassium (e.g., by eating lots of bananas)

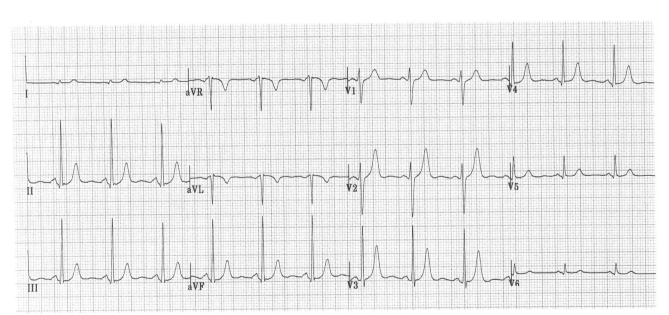

Figure 6-1 ECG with peaked T waves. (Reproduced with permission from Taylor GJ. 150 Practice ECGs: interpretation and review. Malden, MA: Blackwell Science, 2002.)

stimulates the production of aldosterone from the zona glomerulosa of the adrenal cortex. Aldosterone stimulates the Na^+/K^+ pump of the principal cells of the cortical collecting tubules, resulting in secretion of potassium. The converse is also true; in potassium depletion (e.g., due to diarrhea), aldosterone production decreases, resulting in decreased potassium secretion. The ability of the kidney to conserve potassium is limited, with an obligatory excretion of 10 mEq/L in the urine even in the presence of hypokalemia.

Transcellular Shifts   The serum concentration of potassium is also regulated by changes in distribution between the ICF and ECF compartments. During acidemic states, hydrogen ions are shifted from the ECF to the ICF in an attempt to maintain a physiologic pH. For every H^+ that enters the cell, a positive ion (K^+) must leave the cell to maintain electroneutrality. If alkalosis is present, potassium is shifted into cells and hydrogen ions out of cells. **Insulin** and **catecholamines** (epinephrine and norepinephrine) cause increased uptake of potassium by cells resulting in decreased serum potassium.

Hyperkalemia   Hyperkalemia is defined as a serum potassium greater than 5 mEq/L. The causes of hyperkalemia can be broadly categorized as follows: decreased renal excretion, increased ingestion, redistribution of potassium due to transcellular shifts, pseudohyperkalemia, or hyperkalemia induced by drugs. Decreased renal excretion occurs with poor renal function and aldosterone deficiency due to adrenal disease. Hyperkalemia due to increased potassium intake occurs with oral or parenteral potassium supplementation. A decrease in serum pH causes a transcellular shift of potassium from the ICF to the ECF, as discussed above. **Pseudohyperkalemia** is seen if significant hemolysis with release of intracellular potassium occurs during the collection of a blood sample. Leukocytosis or thrombocytosis can also create spurious hyperkalemia by releasing intracellular potassium into the serum collected for testing. Drugs such as ACEIs and potassium-sparing diuretics can lead to hyperkalemia. ACEIs result in decreased aldosterone production and increased serum potassium. Potassium-sparing diuretics include spironolactone, triamterene, and amiloride. Spironolactone antagonizes the effects of aldosterone in the distal nephron. Triamterene and amiloride act directly on sodium channels in the distal renal tubules causing both sodium and potassium retention.

An increased serum potassium causes a less electronegative resting potential, and cells become more excitable. This causes conduction disorders in cardiac muscle and may result in the electrocardiographic pattern seen in the patient on the previous page. ECG changes seen in hyperkalemia include peaked **T waves, a widened QRS complex, prolonged PR interval,** and may result in cardiac arrest.

The treatment of hyperkalemia includes increasing the movement of potassium into cells with insulin (preceded by glucose administration to avoid hypoglycemia) and β-adrenergic agonists such as inhaled albuterol, and alkalinizing the serum with sodium bicarbonate so as to increase transcellular shifts with H^+. To protect the heart from dangerous arrhythmias, intravenous calcium is given to antagonize the effects of hyperkalemia on cell membrane potential. Actual removal of potassium can be accomplished through forced diuresis, elimination from the gastrointestinal tract with an ion exchange resin such as sodium polystyrene sulfonate or hemodialysis.

Hypokalemia   Hypokalemia is defined as a serum potassium of less than 3.5 mEq/L. It may reflect a reduction in total body potassium or it may result from redistribution of potassium in patients with normal or even increased total body potassium. The causes of hypokalemia include dietary deficiency, redistribution with increased entry of potassium into cells, diarrhea, diuretics, aldosterone excess, and hypomagnesemia.

The clinical manifestations of hypokalemia are a result of increased negativity of the resting membrane potential and decreased sensitivity of cell membranes. Skeletal muscles may be weakened, resulting in paresis and rhabdomyolysis. Hypokalemia also causes decreased motility of smooth muscle, leading to decreased intestinal motility and paralytic ileus. ECG changes seen in hypokalemia include decreased T wave amplitude, prolonged QT interval, and a prominent **U wave** (a finding not correlated with the cardiac cycle), and may lead to cardiac arrest.

The cause of hypokalemia should be investigated and treated. Potassium should be replaced according to the degree of hypokalemia using oral or parenteral potassium.

Case Conclusion   The patient is volume depleted due to poor nutrition which is exacerbated by his continuing to take his diuretic. Kidney perfusion is diminished, and substances such as potassium that are normally cleared by the kidney have accumulated. His ability to excrete organic acids is diminished, leading to acidemia and elevated serum K^+ as potassium shifts into the ECF. The patient is hospitalized, rehydrated, and treated with sodium bicarbonate, glucose followed by insulin, and inhaled albuterol, which all shift potassium into cells. To prevent potassium uptake from his gastrointestinal tract, he is given the exchange resin sodium polystyrene sulfonate. His serum potassium and ECG findings normalize over the next few hours and his renal function slowly returns over the next few days.

Thumbnail: Renal Physiology—Hyperkalemia vs. Hypokalemia

	Hyperkalemia	Hypokalemia
Etiology	Renal failure Hypoaldosteronism Drug induced Tubular defects Ingestion Acidemia Insulin deficiency	Dietary deficiency Hyperaldosteronism Renal losses Diarrhea Alkalemia
Clinical manifestation	Weakness Fatigue Cardiac arrhythmias	Weakness Fatigue Cardiac arrhythmias Hyporeflexia Paralytic ileus
ECG findings	Peaked T waves Decreased P wave amplitude PR lengthening QRS widening	Flattened T waves Prominent U wave ST depression Prolonged QT

Key Points

▶ Aldosterone, acting on the cortical collecting ducts, is the main determinant of serum potassium concentration.

▶ A low serum pH shifts potassium from the ICF to the ECF, and a high pH shifts potassium from the ECF to the ICF.

▶ Insulin, catecholamines, and sodium bicarbonate cause potassium to shift from the ECF to the ICF.

▶ Both hyperkalemia and hypokalemia can cause weakness and cardiac arrhythmias, leading to cardiac arrest.

▶ Potassium-sparing diuretics: potassium STAys in = **S**pironolactone, **T**riamterene, **A**miloride.

Questions

1. A patient with known renal failure on hemodialysis presents to the ED in congestive heart failure and is found to have a potassium of 7.0 mEq/L. Which of the following can be used in the ED to treat him prior to initiating dialysis?

   A. Calcium chloride
   B. Insulin
   C. Sodium bicarbonate
   D. Albuterol
   E. All of the above

2. A 60-year-old woman presents to your office with weakness and a heart rate of 38 beats per minute. Her chemistry panel is significant for a potassium of 2.0 mEq/L. Which of the following conditions could be the cause of her hypokalemia?

   A. Hypoaldosteronism
   B. Furosemide
   C. Spironolactone
   D. Metabolic acidosis
   E. Hyperthyroidism

3. A 72-year-old woman was recently started on both triamterene and an ACEI for control of her blood pressure. At her office checkup 2 weeks later, which of the following might be seen on her electrocardiogram?

   A. Peaked T waves
   B. Decreased P wave amplitude
   C. PR lengthening
   D. QRS widening
   E. All of the above

HPI: CD, a 47-year-old woman with human immunodeficiency virus (HIV), was unable to provide a history, as she had been intubated in the ED. Her husband reports that she has been suffering from a cough for the last 2 days. Her HIV is well controlled by antiretroviral therapy and she has never suffered from any opportunistic infections.

PE: T 39°C (rectal) Pulse 110 BP 90/40 RR 40 SaO_2 97% on 100% oxygen
The physical examination is significant for crackles over both lung bases. The patient's extremities are cool and her lower legs have a mottled appearance.
Chest x-ray: Dense infiltrates in the lower lobes bilaterally, cardiac silhouette within normal limits, endotracheal tube present and in proper position.

Labs: A blood gas prior to intubation has the following values: pH 7.27, PCO_2 8 mm Hg, PO_2 50 mm Hg, oxygen saturation 82%, bicarbonate 12 mEq/L. A basic metabolic panel shows the following: Na^+ 130 mEq/L, K^+ 5.5 mEq/L, Cl^- 90 mEq/L, HCO_3^- 14 mEq/L, BUN 37 mg/dL, creatinine 3.0 mg/dL. Her serum lactate is elevated at 8.1 U/L. A complete blood count (CBC) is significant for white blood cell count (WBC) 15,000 cells/μL, hemoglobin 10 g/dL, and platelets 113,000 cells/μL.

Thought Questions

■ What is the renal regulation of acids and bases?

■ What is the renal compensation for deranged serum pH?

■ What are the acid-base disorders?

■ What is an anion gap?

■ What is the acid-base disturbance in our patient?

Basic Science Review and Discussion

The body produces hydrogen ions as a result of the metabolic degradation of glucose, protein, and fatty acids. Under normal circumstances the buffering systems of the blood (bicarbonate and hemoglobin), the exhalation of carbon dioxide (CO_2, a volatile acid), the reabsorption of bicarbonate (HCO_3^-, a base), and excretion of ammonium and phosphoric acid (nonvolatile acids) by the kidney maintain our physiologic pH at approximately 7.4. Blood pH can be determined by blood gas analysis. Normal blood gas values are pH 7.35 to 7.45, PCO_2 35 to 45 mm Hg, PO_2 90 to 100 mm Hg, and a HCO_3^- 20 to 24 mmol/L. The buffering systems of the blood and the lungs are limited by the amount of buffer in the blood and the ability of patients to increase or decrease their respiratory rate. Thus, the kidney must compensate for acid-base disturbances by either reabsorbing or excreting bicarbonate or excreting protons. The major buffers of the urine include bicarbonate, ammonia, and phosphate. When the blood pH falls below 7.4, the urine becomes more acidic to rid the body of excess acid, and when the blood pH exceeds 7.4, the urine becomes more alkaline.

The reabsorption of bicarbonate occurs primarily at the PCT and ensures there is no loss of bicarbonate from the filtered plasma. This mechanism is highly efficient, and, in general, the kidney reabsorbs all of the filtered bicarbonate. Within renal tubular cells, carbon dioxide is hydrated to form carbonic acid, which is then broken down by the enzyme carbonic anhydrase to hydrogen and bicarbonate [$H_2O + CO_2 \leftrightarrow H_2CO_3 \leftrightarrow H^+ + HCO_3^-$]. The bicarbonate ion is reabsorbed down its electrochemical gradient into the blood. The hydrogen ion is excreted into the tubular lumen by countertransport with sodium (this active transport mechanism allows the hydrogen ion to use energy released when sodium moves down its electrochemical gradient created by the basolateral Na^+/K^+ ATPase). The hydrogen ion derived from bicarbonate combines with the filtered bicarbonate, which is then converted by carbonic anhydrase to water and carbon dioxide, both of which readily diffuse into the renal tubule cell. By this mechanism there is no excretion of either bicarbonate or hydrogen ions, but the efficient use of hydrogen ions to conserve bicarbonate. Bicarbonate reabsorption occurs to a great extent (80% to 90%) at the PCT because carbonic anhydrase is active in the extensive PCT cell brush border.

When hydrogen combines with any buffer other than bicarbonate and is excreted, the body rids itself of excess acid. The kidneys compensate for a sustained acidosis by combining hydrogen ions with ammonia and phosphate. Ammonia (NH_3) is formed from the breakdown of glutamine within renal tubule cells. As a neutral molecule, ammonia can diffuse across the cells of the tubular lumen, where it combines with hydrogen to form a positively charged, hydrophilic ammonium ion (NH_4^+), which is trapped in the urine as it can no longer diffuse across the cell membrane (Figure 7-1). Up-regulation of ammonia synthesis and subse-

Urine   PCT   Blood

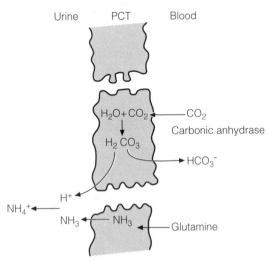

Figure 7-1 Generation of ammonium.

quent **diffusion-trapping** of ammonium ions occurs when blood pH is acidotic for any length of time and is the main mechanism by which the kidney compensates for acidosis. It occurs primarily in the later segments of the nephron after most of the bicarbonate has been reabsorbed in the PCT. Phosphate, the other major urinary buffer, is largely reabsorbed by the kidney; thus a limited amount is available to buffer urinary acid.

Disruptions in Acid-Base Homeostasis   Changes in the concentration of the acid-base buffer components cause disturbances in acid-base balance. The acid-base disorders are divided into two categories: metabolic and respiratory. They can be further subdivided into metabolic acidosis, metabolic alkalosis, respiratory acidosis, and respiratory alkalosis.

Metabolic Acidosis   A serum pH of less than 7.35 with normal or low Pco_2 is diagnostic of a metabolic acidosis and is caused by a decrease in blood bicarbonate. Hyperventilation is the compensatory response, resulting in hypocapnia. The possible etiologies include loss of bicarbonate through the gastrointestinal tract or kidneys, an increase in hydrogen ion load from endogenous or exogenous sources, and a decrease in the renal excretion of hydrogen or production of bicarbonate.

An anion gap is important in the diagnosis of the etiology of metabolic acidosis. The anion gap is the mathematical difference between the concentration of the measured major cations and anions in the serum.

$$\text{Anion gap} = Na^+ - (Cl^- + HCO_3^-)$$

Normally this difference is approximately 12 mEq/L. It is an estimation of the unmeasured anions in the serum such as phosphate, sulfate, and proteins. Although measurable, by convention, potassium, magnesium, and calcium are not included in the formula above. If the anion gap is elevated, it is an indication that an acidic anion (either exogenous or endogenous) is present. The mnemonic **MUD PILES** summarizes the causes of an elevated anion gap: **m**ethanol, **u**remia, **d**iabetic ketoacidosis, **p**araldehyde, **i**soniazid, **l**actate, **e**thanol, **e**thylene glycol, and **s**alicylates.

It is also possible to have an acidosis without an anion gap, also known as a nongap or hyperchloremic acidosis. The etiology is usually a loss of bicarbonate necessitating that sodium be reabsorbed with chloride. Causes of a nongap acidosis are summarized with the mnemonic **HEART CCU**: **h**ypoaldosteronism, **e**xpansion (volume expansion), **a**limentation (parenteral nutrition), **r**enal tubular acidosis, **t**rots (diarrhea), **c**holestyramine, **c**arbonic anhydrase inhibitors (acetazolamide) **u**reterosigmoidostomy.

Metabolic Alkalosis   Metabolic alkalosis, characterized by a pH greater than 7.45, is caused by an increase in serum bicarbonate. The resultant alkalemia decreases the respiratory rate causing compensatory hypercapnia. Alkalemia is caused by loss of acid from vomiting or consumption of alkali, e.g., antacids. Vomiting and/or the use of diuretics leads to hypovolemia, necessitating uptake of sodium. Bicarbonate is absorbed alongside sodium in the place of chloride to maintain electroneutrality. Mineralocorticoid excess leads to a loss of hydrogen ions as aldosterone increases the H^+ pump in the distal convoluted tubule causing alkalemia. The factors that maintain the disturbance include renal failure with the inability to excrete bicarbonate, decreased availability of chloride and the reabsorption of sodium with bicarbonate to compensate, continuing mineralocorticoid excess, and hypokalemia. In hypokalemia, hydrogen ions shift from the intracellular compartment to the extracellular compartment in exchange for potassium, to maintain electrochemical neutrality. These "excess" hydrogen ions are then excreted into the urine in exchange for the reabsorption of potassium, thereby maintaining the alkalosis.

Compensatory Changes   It is not possible to completely compensate or overcompensate for an acid-base disturbance. The compensatory response to the primary disorder only results in partial correction of the disorder, and the change in pH will reflect the primary disorder. If the pH does not fall within the limits of the primary disorder, one should consider a mixed disorder. The compensatory responses of the various disorders are shown on the next page (see Thumbnail).

Case Conclusion This patient has an elevated anion gap metabolic acidosis with an anion gap of 26 mEq/L. She is hypoxic due to *Streptococcus pneumoniae* pneumonia, and her cells are metabolizing glucose via anaerobic respiration, producing lactate. She is attempting to compensate for the production of this endogenous acid by increasing her respiratory rate to rid her body of CO_2. She is treated with antibiotics, improves over the course of several days, is successfully extubated, and recovers quickly.

Thumbnail: Renal Pathophysiology

Renal compensation for changes in pH			
	Primary disorder	**Compensatory response**	**Result**
Metabolic			
Acidosis	↓ HCO_3^-	↓ P_{CO_2}	↓ pH
Alkalosis	↑ HCO_3^-	↑ P_{CO_2}	↑ pH
Respiratory			
Acute acidosis	↑ P_{CO_2}	+/− ↓ HCO_3^-	↓ pH
Chronic acidosis	↑ P_{CO_2}	↑↑ HCO_3^-	↓ pH
Acute alkalosis	↓ P_{CO_2}	+/− ↑ HCO_3^-	↑ pH
Chronic alkalosis	↓ P_{CO_2}	↑ HCO_3^-	↑ pH

Key Points

▶ **Carbonic anhydrase** is the enzyme responsible for each step of the following reaction: $H_2O + CO_2 \leftrightarrow H_2CO_3 \leftrightarrow H^+ + HCO_3^-$.

▶ Reabsorption of bicarbonate occurs primarily at the proximal convoluted tubule.

▶ Regulation of bicarbonate reabsorption is how the kidney compensates for acidosis in the short- and long-term.

▶ Up-regulation of ammonia synthesis and **diffusion-trapping** of the ammonium ion (NH_4^+) is the kidney's main compensation for prolonged acidosis.

▶ Anion gap = $Na^+ - (Cl^- + HCO_3^-)$. An anion gap acidosis is present if the gap is greater than the normal gap of 12, indicating the presence of an unmeasured anion.

▶ A **nongap acidosis** is also known as a **hyperchloremic** acidosis.

Questions

1. A 62-year-old man arrives for his first checkup in 20 years. He is a smoker who received a diagnosis of hypertension many years ago, but did not take medication or return to his primary care physician. On physical examination, his blood pressure is 180/105. He is well-appearing but overweight. His laboratory examination is significant for sodium 138 mEq/L, potassium 5.8 mEq/L, chloride 104 mEq/L, bicarbonate 20 mEq/L, BUN 60 mg/dL, creatinine 2.8 mg/dL, and glucose of 230 mg/dL. What is the most likely cause of his decreased bicarbonate?

    A. Diabetic ketoacidosis
    B. Hypertension
    C. Renal insufficiency
    D. Diarrhea
    E. Chronic obstructive pulmonary disease

2. An elderly homeless woman is found unresponsive in the street, breathing rapidly. A blood gas analysis is performed with these results: pH 7.29, Pco_2 18 mm Hg, Po_2 100 mmHg, O_2 saturation 99%, Na^+ 145 mEq/l, Cl^- 90, HCO_3^- 12. A likely cause of her acidosis is which of the following?

    A. Hypoxia
    B. Diarrhea
    C. Methanol
    D. Vomiting
    E. Chronic obstructive pulmonary disease

3. A young man is brought in by ambulance after attempting suicide. He admits to being severely depressed and trying to end his own life by taking a bottle of aspirin. What abnormalities can we expect to see on his arterial blood gas?

    A. Hypercapnia and hypoxia
    B. Hypocapnia and hypoxia
    C. Hypocapnia and decreased bicarbonate
    D. Hypercapnia and decreased bicarbonate
    E. Hypoxia and increased bicarbonate

4. A teenage girl visits her primary care physician for her annual checkup. The astute family physician notices several worrisome physical signs including red puffy eyes, swollen parotid glands, and erosion of her tooth enamel. Her basic metabolic panel is as follows: Na^+ 123 mEq/L, K^+ 2.9 mEq/L, HCO_3^- 32 mEq/L. Which of the following is the likely cause of her metabolic abnormalities?

    A. Hyperventilation
    B. Ingestion of calcium carbonate
    C. Renal failure
    D. Vomiting
    E. Polydipsia

HPI: LM is a 70-year-old woman with type 2 diabetes and hypertension who presents to the ED complaining of lack of appetite, a dull, constant ache over her entire abdomen, and constipation for the last week. She is recovering from a bout of influenza diagnosed by her primary care physician 2 weeks ago, and has not been eating or drinking well since the onset of her illness. She has also had a headache and difficulty concentrating for the last several days. Her diabetes and hypertension are well controlled, and she has continued to take her medications, which include hydrochlorothiazide, lisinopril, glipizide, and metformin.

PE: BP 100/60 HR 60 RR 12/min T 36.7°C
Her oral mucosa is dry. Her heart rate is bradycardic and regular, and her lungs are clear to auscultation. Her abdomen is protuberant and soft, with few bowel sounds and no tenderness to palpation. She is somnolent and easily aroused, but falls back to sleep immediately and cannot state where she is.

Labs: Na^+ 139 mEq/L, K^+ 5.5 mEq/L, Cl^+ 98 mEq/L, HCO_3^- 29 mEq/L, BUN 65 mg/dL, Cr 3.4 mg/dL, glucose 200 mg/dL, Ca^{2+} 15 mEq/dL, phos 4.2 mEq/L.

Thought Questions

- How does the kidney contribute to calcium and phosphate homeostasis?

- How is vitamin D involved in calcium and phosphate regulation?

- What are the causes of and symptoms associated with hyper- and hypocalcemia? Hyper- and hypophosphatemia?

- What is the pathophysiology of our patient's condition?

Basic Science Review and Discussion

Homeostasis of both calcium and phosphate can be discussed together because serum levels of both ions are dependent on renal excretion, intestinal absorption, the action of PTH, and regulation of bone metabolism.

Calcium Homeostasis Calcium is a very important ion in both the physiology and the structure of the body. It is a rapidly fluctuating intracellular messenger, induces microtubule and muscle contraction, enables neurotransmitter release, is an important cofactor in the coagulation cascade, and is a component of the bony skeleton. It is the most abundant electrolyte in the body and most of it is found in the skeleton. The normal serum calcium concentration ranges from 8.5 to 10.0 mg/dL, with approximately 40% to 50% bound to albumin. **For every 1 g/dL fall in plasma albumin concentration, there is a 0.8 mg/dL reduction in serum calcium concentration.** The active form of calcium is the ionized portion, which accounts for 45% to 50% of serum calcium. The percentage of calcium bound to protein changes with changes in blood pH; binding increases with increased pH.

Ionized calcium is filtered at the glomerulus and approximately 65% is reabsorbed at the proximal tubule and 20% at the thick ascending loop of Henle. **PTH,** the most impor-tant regulator of ionized calcium concentration, increases the reabsorption of calcium in the distal convoluted tubule (DCT). Diuretics have a variable effect on calcium excre-tion, with furosemide increasing calcium excretion and hydrochlorothiazide decreasing calcium excretion. Oppos-ing PTH and of lesser significance in normal calcium homeo-stasis is **calcitonin,** released by the parafollicular cells (C cells) of the thyroid, which decreases bone reabsorption of calcium, resulting in decreased serum ionized calcium.

The most important regulator of calcium absorption from the gut is **1,25-(OH) vitamin D** (Figure 8-1). The precursor to vitamin D, 7-dehydrocholesterol, is converted in the skin in the presence of ultraviolet radiation to cholecalciferol. Cholecalciferol is then hydroxylated in the liver to 25-hydroxycholecalciferol and then further hydroxylated in the kidney to produce the active form 1,25-dihydroxycholecal-ciferol, which stimulates gastrointestinal absorption of calcium. PTH directly stimulates α-1-hydroxylase. PTH is syn-thesized and released from the parathyroid gland in response to a lowered serum ionized calcium level. Vitamin D negatively feeds back on 1-α-hydroxylase at the level of the kidney and inhibits the production of PTH thereby regu-lating the intestinal absorption of calcium.

Hypercalcemia Hypercalcemia results from several mecha-nisms including increased mobilization of calcium from bone, increased gastrointestinal absorption, and decreased urinary excretion. Under normal circumstances, PTH in-creases mobilization of ionized calcium from bone, and in certain malignancies and hyperparathyroidism increased mobilization occurs to an extreme degree, resulting in hypercalcemia. Squamous cell lung cancer produces PTH-related peptide and causes the paraneoplastic syndrome of hypercalcemia. Osteoblastic metastases from breast cancer and osteolytic lesions due to multiple myeloma may also precipitate hypercalcemia, especially in immobile patients. **Primary hyperparathyroidism** is usually due to a single,

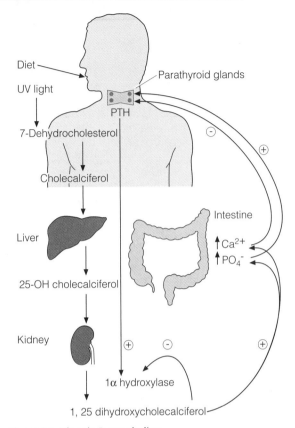

Figure 8-1 Vitamin D metabolism.

hyperfunctioning adenoma in one of the four parathyroid glands. Long-standing renal insufficiency may lead to chronically elevated levels of parathyroid hormone and hypercalcemia, termed **secondary hyperparathyroidism.** Secondary hyperparathyroidism may progress until the parathyroid glands autonomously hyperfunction, leading to **tertiary hyperparathyroidism** and hypercalcemia that can only be corrected by parathyroidectomy. Other causes of hypercalcemia include thiazide diuretics and granulomatous diseases. Thiazide diuretics increase the sodium gradient used for the reabsorption of calcium in the DCT and thus elevate serum calcium levels. Granulomatous diseases such as sarcoidosis may cause hypercalcemia because macrophages convert vitamin D precursors to the active form of vitamin D. A complete list of etiologies of hypercalcemia is given below (see Thumbnail).

Symptoms of hypercalcemia include anorexia, nausea, abdominal pain, polydipsia, polyuria, headache, impaired concentration, loss of memory, confusion, hallucinations, and muscle weakness. Hypercalcemia induces a nephrogenic diabetes insipidus (DI) that impairs the kidney's ability to concentrate urine, resulting in dehydration. Hypercalcemia may result in nephrocalcinosis and nephrolithiasis. The treatment of hypercalcemia is aimed at hydration with normal saline, forced diuresis with furosemide, and bisphosphonates to bind calcium to bone. Hemodialysis may be necessary.

Hypocalcemia The causes of hypocalcemia include hypoparathyroidism, decreased calcium mobilization from bone, and reduced absorption of calcium from the gut. Long-standing renal insufficiency may contribute to hypocalcemia due to the lack of nephron mass available to hydroxylate vitamin D. Hypocalcemia may be seen in association with hypomagnesemia because low magnesium levels inhibit PTH release. A complete list of etiologies is given on the next page (see Thumbnail).

Symptoms of hypocalcemia include paresthesias such as perioral or acral (fingertip) tingling and muscle cramps. Classic physical examination signs of hypocalcemia include **Chvostek's sign,** a twitching of the lip brought about by tapping on the facial nerve just anterior to the ear below the zygomatic bone, and **Trousseau's sign,** carpal spasm after the inflation of a blood pressure cuff for 2 minutes. Severe hypocalcemia may precipitate **tetany** due to increased neuromuscular excitability including laryngospasm. Treatment of hypocalcemia includes the administration of calcium and vitamin D.

Phosphate Homeostasis Phosphate is present in various forms in the body. In its ionic form (PO_4^{3-}) it is an important intracellular anion [many essential reactions use the breaking of the high energy phosphate bonds in adenosine triphosphate (ATP) for energy]; in its organic form it is a component of all body tissues, as it forms the backbone of all nucleic acids. Urinary phosphate buffers protons in the urine.

Normal serum phosphorus levels range from 3.5 to 4.5 mg/dL. Serum phosphate concentration is determined by both intestinal absorption and renal excretion, with renal excretion being most important. In the kidney, approximately 90% of the filtered phosphorus is reabsorbed in the proximal tubule. Vitamin D increases absorption of phosphorus in the gut.

Hyperphosphatemia Hyperphosphatemia is caused by decreased renal excretion, increased cell turnover, acidosis, exogenous administration of phosphorus or vitamin D, and magnesium deficiency. A complete list of etiologies is given on the next page (see Thumbnail). Phosphate inhibits renal hydroxylation of vitamin D; thus, elevated phosphorus levels may lead to hypocalcemia. Hyperphosphatemia in the presence of a normal calcium level may result in metastatic calcification as phosphate complexes with calcium and deposits in the tissues.

The treatment of hyperphosphatemia includes using phosphate binders such as calcium carbonate or calcium acetate, alkalization of the urine with a carbonic anhydrase inhibiting diuretic, or dialysis.

Hypophosphatemia Hypophosphatemia is due to renal loss, decreased intestinal absorption, or redistribution during various conditions. A complete list of etiologies is given below (see Thumbnail). Clinical manifestations may include anorexia, confusion, paresthesias, and bone pain due to skeletal abnormalities. The treatment is a high phosphate diet and oral or parenteral phosphate.

Case Conclusion The patient has many of the symptoms of hypercalcemia: anorexia, constipation, impaired concentration, and abdominal pain. Symptoms of hypercalcemia are often referred to as **moans (abdominal pain), groans (bone pain), stones (kidney stones), and psychic overtones (mental status changes).** During the patient's illness, her oral fluid intake decreased while she continued to take her thiazide diuretic. Her hypercalcemia was precipitated by dehydration, worsened by renal insufficiency, and exacerbated by immobilization. Her increased serum calcium further impaired her kidney's ability to concentrate urine, worsening her dehydration. Following rehydration and discontinuation of hydrochlorothiazide, her serum calcium levels slowly normalized and her kidney function returned.

Thumbnail: Renal Pathophysiology—Calcium and Phosphate Abnormalities

	Etiology	Symptom	Sign

Hypercalcemia	Malignancy
	Hyperparathyroidism
	  Primary
	  Secondary
	  Tertiary
	Renal disease
	Thiazide diuretics
	Hyperthyroidism
	Vitamin D intoxication
	Vitamin A intoxication
	Hypophosphatemia
	Immobilization
	Granulomas
	Sarcoidosis
	Milk alkali syndrome
		Fatigue
		Muscle weakness
		Abdominal pain
		Constipation
		Anorexia
		Nausea
		Polydipsia
		Polyuria
		Headache
		Impaired concentration
		Loss of memory
			Lethargy to coma
			Seizure
			Dilute urine
			Metastatic calcification
			Arrhythmia
			Paralytic ileus
			↓ QT segment

Hypocalcemia	Hypoparathyroidism Post-thyroidectomy Chronic magnesium deficiency Vitamin D deficiency Pseudohypoparathyroidism Hyperphosphatemia Pancreatitis Alcohol withdrawal	Muscle cramps Tetany Paresthesias	Carpal spasm Pedal spasm Laryngospasm Arrhythmia ↑ QT segment
Hyperphosphatemia	Renal failure Hypoparathyroidism Pseudohypoparathyroidism Lysis of cells with chemotherapy Hemolytic anemia Rhabdomyolysis Acidosis Vitamin D intoxication Magnesium deficiency	Symptoms of hypocalcemia Weakness Fatigue Anorexia Nausea	Decreased urine volume Arrhythmias Paralytic ileus Heart failure
Hypophosphatemia	Hyperparathyroidism Hypomagnesemia Corticosteroids Malabsorption Alcoholism Phosphate binders Vitamin D deficiency Sepsis Salicylate poisoning Alkalosis Refeeding syndrome	Bone pain Weakness Anorexia Lethargy Confusion Paresthesias	Seizures Coma Reduced GFR Heart failure

Key Points

▸ The renal contribution to calcium homeostasis is the production of vitamin D and, via the influence of PTH, the renal absorption of calcium.

▸ The primary regulation of serum phosphate levels is via renal excretion of phosphate.

▸ Long-standing renal disease results in hypocalcemia and hyperphosphatemia.

Questions

1. A healthy 27-year-old woman presents to your office for a routine examination and is found to have a serum calcium level of 12 mEq/L and a phosphorus level of 2.2 mEq/L. What is the most likely diagnosis?

   A. Renal insufficiency
   B. Familial hypocalciuric hypercalcemia
   C. Hyperparathyroidism
   D. Pseudohypoparathyroidism
   E. Excessive use of vitamin D

2. A patient of yours has suffered for many years from severe chronic renal insufficiency due to hypertension. His blood pressure is well controlled with a combination of an ACEI and a beta-blocker. Which of the following electrolyte abnormalities is he most likely to have?

   A. Hypercalcemia and hyperphosphatemia
   B. Hypercalcemia and metabolic alkalosis
   C. Hypercalcemia and hypophosphatemia
   D. Hypocalcemia and hyperphosphatemia
   E. Hypercalcemia and metabolic acidosis

3. A very anxious medical student complains of anxiety attacks characterized by tingling of his hands and around his mouth. Which of the following is the pathophysiology of his complaint?

   A. Hypercalcemia
   B. Hypocalcemia
   C. Hyperphosphatemia
   D. Metabolic acidosis
   E. Metabolic alkalosis

> **HPI:** DB, a 40-year-old African-American man, presents to his primary care provider's office for an annual physical. He has not seen a doctor for some time, and has no complaints, but wants to have his cholesterol checked because his 48-year-old brother just had a heart attack. He jogs and plays basketball to stay in shape but knows he doesn't eat the right foods. Both his father and his mother have hypertension.
>
> **PE:** BP 154/92 Pulse 72
> The patient has an athletic build. His fundi are within normal limits. His heart has a regular rate and rhythm with an S_4 present. His lungs are clear to auscultation.

Thought Questions

- What is essential hypertension and what mediates it?

- What are the consequences of hypertension on the kidney?

- What is accelerated/malignant hypertension?

- What are the causes of renovascular hypertension and when should we suspect them?

- How can we best treat this patient?

Basic Science Review and Discussion

Essential hypertension is an elevation in blood pressure, without a proximate cause, above an ambiguously defined "normal level." Current guidelines are listed in Table 9-1.

No single value should be considered proof of high blood pressure. Blood pressure values should be well established over several visits. The definitions of hypertension are changing because it is now apparent that lower blood pressures significantly reduce cardiovascular morbidity and mortality and are renal protective.

Although the etiology of essential hypertension is unclear, there are endocrine, neural, genetic, and environmental factors responsible for the apparent upward resetting of blood pressure homeostatic set points. It is likely that many different, interrelated factors contribute to the development of hypertension in susceptible individuals.

Table 9-1 Current guidelines for assessing blood pressure

Blood pressure stage	Systolic (mm Hg)	Diastolic (mm Hg)
High normal	139	89
Mild hypertension	140–159	90–99
Moderate hypertension	160–179	100–109
Severe hypertension	> 180	> 110

The prevalence of essential hypertension varies among the population. It is estimated that 10% to 15% of Caucasian adults and up to 30% of African Americans have blood pressures greater than 140/90. For unclear reasons, African Americans have a more serious form of the disease. The incidence of hypertension increases with age. Women have a lower incidence of hypertension until menopause when the incidence of hypertension rapidly approaches that of men. The incidence of **secondary hypertension,** attributed to causes such as renal artery stenosis, fibromuscular dysplasia, pheochromocytoma, primary hyperaldosteronism, Cushing's disease, and coarctation of the aorta comprise only 2% to 5% of all cases of hypertension. It is particularly important to suspect secondary hypertension in young adults.

Etiologies of Hypertension

Renin-angiotensin-aldosterone axis   The renin-angiotensin-aldosterone hormonal axis (Figure 9-1) is an important determinant of blood pressure. **Renin** is an enzyme produced and secreted from the juxtaglomerular cells of the kidney. Its substrate, angiotensinogen, is an α-globulin produced in the liver, and cleaved by renin to produce angiotensin I. **Angiotensin I** is cleaved by angiotensin converting enzyme, found on the surface of endothelial cells, primarily in the lung, to angiotensin II. **Angiotensin II** is a potent vasoconstrictor and stimulates the production of aldosterone from the adrenal cortex. **Aldosterone,** a steroid hormone, is produced in the zona glomerulosa of the adrenal cortex. Its main actions are increased sodium reabsorption, potassium secretion, and hydrogen ion secretion. Aldosterone acts on the principal cells of the cortical collecting duct to increase the permeability of luminal sodium channels and increase the activity of the sodium-potassium pumps in the basolateral membrane, facilitating the uptake of sodium and the secretion of potassium.

Another determinant of blood pressure is **sympathetic tone** mediated by the catecholamines of the adrenal medulla. This is often termed the neural hormonal axis as atrial baroreceptors are activated by a decrease in blood pressure

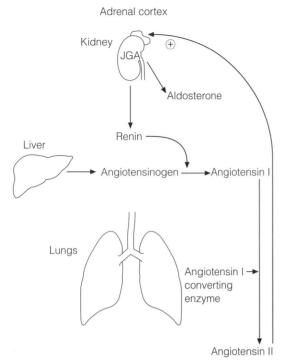

Figure 9-1 The renin-angiotensin-aldosterone axis.

to stimulate the adrenal medulla to release epinephrine and norepinephrine. These vasoactive substances vasoconstrict both arteries and veins, stimulate heart rate and contractility, and increase renin secretion.

A drop in blood pressure results in renal hypoperfusion and increased renin secretion from the cells of the juxtaglomerular apparatus. Decreased blood pressure is also sensed by the cardiac baroreceptors and stimulates epinephrine and norepinephrine release from the adrenal medulla. Renin secretion is further stimulated by epinephrine and norepinephrine. Increased plasma renin results in increased levels of angiotensin I, which is converted to angiotensin II in the lungs. Renin also stimulates the adrenal cortex to produce aldosterone, resulting in increased salt and water reabsorption from the kidney, thereby increasing intravascular volume. The combination of angiotensin II-mediated vasoconstriction and an aldosterone-mediated increase in salt and water reabsorption is the mechanism by which normal blood pressure is maintained. Increased blood pressure and plasma volumes negatively feed back to the kidney to lower renin levels.

Both an overactive renin-angiotensin-aldosterone axis and a tonically active sympathetic nervous system have been postulated to cause hypertension, but neither etiology can fully explain the pathogenesis of hypertension. Only 15% of patients with essential hypertension have elevated renin levels. Increased sympathetic activity has been linked with transient elevations in blood pressure but cannot account for the sustained hypertension seen in essential hypertension.

Other etiologies of hypertension Noninherited factors that increase blood pressure include a high-sodium diet, obesity, and alcohol ingestion. The mechanism for sodium-sensitive hypertension is not clear, and only 40% to 60% of hypertensives respond to a reduction in dietary salt. In these patients, sodium restriction and diuretics decrease plasma volume and aid in blood pressure reduction. **Syndrome X** is a triad of insulin resistance, hypertension, and hypercholesterolemia found in patients with centripetal obesity. Alcohol is also associated with hypertension by an unclear mechanism, and a reduction in blood pressure is seen with the cessation of alcohol consumption.

Renal artery stenosis is one cause of secondary hypertension. It is found in older patients with atherosclerotic vascular disease and suggested by an abdominal bruit. It usually causes severe hypertension and may present as a rapid rise in blood pressure in a patient with hypertension that was previously well controlled. Renal artery stenosis can be bilateral or unilateral and may cause hypertension by activation of the renin-angiotensin cascade in response to kidney hypoperfusion. The gold standard for diagnosis is an angiogram.

Fibromuscular dysplasia is another cause of secondary hypertension in younger patients. Most commonly the disease affects young women who have dysplasia or hyperplasia of the media of many different vessels. The characteristic appearance of the renal arteries on angiogram is a **"string of beads."** The bead-like appearance is due to areas of arterial wall hyperplasia alternating with normal-appearing segments.

Genetic factors clearly play a role in hypertension, although a specific gene (or set of genes) has not been identified. Patients with one or two hypertensive parents are two to three times more likely to develop hypertension than patients with a family history negative for hypertension.

Effects on the Kidneys Hypertension is a chronic illness that can result in cumulative injury to the kidney if left untreated. The typical course of renal damage is a slow decline in renal function, with sclerosis of the glomerular arteries and arterioles, cortical glomeruli being most affected. Sclerotic glomeruli are thickened and hyalinized decreasing renal perfusion. Eventually the tubules and supportive stroma atrophy, leading to shrunken and scarred kidneys bilaterally.

An accelerated form of hypertension also occurs and leads to acute renal failure. **Malignant hypertension,** more correctly referred to as **accelerated hypertension,** is associated with diastolic blood pressures above 130 mm Hg. It often occurs in patients with long-standing hypertension who have stopped taking their medications. Blood pressures in this range are an urgent matter and become an emergent matter when associated with renal failure, retinal hemorrhages and exudates, papilledema, encephalopathy, congestive heart failure, myocardial infarction, or aortic dissection. A diagnosis of hypertensive emergency does not depend on the absolute value of the patient's blood pressure but on the rapidity of the rise and the patient's associated symptoms. The renal failure causes glomerular damage and is thus associated with proteinuria and dysmorphic red blood cells seen on urinalysis. The histologic lesions are cortical petechial hemorrhages, fibrinoid necrosis of the small vessels, and **"onion skinning"** of the arterioles due to intimal hyperplasia. When seen together, the above findings are termed **malignant nephrosclerosis.**

Case Conclusion   DB had two repeat blood pressures of 146/96 and 158/101. After education about the risks of hypertension including stroke, renal failure, heart failure, and retinopathy, the patient was started on a thiazide diuretic and a beta-blocker. He was also referred to a nutritionist for counseling and began to eat a low-sodium diet. He remains physically active and his hypertension is well controlled on this regimen.

Thumbnail: Renal Pathophysiology—Essential vs. Renovascular Hypertension

	Essential hypertension	vs	**Renovascular hypertension**
Etiology	Idiopathic		Renal artery stenosis
Age	More than 40		Less than 30 or more than 50
Gender	Males more than female		Female in fibromuscular dysplasia
With Rx	Responds to treatment		Refractory to treatment
Clues	No atherosclerosis		Atherosclerosis likely
			Accelerated hypertension
			Pulmonary edema
			Flank bruit

Key Points

▶ Essential hypertension is far more common than secondary hypertension.

▶ Accelerated hypertension is high blood pressure associated with neural, renal, and cardiovascular compromise.

▶ Secondary causes of hypertension include renal artery stenosis, pheochromocytoma, primary hyperaldosteronism, Cushing's disease, and coarctation of the aorta.

▶ Good blood pressure control reduces the risk of stroke, heart attack, retinopathy, and kidney damage.

Questions

1. A 67-year-old man with a history of myocardial infarction, diabetes, and hypertension is started on lisinopril. What are the potential complications?

   A. Acute renal failure
   B. Hyperkalemia
   C. Hypotension
   D. Angioedema
   E. All of the above

2. A 29-year-old woman presents to your office for a general checkup. She has not seen a doctor other than to have Pap smears for many years. Her blood pressure is found to be 200/140. On physical exam she has narrowing of her retinal arteries, a carotid bruit, and an S_4. She has no family history of hypertension. Her most likely diagnosis is which of the following?

   A. Hyperaldosteronism
   B. Cushing's syndrome
   C. Fibromuscular dysplasia
   D. Pheochromocytoma
   E. Atherosclerotic renal disease

3. A 61-year-old woman in otherwise good health has hypertension. In your office today her blood pressure is 180/100. Her blood pressure has been well controlled with medication in the past but she refuses to take medication because she feels well. Which of the following is she at risk for?

   A. Renal failure
   B. Retinopathy
   C. Left ventricular failure
   D. Stroke
   E. All of the above

> **HPI:** LR is an 8-year-old girl with fever, nausea, oliguria, and dark-colored urine. At about 10 A.M. this morning, the patient began feeling and looking ill. Her mother noticed that she was urinating infrequently and that when she did urinate, it looked like "Coca-Cola." Her mother is also concerned about the swelling around her eyes. The mother states that her daughter is generally a healthy child and has never had similar symptoms. Upon further questioning, she admits her daughter was recently (~2 weeks ago) out of school for a few days with a sore throat, which resolved on its own. LR lives with her mother and older brother. Her father shares custody and sees her on weekends. She attends Stuart Day School and is in the third grade.
>
> **PE:** The patient is febrile with a temperature of 39.0°C, moderately elevated blood pressure at 117/78, and normal pulse and respirations. She has periorbital edema.
>
> **Labs:** Serum evaluation reveals a slightly elevated serum BUN and creatinine, depressed C3 concentration, cryoglobulins, and an elevated antistreptolysin O (ASO) titer. Urinalysis and urine cytology reveals mild proteinuria and red cell casts.

Thought Questions

- Describe the pathophysiology and the associated microscopic and immunofluorescence findings of the glomerular diseases.

- How is the immune system involved in the etiology of glomerular diseases?

- What is the difference between nephritic and nephrotic syndrome?

Basic Science Review and Discussion

There are many glomerular diseases, and the task of keeping them straight is overwhelming. However, there are a few guiding principles that help with organization. There are two ways to approach these diseases, either pathophysiologically or clinically. The pathophysiology of most glomerulonephritis (GN) is immune related, through the formation of antigen-antibody (Ag-Ab) complexes. Nonimmune mechanisms include hereditary defects in the glomerular basement membrane (GBM) and the pathologic processes involved in systemic diseases like amyloidosis and diabetes. Glomerular diseases present with different clinical syndromes including nephritic syndromes, discussed in this case, and nephrotic syndromes, discussed in the subsequent case.

Pathophysiology

Immune-complex GN Ag-Ab complexes can form when antibodies attach themselves to antigens that constitute the normal glomerular basement membrane, as in **Goodpasture's syndrome/anti-GBM disease**. As a result, antibodies and complement line up along the GBM, forming linear patterns on immunofluorescence (IF). There are no **circulating** immune complexes to form lumpy deposits.

Alternately, Ag-Ab complexes can form when circulating antigens are bound by circulating antibodies, and then deposit in the glomeruli because of their physical or chemical properties. In this case, antigens are either endogenous, as in **lupus GN,** or exogenous, as in **poststreptococcal GN.** Once these Ag-Ab complexes have deposited in the glomerulus, they activate the alternate complement pathway, causing inflammation and injury to the glomerular filtration apparatus, leading to proteinuria and hematuria. Leukocytes infiltrate and mesangial cells proliferate in an attempt to repair the injury. Immune complexes appear as electron dense deposits in the **mesangium** [as in **immunoglobulin A (IgA) nephropathy**], between the *endo*thelium and the GBM (**sub*endo*thelial** deposits as in **membranoproliferative GN**), or between the outer surface of the GBM and the podocytes of the glomerular *epi*thelial cells (**sub*epi*thelial** deposits as in **poststreptococcal GN**). The charge and size of the Ag-Ab complexes determine where they get lodged.

Another variant of immune-complex associated GN is **anti-neutrophil cytoplasmic autoantibodies (ANCA)-associated GN. Wegener's granulomatosis, Churg-Strauss syndrome,** and **microscopic polyangiitis** are small vessel vasculitides and, as such, impact the glomerular capillary tuft. They are associated with the ANCA that bind endothelial cells. However, the mechanism of glomerular injury is not simply immune-complex deposition since antibodies are not seen on immunofluorescence (these are sometimes referred to as "pauci-immune GNs").

Hereditary GN **Alport's syndrome** is a primarily X-linked dominant mutation in the gene encoding part of collagen IV, which composes the GBM. It presents with hematuria and, rarely, nephrotic syndrome. It frequently progresses to renal failure over 20 to 30 years and is associated with nerve deafness and eye problems. **Thin basement membrane disease** (benign familial hematuria) also results from hereditary defects in type IV collagen. However, it presents with asymptomatic hematuria, requires no treatment, and never causes renal failure.

Clinical Syndromes Clinically, glomerular diseases can be divided into those that present with *nephrotic* syndrome and those that present with *nephritic* syndrome. **Nephrotic syndrome** ("o" for pr**o**teinuria) is characterized by heavy proteinuria (>3.5 g/d) with resulting hypoalbuminemia and edema, hyperlipidemia and lipiduria. **Nephritic syndrome** is characterized by hematuria, red cell casts in the urinary sediment, azotemia (increase in serum nitrogenous compounds including BUN), oliguria, mild to moderate hypertension, and only mild edema/proteinuria. Another clinical syndrome, **rapidly progressive (crescentic) GN** is a final common pathway of rapid progression to renal failure in weeks to months. It is often associated with Goodpasture's, ANCA-associated vasculitides, or systemic lupus erythematosus.

Definitions Lesions can be described as:

Focal: involves < 50% of the glomeruli

Diffuse: involves > 50% of the glomeruli

Segmental: involves *part* of the individual glomerular tuft

Global: involves *all* of the individual glomerular tuft

Proliferative: involves increase in glomerular cell number (either WBCs or local proliferation of glomerular cells)

Crescentic: half-moon shaped collection of cells in Bowman's space

Membranous: expansion of the GBM by immune deposits

Sclerotic: increase in extracellular material

Fibrotic: deposition of type I and II collagen; consequence of healing inflammation

Immune-complex deposits can be described as:

Subendothelial: between the *endo*thelium and the GBM

Mesangial: in the mesangium

Subepithelial: between the GBM and the podocytes of the glomerular *epi*thelium

---

Case Conclusion After arriving at a clinical diagnosis of poststreptococcal GN, you admit the child to the hospital. Treatment includes antibiotics to eliminate any remaining streptococci, bed rest, diuretics and antihypertensives to control blood pressure, and careful monitoring and correcting of fluid and electrolyte abnormalities. You reassure the patient's parents that she has an excellent prognosis, with 95% recovery and recommend regular follow-up appointments for 1 year to ensure that the hematuria resolves.

Thumbnail: Renal Pathophysiology—Nephritic Syndromes

Disease	Most common clinical presentation and findings	Pathogenesis	Pathology
Postinfectious GN	Acute nephritis • 2 weeks post-pharyngitis/impetigo • Children; self-resolving • Group A β-hemolytic strep (elevated ASO titers)	Trapped Ag-Ab complexes	LM: Diffuse proliferation IF: IgG + C3, granular EM: **subepithelial humps**
IgA nephropathy (Berger's disease) and Henoch-Schönlein purpura	Hematuria • Associated w/upper respiratory or gastrointestinal infection	Unknown	LM: focal/mesangial proliferation IF: **IgA**, (+/−IgG, IgM, C3) EM: mesangial deposits
Goodpasture's syndrome/ anti-GBM GN	**Rapidly progressive GN** • Young men • Goodpasture's if also with pulmonary hemorrhage	Abs against fixed Ags in GBM	LM: crescents IF: IgG + C3, linear along GBM EM: widening of BM
ANCA-associated GN (pauci-immune GN)	**Rapidly progressive GN** • Wegener's granulomatosis, Churg-Strauss syndrome, microscopic polyangiitis • Systemic involvement common	Unknown	LM: crescents IF: **No Ig** EM: No deposits
Alport's syndrome	Hematuria • Most cases **X-linked** dominant • < 20 years old • Associated w/deafness and eye disorders	Structural defect in type IV collagen leads to leaky GBM	EM: **GBM splitting**
Thin basement membrane disease (benign familial hematuria)	Hematuria • Asymptomatic • Familial	Defect in type IV collagen	EM: diffusely thin GBM

LM, light microscopy; IF, immunofluorescence; EM, electron microscopy.

Key Points

▸ **Nephritic syndrome** is characterized by hematuria, red cell casts, azotemia, oliguria, and hypertension.

▸ Nephritic syndromes result from defects in the GBM caused by:
  1. Immune responses initiated by deposition of circulating Ag-Ab complexes or Ab attack of GBM components.
  2. Hereditary defects in components of the GBM.

Questions

1. A 6-year-old boy presents with gross hematuria and no other symptoms 2 days after a sore throat. A kidney biopsy reveals mesangial proliferation on light microscopy and IgA deposits on immunofluorescence. What is his likely diagnosis?
   A. Poststreptococcal GN
   B. Henoch-Schönlein purpura
   C. Alport's syndrome
   D. Benign familial hematuria
   E. IgA nephropathy

2. A 24-year-old man presents with hemoptysis and hematuria. A renal biopsy reveals crescents on light microscopy, and linear IgG on immunofluorescence. What is the inciting event in the pathophysiology of the implicated disease?
   A. Circulating endogenous antigens are trapped by circulating antibodies and lodge along the GBM in a linear pattern.
   B. There is an autosomal-dominant mutation in a component of Type IV collagen in the GBM and lung endothelium.
   C. Exogenous circulating antigens bind to local stationary antibodies as they pass through the glomerulus and lung endothelium.
   D. Autoimmune antibodies bind to normal components of the lung and kidney endothelium.
   E. The pathophysiology is unknown.

3. A 45-year-old woman with a history of adult-onset asthma presents with microscopic hematuria, hypertension, and acute renal failure as evidenced by significantly increased BUN and creatinine. Her renal biopsy reveals eosinophil infiltration in the mesangium but no evidence of Ag-Ab complex deposition on light microscopy or immunofluorescence. Serum evaluation is ANA negative but ANCA positive. What is her likely diagnosis?
   A. Wegener's granulomatosis
   B. Churg-Strauss
   C. Amyloidosis
   D. Minimal change disease
   E. Thin basement membrane disease

4. A 17-year-old boy with deafness and near-blind vision is referred to a research nephrologist by his primary care doctor, who is concerned about the microscopic hematuria discovered during a routine physical exam. His father was also deaf but was adopted, so no other family history is available. This nephrologist has easy access to electron microscopy (EM) and finds splitting of a thick GBM. What is the likely diagnosis?
   A. Goodpasture's syndrome
   B. Alport's syndrome
   C. Berger's syndrome (IgA nephropathy)
   D. Type IV lupus GN
   E. Type I membranoproliferative GN

HPI: LM is a 6-year-old boy with sudden-onset lower extremity edema. Over the past 4 days, the patient's father noticed significant and worsening swelling that began in the patient's feet and seems to be moving up his legs. The father reports his son is urinating infrequently, but there is no gross blood in the urine. The patient recently recovered from an upper respiratory infection 2 weeks ago. The patient lives with his parents and younger sister, attends the local public school, and is in the first grade.

PE: The patient is afebrile and his vital signs are normal. There is no periorbital edema; however, he has pitting edema to his knees.

Labs: Urinalysis and urine cytology reveal significant proteinuria (albumin only), with no red cells or casts. Serum evaluation reveals a serum BUN and creatinine at the upper limits of normal.

Thought Questions

■ Proteinuria represents a failure of the glomerular filtration apparatus. Describe the elements of the glomerular filtration apparatus.

■ What is the difference between the nephritic and nephrotic syndromes?

■ What are the nephrotic syndromes? Describe the general pathophysiology, and the associated microscopic and immunofluorescence findings.

Basic Science Review and Discussion

Glomerular Filtration Apparatus The glomerular filtration apparatus (Figure 11-1) is composed of three layers: the **endothelium** of the glomerular capillary, the **basement membrane,** and the Bowman's capsule (BC) **epithelium.** The capillary endothelium is fenestrated with 50- to 100-nm fenestrations, providing a *size* barrier to filtration. The basement membrane is thicker than most, is secreted by the BC epithelium, consists of collagen, glycoproteins, and mucopolysaccharides, and is negatively charged, thus providing a *charge* barrier to filtration. Finally, the BC epithelial cells, "podocytes," have foot processes that embrace the capillary basement membrane. These processes are coated with and bridged by a negatively charged glycocalyx, providing another mechanical and charge barrier to filtration. The end result is that size, electrical charge, and molecular configuration determine the permeability of the filter to macromolecules. Molecules smaller than molecular weight (MW) 65,000 can pass (e.g., free hemoglobin), but molecules larger than MW 68,000 are blocked (e.g., albumin). Negatively charged molecules (e.g., albumin) are blocked by the filter's strong electronegativity. Molecules that are trapped on the epithelial side of the basement membrane are phagocytosed by podocytes, and those trapped on the endothelial side are phagocytosed by mesangial cells.

Nephrotic Syndrome Nephrotic syndrome is characterized by excretion of protein in the urine greater than 3.5 g/day, which leads to **hypoalbuminemia.** This decrease in oncotic pressure in the vasculature leads to fluid extravasation into the surrounding tissues, leading to **edema.** The drop in oncotic pressure also leads to increased hepatic production of lipids and **hyperlipidemia.** This in turn leads to **hyperlipiduria or oval fat bodies** (grape-like clusters) in the urine, seen as **maltese crosses** when the urinary sediment is examined under polarized light microscopy. This is in contrast to *nephritic* syndrome, which is characterized by hematuria, red cell casts in the urinary sediment, azotemia, oliguria, mild to moderate hypertension, and only mild edema and proteinuria.

Nephrotic syndrome results from deposition of immune complexes, as a complication of a systemic illness, or idiopathically (with unknown pathophysiology). The most common nephrotic syndrome in adults is **membranous nephropathy.** It is characterized by basement membrane

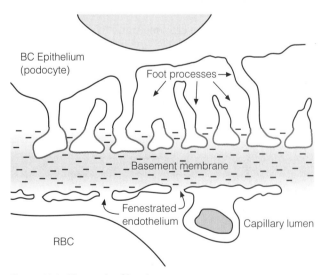

Figure 11-1 Glomerular filtration apparatus.

thickening forming a "**spike and dome**" pattern between subepithelial immune-complex deposits. Immunofluorescence reveals granular IgG and C3 lining capillary loops. It is usually secondary to other diseases such as systemic lupus erythematosus or hepatitis B, or drugs such as gold and penicillamine.

The most common nephrotic syndrome in children 2 to 6 years old is **minimal change disease** (aka lipoid nephrosis). It is characterized by the effacement of foot processes of podocytes. Electron microscopy is required for definitive diagnosis since there are no unusual findings on light microscopy (thus "*minimal* change"). Edema is the usual presenting symptom. Other symptoms such as renal failure and hypertension are less common, particularly in children. As with other nephrotic syndromes, laboratory studies reveal severe proteinuria (in this case, selective for albumin) with rare hematuria, and an elevation of the total cholesterol and triglycerides. Fortunately, more than 90% of children respond dramatically to steroid treatment (e.g., prednisone).

Like minimal change disease, **focal segmental glomerulosclerosis (FSGS)** is characterized by effacement of foot processes on electron microscopy but normal findings on light microscopy and no immunoglobulin deposition on immunofluorescence. In FSGS, there is sclerosis in a proportion of the glomeruli (thus it is *focal*) and each affected glomeruli is only partly sclerosed (thus it is *segmental*). FSGS is often associated with HIV infection, heroin abuse, sickle cell disease, and morbid obesity. It is grouped with the

nephrotic syndromes because of significant proteinuria, though it does present with microscopic hematuria as well. Treatment is with steroids. Unlike minimal change disease, it has a poor prognosis, with 50% progressing onto end-stage renal disease in 5 to 10 years.

Nephrotic Glomerular Diseases Secondary to Systemic Disorders **Amyloidosis** is a systemic disease characterized by deposits of one of many types of insoluble fibrous proteins (e.g., monoclonal Ig light chains) in multiple organ systems. These deposits stain positive with **Congo red** and show **apple green birefringence** under polarized light, and lead to nephrotic syndrome and ultimately renal failure when they deposit in the glomerulus.

Diabetes is a systemic disease with macrovascular and microvascular impact. The afferent and efferent arterioles lose their ability to regulate GFR as they undergo **hyaline arteriosclerosis.** The basement membrane of the smaller glomerular capillaries becomes thickened as a result of hyperfiltration that occurs in diabetic nephropathy. There is diffuse or nodular (**Kimmelstiel-Wilson nodules**) glomerulosclerosis, which slowly progresses to renal failure.

Systemic lupus erythematosus may present with nephrotic syndrome, nephritic syndrome, or a combination. The World Health Organization (WHO) has developed a classification schema to represent the five patterns seen on biopsy. The important point is that **WHO IV (diffuse proliferative)** has the worst prognosis, and **wire-loop** lesions are seen on IF.

Case Conclusion Based on the findings of edema and albuminuria in the absence of hematuria or systemic disease, minimal change disease tops the differential diagnosis list for this 6 year old. LM's parents will be reassured by the likelihood that LM will improve quickly with a long-term course of prednisone.

Thumbnail: Renal Pathophysiology—Diseases with Nephritic and Nephrotic Elements

Disease	Clinical presentation and associated findings	Pathogenesis	Pathology
Lupus GN	• Five WHO patterns, each with proliferation in different parts of the glomerulus and with different degrees of nephrotic and nephritic syndromes. • ANA and anti–double-stranded DNA (dsDNA) associated	Trapped Ag-Ab complexes	LM: crescents; "wire loop" appearance in **type IV** IF: IgG, IgM + C3, granular EM: subepithelial, subendothelial, mesangial deposits (anywhere)
Membranoproliferative GN	Type I: Nephrotic • Recent upper respiratory infection • < 30 y.o. Type II: hematuria, CRF	Ag-Ab complexes	LM: mesangial proliferation IF: IgG, IgM + C3/C1/C4 granular EM: splitting of GBM; "train track" appearance LM: mesangial proliferation IF: C3 only EM: dense subendothelial deposits

LM, light microscopy; ESRD, end-stage renal disease; C3, complement; IF, immunofluorescence; RTA, renal tubular acidosis; GN, glomerulonephritis; EM, electron microscopy; GBM, glomerular basement membrane.

Thumbnail: Renal Pathophysiology—Nephrotic Syndromes

Disease	Clinical presentation and associated findings	Pathogenesis	Pathology
Minimal change disease (lipoid nephrosis)	Nephrotic syndrome • **Leading cause in children** • Albumin selectively secreted • Idiopathic; also associated w/allergy, Hodgkin's • Responds well to steroids	Unknown	LM: normal IF: negative/normal EM: **fusion of podocytes;** no deposits
Membranous nephropathy	Nephrotic syndrome • **Leading cause in adults** • Sudden lower extremity edema • Associated w/hepatitis B, malignancy, gold therapy, lupus GN type V	In situ Ag-Ab complex formation	LM: thickened GBM with **"spike and dome"** pattern **IF: IgG** + C3, granular, along capillary loops EM: **subepithelial** deposits
Focal segmental glomerulosclerosis	Nephrotic syndrome +/− hematuria • Associated w/heroin, HIV, obesity, sickle-cell • 50% to ESRD	Unknown	LM: focal segmental sclerosis IF: IgM + C3 in sclerotic parts EM: fusion of podocytes
Diabetic nephropathy	Nephrotic syndrome • Associated w/retinopathy, type IV RTA • 10–20 years after onset of diabetes	Unknown	LM: nodular (**Kimmelstiel-Wilson nodules**) or diffuse sclerosis; hyaline arteriosclerosis of afferent and efferent arterioles IF: No Ig EM: No deposits
Amyloidosis	Nephrotic syndrome • > 60 y.o. • Associated w/multiple myeloma, etc.	Deposition of light chains	LM: **Congo red** staining mesangial deposits; **apple green birefringence** w/ polarized light

Key Points

▶ **Nephrotic syndrome** is characterized by proteinuria, hypoalbuminemia, edema, hyperlipidemia, and lipiduria.

▶ **Nephritic syndrome** is characterized by hematuria, red cell casts, azotemia, oliguria, and hypertension.

Questions

1. A 45-year-old male homeless HIV+ IV drug user comes to the ED for gross hematuria and peripheral edema. A urinalysis with cytology reveals significant proteinuria and oval fat bodies, but few red cells and no casts. Serum analysis reveals hypoalbuminemia. ED doctors diagnose a nephrotic syndrome. This patient has a disease that requires electron microscopy for definitive diagnosis. Which one of the following is his likely diagnosis?

    A. Membranous glomerulonephritis
    B. Focal segmental glomerulosclerosis (FSGS)
    C. Lupus glomerulonephritis
    D. Diabetic nephropathy
    E. Minimal change disease

2. A 52-year-old woman is being treated by her primary care doctor for a chronic illness. At this year's annual checkup, her BUN and creatinine are significantly elevated and she has 3+ proteinuria on urine dipstick. A renal biopsy reveals + Congo red staining and apple green birefringence under polarized light. Which chronic disease does this patient have?

    A. Lesch-Nyhan syndrome (a syndrome of hyperuricemia)
    B. Diabetes mellitus, type 2
    C. Diabetes insipidus
    D. Systemic lupus erythematosus
    E. Amyloidosis

HPI: CC is a 16-year-old girl with right flank pain, fever, chills, nausea, and vomiting for the past 24 hours. Ten days prior to presentation, she began having pain and burning with urination, increased frequency of urination, urinating several times at night, and she noticed streaks of blood on the toilet tissue after urinating. She thought these symptoms were related to her new sexual partner and was afraid if she went to see a doctor that her parents would find out when the insurance bill arrived. So she took an over-the-counter analgesic for "pain with urination" and hoped it would resolve with time. She has no known medical problems or allergies. She lives with her parents and twin brother and attends a magnet high school in a nearby city. She smokes one pack of cigarettes per week and drinks about three beers each Friday and Saturday night. She has been sexually active since age 15, has had a total of three sexual partners, and has been with her current partner for 2 weeks.

PE: T 40.0°C (104°F) BP 110/65 Pulse 101 RR 19 SaO$_2$ 99% at room air
The patient is diaphoretic, flushed, and ill-appearing, has right flank pain at the costovertebral angle, and a soft, nondistended abdomen. She also has mild to moderate suprapubic tenderness.

Labs: Urine analysis (UA): positive nitrites, blood, and leukocyte esterase, leukocytes, red blood cells, and white cell casts. CBC: Leukocytosis and left shift (↑ immature neutrophils). Urine and blood cultures: results pending.

Thought Questions

- How can one differentiate between a simple urinary tract infection (UTI) and pyelonephritis?

- Which organisms are most commonly responsible for UTIs? What about UTIs in special populations (e.g., hospitalized patients)?

- What drugs are used to treat UTIs?

Basic Science Review and Discussion

Acute cystitis (a "bladder infection") is characterized by **dysuria** (pain or burning with urination), increased **frequency** and **urgency** of urination, gross **hematuria** (50%), **pyuria** (pus in the urine), and suprapubic pain. Fever, chills, and nausea or vomiting are *not* characteristic of a lower UTI. Before diagnosing simple cystitis, one must also consider candidal vulvovaginitis in women and prostatitis in men. Cystitis may also occur secondary to chemotherapy (cyclophosphamide is notorious for causing hemorrhagic cystitis), radiation or viral infection (e.g., adenovirus), bladder cancer, interstitial cystitis, voiding dysfunction disorders, and psychosomatic disorders (diagnoses of exclusion). UTIs are far more common in women, affecting about 8% of the adult female population each year. Cystitis in men is rare, occurring mainly in boys with genitourinary abnormalities or in older men with prostate enlargement and urinary stasis. Therefore, when cystitis occurs in men, a further work-up is required.

The most common route of UTI infection is ascension from the urethra to the bladder. The most common organisms involved in UTIs are the coliforms (colonic flora). *Escherichia coli* is the most common culprit, causing over 90% of first infections and 80% of infections overall. Uropathic strains of *E. coli* have adhesive pili that bind to receptors on the urinary tract epithelium. *Serratia, Enterobacter, Klebsiella, Proteus,* and *Pseudomonas* are found in hospitalized patients. *Proteus* is associated with recurrent infections in patients with struvite stones, and *Staphylococcus saprophyticus* is a gram-positive cocci that causes 10% to 15% of UTIs in young sexually active women. UTI risk factors include being female (short urethra), penetrative sexual activity (the vagina is often colonized with fecal flora), bladder instrumentation such as in-dwelling Foley catheters, diaphragm use, pregnancy, urinary stasis from obstruction (e.g., prostatic hyperplasia) or a neurogenic bladder, infected kidney stones, and an immunecompromised state.

Pyelonephritis is an upper UTI characterized by flank pain or **costovertebral angle (CVA) tenderness,** the triad of **dysuria/frequency/urgency, fever and chills,** and **nausea and vomiting.** Since pyelonephritis usually results from ascending bladder infections, pyelonephritis risk factors are the same as lower UTI risk factors, with the addition of vesicoureteral reflux. When the ureter enters the bladder at a less oblique angle, it is not compressed during urination and there is opportunity for retrograde flow up the ureter. If severe and untreated, this can progress to chronic pyelonephritis and irreversible renal damage.

UTIs are diagnosed by UA followed by a urine culture. In the UA, positive nitrites, blood, and leukocyte esterase suggest the presence of a UTI. White blood cells and bacteria on microscopy are suggestive of lower UTI, while white cell *casts* suggest pyelonephritis (implies the infection is occurring in the renal tubules, which form the casts). In the urine culture (which takes 24 to 48+ hours to grow), we look for bacterial growth measured in colony-forming units (CFUs).

The drugs used to treat cystitis include **trimethoprim-sulfamethoxazole** (both interfere with purine synthesis), **cephalexin** (a first generation cephalosporin), nitrofurantoin, or a **quinolone** (e.g., ciprofloxacin). For pyelonephritis, admission to the hospital for close monitoring and IV antibiotics is often required.

Case Conclusion   As this patient is ill-appearing and tachycardic with a significantly elevated temperature, her physician decides to admit her to the hospital for IV antibiotics, hydration, and close observation. She is given IV ciprofloxacin and does well overnight. She is afebrile in the morning and is able to finish her antibiotics at home. Prior to leaving the hospital, she is given information about contraceptive options and safe sex and is referred to the local teen clinic, where she can receive free treatment without the need for parental involvement or consent.

Thumbnail: Renal Pathophysiology—The EKES PPS! bugs

Microbes	Characteristics	Clinical setting
E. coli	G−; metallic sheen on EMB agar	#1 cause
Klebsiella	G−; large mucoid capsule; viscous colonies	Nosocomial
Enterobacter	G−	Nosocomial
Serratia	G−; red colonies	Nosocomial
Pseudomonas	G−; blue-green colonies; fruity odor	Nosocomial
Proteus	G−; swarming on agar; urease-producing	Struvite stones
Staphylococcus saprophyticus	G+	#2 cause in sexually active young women

EMB, eosin methylene blue agar.

Key Points

▶ Cystitis is characterized by dysuria, increased urgency and frequency of urination, hematuria, and suprapubic pain.

▶ Pyelonephritis may be characterized by all of the above plus costovertebral angle tenderness, fever and chills, and nausea and vomiting.

▶ The microbes responsible for upper and lower UTIs are the EKES PPS! bugs, described in the Thumbnail above.

Questions

1. The lab technician calls to inform you that the urine culture from your patient is growing a single organism with a green sheen on EMB agar. These colonies are lactose-fermenting but do not ferment sorbitol. The colony count is 10^6 CFU/mL. What organism is this?

   A. *E. coli* (O157:H7)
   B. *Staphylococcus saprophyticus*
   C. *E. coli* (O1)
   D. *Serratia*
   E. *Enterobacter*

2. A 16-year-old girl comes to your clinic with dysuria, increased urinary frequency, urgency, and suprapubic pain. She has recently become sexually active. What is the one gram-positive organism associated with UTIs in this type of patient?

   A. *Staphylococcus aureus*
   B. *Chlamydia trachomatis*
   C. *Neisseria gonorrhoeae*
   D. *Staphylococcus saprophyticus*
   E. *E. coli*

3. A woman comes to your clinic with dysuria, increased urinary frequency, and suprapubic pain. She has had symptoms like this many times in the past and is demanding a more thorough work-up. What is a possible cause of recurrent UTIs in this patient?

   A. Struvite kidney stones
   B. Imperforate hymen
   C. Calcium oxalate kidney stones
   D. Systemic lupus erythematosus
   E. Phimosis

4. An 18-year-old woman comes to your clinic with dysuria and suprapubic pain. She gets these symptoms predictably every time she visits her long-distance boyfriend. Which of the following would minimize her chance of developing recurrent UTIs?

   A. Drinking lots of cranberry juice
   B. Urinating after intercourse
   C. Switching from a diaphragm to condoms
   D. Taking prophylactic antibiotics before, during, and after each visit
   E. All of the above

HPI: AL, a 28-year-old Caucasian man, presents to the ED with colicky left-sided pelvic pain and hematuria. The pain began suddenly at 4 A.M., awakening him from sleep. It began in his left flank and traveled downward toward the left testis over 40 minutes, becoming increasingly severe (now 9/10 pain). He has vomited twice and complains of severe nausea. The pain is intermittent/colicky. He has not experienced dysuria, increased urination, fever, or chills. There is no history of trauma. Over the past several months, he has been experiencing significantly increased stress while working on his Ph.D. dissertation in Russian history, spending endless hours in his library carrel, living on coffee and leftover pepperoni pizza. He claims that whenever his stress level increases, his heartburn does, too, and he's been popping Tums and multivitamins to avoid getting sick. His family history is pertinent for kidney stones in his father and paternal grandfather, and hypertension in his mother. He lives with his girlfriend and two roommates. He drinks one to two six-packs per week and denies intravenous drug use.

PE: T 37.0°C RR 22/min BP 145/90 Pulse 100
The patient is in constant motion and appears to be in significant distress. His physical exam is significant only for LLQ and flank tenderness.

Labs: His blood is drawn and his urine is sent for UA. Electrolytes, including Ca^{2+} are entirely normal, but his UA shows 50 RBC/hpf (gross hematuria).

Thought Questions

- What is the pathophysiology of nephrolithiasis?

- How do you diagnose nephrolithiasis?

- How do you treat nephrolithiasis?

Basic Science Discussion and Review

Colicky, severe flank pain accompanied by hematuria is a classic presentation of nephrolithiasis (kidney stones). The pain is often referred to the testes (or labia). Associated symptoms can include nausea, vomiting, or fever. The patient is classically in constant motion, nicely distinguishing nephrolithiasis from other causes of an acute abdomen where patients tend to remain completely still to minimize pain. Pyelonephritis must be considered as it also presents with flank pain and hematuria. Since pain from kidney stones often radiates to the groin, in males it is important to consider testicular torsion and epididymitis in the differential diagnosis, both of which can present with testicular pain and hematuria.

There are several types of kidney stones. **Calcium stones** are associated with increased urinary excretion of calcium, uric acid, or oxalate, or decreased urinary excretion of citrate. These alterations are the result of altered gastrointestinal absorption or renal reabsorption and/or secretion of these substances, or they are idiopathic. **Struvite** stones are formed from the precipitation of magnesium ammonium phosphate salts in urine made alkaline by infection with urea-splitting bacteria like *Proteus*. **Uric acid** stones are found in patients with states of increased cell lysis (leukemia, chemotherapy) or hyperuricemia (gout, Lesch-Nyhan syndrome). **Cystine** stones are rare and are associated with genetic defects of renal tubular amino acid reabsorption.

Kidney stones are unilateral in 80% of patients and they tend to form in the renal pelvis or bladder; 50% to 60% of patients have stones that recur every 2 to 3 years. Nephrolithiasis affects men more than women (4:1) and the first episode tends to occur in the patient's 20's or 30's. Certain lifestyles increase the risk of nephrolithiasis. As we see with our coffee-slurping, pepperoni pizza-chomping patient, dehydration and increased sodium intake, increased protein intake, and *rarely* increased calcium intake predispose to stone formation. Increased sodium intake causes increased sodium and calcium excretion, leading to hypercalciuria, a prerequisite for *calcium* stone formation. Stones are also increased in those with sedentary lifestyles and in those with a positive family history.

An abdominal plain film is the least expensive method of diagnosis since approximately 92% of stones are radiopaque. A renal ultrasound diagnoses most other stones and evaluates for hydronephrosis, a common complication of ureteral obstruction. Further tests are indicated if the situation is complicated by obstruction or severe pain; a computed tomography (CT) scan can diagnose a ruptured calyx and an intravenous pyelogram (IVP) or CT can assess the degree of obstruction and size of the stone.

The UA is an important test in evaluating kidney stones. The only consistent finding on dipstick or microscopy is the presence of red blood cells. Since calculi are frequently associated with infection, always look for signs and symptoms of UTI and/or pyelonephritis. Urinary pH is associated with certain types of stones. A pH less than 5.0 suggests uric acid or cystine stones, and pH greater than 7.0 suggests struvite stones; pH is uninformative in diagnosing calcium stones. If the kidney stone is successfully "passed" or surgically removed, its composition should be analyzed to determine its etiology to guide treatment.

Acutely, treatment of small stones involves hydration, pain management, and bed rest to allow stone passage with ureteral and urethral peristalsis. Most stones pass within 24 hours. Stones must be removed surgically or dissolved with shock waves in cases of severe obstruction, concurrent infection, intractable pain, or severe bleeding.

If stones are recurrent, a metabolic analysis of serum and urine is warranted, as there are many complex etiologies for calcium and other stones, and etiology guides treatment. For example, in calcium nephrolithiasis, some subtypes are treated by restricting calcium intake, some by increasing calcium intake, some with thiazide diuretics (which decrease renal calcium excretion), and some with allopurinol (which decreases uric acid). *All* patients with recurrent stones should at least double their fluid intake as dehydration is a common precipitating factor.

Thumbnail: Types of Kidney Stones

Composition	Calcium oxalate (hydroxyapatite) or calcium phosphate	Struvite (magnesium ammonium phosphate)	Uric acid	Cystine
Frequency	**80%** of stones	12% of stones	7% of stones	Uncommon
High-risk group	Men 20–30 years old	Women	Men	Genetic
Risk factors	• Previous stones • Positive FH • Hypercalcemic states (hyperparathyroidism, metastatic cancer, increased vitamin D, milk-alkali syndrome)	• Catheters • Recurrent UTIs (especially w/urease-producing *Proteus*, which makes urine alkaline)	• Gout • States of cell lysis (chemotherapy, leukemia/myeloproliferative disorders) • Diet high in **purines** (organ meats)	• Secondary to **cystinuria** (autosomal-recessive disorder w/ defective amino acid transport) • Positive FH • Most common stone in **kids**
Seen on X-ray?	Densely radiopaque	Radiopaque **Staghorn**	**Radiolucent**	Radiopaque
pH	pH varies	**pH > 7.5**	pH < 5.0	pH < 5.0
Crystals	Weak/no birefringence under polarized light	Coffin-shaped	Often red, shows strong birefringence	Flat, hexagonal

Case Conclusion The patient is given narcotic medications to control his pain and is sent for a CT scan. A small stone is visualized in the lower third of the left ureter. The upper ureter is not dilated and the kidneys are normal size. There is no evidence of obstruction, his pain is adequately treated with the narcotics, and there is no evidence of infection or severe bleeding, so the patient is discharged home with narcotic analgesics. He is instructed to strain his urine to trap any stones for evaluation. Subsequent analysis of the stone reveals a calcium oxalate stone, the most common type. This is not surprising, given this patient's positive family history. Since this patient is likely to have recurrent stones, we advise him to consult with a urologist to determine the precise etiology of his tendency to nephrolithiasis.

Key Points

▶ Nephrolithiasis classically presents with acute-onset colicky, severe flank pain, and hematuria.

▶ There are four types of stones—calcium, struvite, uric acid, and cystine—each with their own etiologies and treatments. In nephrolithiasis, etiology guides treatment.

▶ Red blood cells and pH are the most useful components of the urinalysis to screen for nephrolithiasis.

Questions

1. A 26-year-old woman presents to her primary medical doctor (PMD) for treatment of her eighth UTI in 2 years. Her PMD refers her to a urologist for a complete evaluation of her recurrent UTIs. The urologist's diagnosis is nephrolithiasis. Which of the following stones is most strongly associated with recurrent urinary tract infections?
   - A. Calcium oxalate
   - B. Cystine
   - C. Calcium phosphate
   - D. Uric acid
   - E. Struvite

2. A 30-year-old man presents to the ED with severe colicky right-sided pelvic pain and hematuria. An ultrasound reveals a large stone lodged in the right ureter-bladder junction, dilation to 1-cm diameter of the R ureter, and evidence of hydronephrosis. His electrolyte panel reveals moderately elevated BUN and creatinine. Which type of acute renal failure is associated with large kidney stones?
   - A. Prerenal
   - B. Renal/parenchymal
   - C. Postrenal
   - D. Nephritic syndrome
   - E. Nephrotic syndrome

3. A 42-year-old man with gout is being treated by a urologist for recurrent kidney stones. He has had six episodes of uric acid stones in the past 15 years. Which of the following is/are complications of kidney stones?
   - A. Recurrent UTIs
   - B. Hydronephrosis
   - C. Pyelonephritis
   - D. Acute renal failure
   - E. All of the above

4. A 12-year-old girl presents with colicky abdominal pain and hematuria. A CT scan reveals hydronephrosis of the right kidney and severe right ureteral obstruction. The patient is taken to the OR for removal of a kidney stone. Which type of stone is associated with disordered amino acid transport?
   - A. Calcium oxalate
   - B. Cystine
   - C. Calcium phosphate
   - D. Uric acid
   - E. Struvite

HPI: JH, a 44-year-old Caucasian man, presents to his primary care physician complaining of back pain that has worsened over the past several months. He cannot recall a precipitating event, though he has been doing more heavy lifting lately. He states he has always been healthy otherwise. His mother began hemodialysis at age 66 and died 5 years later of renal failure; his brother died suddenly at age 48 from "an aneurysm"; and his maternal grandfather died at age 62 from a heart attack. He lives with his wife, teenage son, and college-age daughter, is a nonsmoker, and works as an accountant. He drinks one gin and tonic each night after work and denies intravenous drug use (IVDU).

PE: T 37.0°C RR 18/min BP 160/94 Pulse 70
His heart has a regular rate and rhythm with a late systolic murmur and faint systolic click best heard at the apex or left lower sternal border. His abdomen is soft, with normoactive bowel sounds. Bilateral large, tender flank masses are felt with very deep palpation. The remainder of his physical exam is noncontributory.

Labs: Na^+ 139 mEq/L, K^+ 4.1 mEq/L, Cl^- 99 mEq/L, HCO_3^- 28 mEq/L, BUN 30 mEq/L, Cr 1.9 mg/dL. Urinalysis: glucose neg, ketones neg, protein +, RBC 12/hpf, WBC 0–1.

Thought Questions

- What is the genetic defect in autosomal-dominant (adult) polycystic kidney disease (ADPKD)?

- What imaging tools help diagnose adult polycystic kidney disease?

Basic Science Review and Discussion

ADPKD is the most common hereditary disease in the U.S. This cystic renal disease is inherited in an autosomal dominant pattern, with full penetrance. A careful genogram reveals many affected individuals on one side. The most common clinical presentation is of flank pain and hematuria. However, isolated kidney problems may not be the presenting problem in every case. ADPKD is associated with **berry aneurysms** in the circle of Willis, which can rupture causing subarachnoid hemorrhage, asymptomatic mitral valve prolapse (25%), asymptomatic liver cysts (50% to 75%), calcium and uric acid kidney stones (20%), hypertension (25% of children and 75% of adults), diverticulosis, and increased incidence of UTIs and pyelonephritis. ADPKD has a prevalence of 1/1000 in the U.S. and accounts for approximately 10% of chronic renal failure necessitating dialysis or transplantation. Fifty percent progress to ESRD by age 60. Perhaps surprisingly, there is no increased risk of renal cell carcinoma in this population.

The primary genetic defect is in one of two genes, *PKD1* on chromosome 16 or *PKD2* on chromosome 4, which code for proteins that make up the polycystin complex. This protein complex is thought to regulate cell–cell and cell–matrix interactions, important in controlling growth and differentiation of tubular epithelium. Cysts result from monoclonal proliferation of this epithelium and cyst enlargement occurs due to fluid secretion by these abnormal epithelial cells. Presumably, the epithelial proliferation that occurs in cyst formation is similar to the proliferation responsible for the extraluminal "pouches" that result in berry aneurysms and diverticulosis.

Other diagnostic considerations in an *adult* include simple renal cysts, acquired renal cysts, and medullary cystic kidney disease. Simple renal cysts are present in 50% of people by age 50 and can be single or multiple. They are usually found along the outer cortex and are asymptomatic unless infected. Acquired renal cysts are associated with chronic hemodialysis, and although these resemble simple cysts, 7% of these cysts develop adenocarcinoma. Medullary sponge kidney is a common benign disorder present at birth in which the collecting ducts are irregularly enlarged and cystic, giving a "Swiss cheese" appearance. In a *child* with renal cysts, one must consider autosomal-recessive (child-

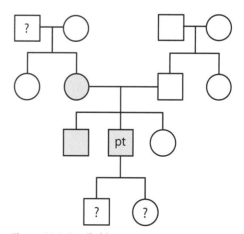

Figure 14-1 Family history genogram.

hood) polycystic kidney disease. These children die in infancy or childhood.

Renal ultrasound is the key to diagnosis; 80% to 90% of patients over 20 years old have cysts, reaching 100% by age 30. There must be more than five cysts in each kidney to confirm the diagnosis. CT scan can confirm uncertain diagnoses. In ADPKD, the kidneys are large with multiple cysts of irregular size scattered throughout the cortex and medulla. This helps to distinguish it from the medullary cystic diseases, which have normal or small-sized kidneys and thousands of tiny medullary cysts.

Case Conclusion   Our careful family history reveals the following genogram (Figure 14-1) with shading of individuals affected with the disease. As we cannot perform renal ultrasound on deceased family members, we must infer that the patient's brother's aneurysm was related to ADPKD. Suspecting ADPKD, our patient is sent for an ultrasound that reveals numerous (more than 15) cysts of varying sizes in each kidney. Our diagnosis confirmed, we take several additional steps. We refer him to cardiology to assess the severity of his mitral valve prolapse. We advise him to double his hydration to decrease the risk of kidney stones and infection. We begin treating his hypertension aggressively to prolong the time to ESRD and minimize other end-organ damage. We offer screening for berry aneurysms, given this patient's positive family history, recognizing that it is a difficult decision to be screened. We refer him and his young-adult children for genetic counseling. Finally, we educate him about the warning signs and symptoms of pyelonephritis/UTI, nephrolithiasis, diverticulitis, subarachnoid hemorrhage, and worsening of his mitral valve prolapse, for which he is at increased risk.

Thumbnail: Renal Pathophysiology—Autosomal Dominant (Adult) PKD and Autosomal Recessive (Childhood) PKD

	Adult PKD	**Childhood PKD**
Pathogenesis	Defect in polycystin complex	Unknown
Incidence	1/300–1000 live births	Rare (1/10,000–40,000)
Age of onset	**Adulthood (20–40)**	**Infancy (less than 1 year old)**
Clinical features	Hematuria Flank pain UTI HTN Renal stones	Congenital hepatic fibrosis HTN Pulmonary hypoplasia
Inheritance pattern	**AD**	**AR**
Implicated genes	*PKD1* on chrom 16 (90% cases) *PKD2* on chrom 4	Chromosome 6
Life span	Adulthood	Infancy/childhood
Gross appearance	Markedly enlarged kidneys Bumpy external appearance Large irregular spherical cysts	Normal/enlarged kidneys Smooth external appearance Small cysts (*spongelike*)

Key Points

▶ Adult PKD is autosomal dominant. A careful family history is key in assessing risk.

▶ Adult PKD is a systemic disease that may present with different manifestations in different family members.

▶ Ultrasound is the key to diagnosis.

Questions

1. A 42-year-old woman is diagnosed with ADPKD following hospitalization for severe pyelonephritis. She has a complex family history of renal and other problems on her father's side. Which of the following would we expect to find in her genogram?

   A. Berry aneurysms in the circle of Willis
   B. Mitral valve prolapse
   C. Colonic diverticular disease
   D. Nephrolithiasis
   E. All of the above

2. You are a primary care doctor who has just picked up a new patient with ADPKD. Which of the following is a chronic complication of ADPKD?

   A. Renal infection
   B. Abdominal pain
   C. Hypertensive heart disease
   D. Chronic renal failure
   E. All of the above

HPI: MM is a 77-year-old Latina sent to the ED after being seen at her local clinic for a regular follow-up appointment. On routine laboratory tests, her BUN and creatinine were significantly increased above her baseline creatinine of 1.1 and her physician was concerned. She is remarkably healthy for her age. Osteoarthritis and hypertension are her only medical problems. Her medications include metoprolol, benazepril, furosemide, and occasional ibuprofen for arthritis pain. Upon further questioning, she reveals that she has been more active lately. She joined a quilting group and has begun gardening again. Her arthritis has been "acting up," and she has been taking significantly more ibuprofen, up to 2400 mg per day.

PE: Her physical exam is significant for moderate pitting bilateral ankle edema.

Labs: Electrolytes: Na^+ 142, K^+ 4.1, Cl^- 101, Bicarb 16, BUN 60, Cr 3.2. Urine dipstick shows negative leukocyte esterase, negative nitrates, a slightly elevated specific gravity, and no protein, ketones, or glucose. Urine microscopy is pending.

Thought Questions

- Define acute renal failure.

- What are the three broad categories of acute renal failure?

- How does a urinalysis help distinguish between causes of acute renal failure?

Basic Science Review and Discussion

Acute renal failure (ARF) is a syndrome characterized by a **decline in GFR** over hours to days (as measured clinically by an increasing creatinine), azotemia, and disturbances in fluid and electrolyte balance. **Azotemia** is an excess of BUN or other nitrogenous compounds in the blood. ARF is initially characterized by nonspecific symptoms like malaise but becomes more seriously symptomatic when BUN exceeds 100 mg/dL. Signs and symptoms include **oliguria,** cardiovascular complications (pericardial effusions, arrhythmias), neurologic abnormalities (asterixis, confusion, seizures), gastrointestinal complications (nausea, vomiting, abdominal pain), electrolyte abnormalities (including an anion gap metabolic acidosis), or bleeding secondary to uremic platelet dysfunction. Fortunately, most ARF is reversible. Although ARF often presents with similar symptoms, it is distinguished from chronic renal failure where the decline in GFR occurs over months to years.

Broadly speaking, ARF may result from problems arising in the kidney itself (*renal* causes ~50%), from inadequate blood flow to the kidney (*prerenal* causes ~45%), or from obstruction downstream from the kidney (*postrenal* causes ~5%).

Prerenal Failure   In prerenal failure, the kidneys themselves function more-or-less normally and the problem lies in the inability of the circulatory system to deliver the proper perfusion to the kidney to produce a normal GFR. This occurs with **hypovolemic** states (hemorrhage, dehydration), impairment of renal **autoregulation** (as seen with cyclooxygenase inhibitors like NSAIDs and aspirin, or angiotensin-converting enzyme (ACE) inhibitors), or **low effective plasma flow** states. Low effective plasma flow states include low cardiac output states (arrhythmias, valvular disease, congestive heart failure), systemic vasodilation (sepsis, antihypertensives), or congestion (cirrhosis with ascites → hepatorenal syndrome). Once the underlying deficit is corrected, the kidneys usually recover rapidly.

Intrinsic Renal Failure   In intrinsic renal failure, the renal parenchyma is itself malfunctioning. The malfunction may be glomerular, vascular, tubular, or interstitial. *Glomerular* causes include glomerular diseases and the thrombotic microangiopathies such as hemolytic-uremic syndrome (HUS), thrombotic thrombocytopenic purpura (TTP), and disseminated intravascular coagulation (DIC). *Macrovascular* causes include narrowing of the renal arteries and arterioles by atherosclerosis, vasculitis, scleroderma, or malignant hypertension.

Acute *interstitial* nephritis (AIN) and acute *tubular* necrosis (ATN) comprise 90% of intrinsic renal ARF. The pathophysiology of AIN is acute hypersensitivity (allergic), infection, or infiltration. **Allergic AIN** is most commonly a reaction to drugs, especially antibiotics or NSAIDs, with onset approximately 2 weeks after exposure. ARF occurs in about 50% of those with AIN and may be accompanied by fever, eosinophilia, rash, and urinary abnormalities such as hematuria and **eosinophils** in the urine. **ATN** may be ischemic or nephrotoxic. **Ischemic ATN** occurs when prerenal conditions of poor perfusion persist so long that renal tubule cells begin dying. **Nephrotoxic ATN** occurs when exogenous (drugs, radiocontrast) or endogenous (myoglobin, hemoglobin) toxins damage the renal tubules. In either case, the necrotic tubular cells slough off, forming **muddy brown casts** in the urine.

In an oliguric patient (less than 500 cc/24 hours), measuring urine electrolytes can help distinguish between prerenal and intrinsic renal failure. In prerenal failure, the urine sodium concentration should be tiny (less than 10 mg/dL) as the kidneys avidly retain sodium and water. The fractional excretion of sodium (FE_{Na+}) compares the clearance of sodium to that of creatinine. An FE_{Na+} less than 1% suggests prerenal failure, while an FE_{Na+} 1% or greater suggests intrinsic renal failure as the kidneys have lost their ability to reabsorb sodium.

$$FE_{Na+} [\%] = \frac{U_{Na+}/P_{Na+}}{U_{Cr}/P_{Cr}} \times 100$$

In addition, BUN is reabsorbed by normally functioning tubules far in excess of creatinine, which is not reabsorbed. Therefore, BUN:Cr greater than 20:1 indicates properly functioning tubules and prerenal failure.

Postrenal Failure Severe urinary tract obstruction is the hallmark of postrenal failure. In men, the most common cause of postrenal failure is prostate enlargement from benign prostatic hyperplasia or prostate cancer. Other causes include obstruction by bladder or cervical cancer, kidney stones (lodged in the urinary tract such that flow from both kidneys is obstructed), phimosis (nonretractable foreskin), and a neurogenic bladder.

Case Conclusion MM's urinalysis and electrolytes shows hyaline casts, an FE_{Na+} less than 1%, and a U_{Na+} of 6 mg/dL, which suggest prerenal failure. MM was dehydrated (secondary to furosemide and decreased intake of fluids with increased activity), and her ACEI and NSAID compromised her kidney's ability to autoregulate to conserve GFR.

ACEIs decrease the production of angiotensin II (A II), a potent constrictor of the efferent arteriole. AII also induces the synthesis of local prostaglandins (PGs), powerful dilators of the afferent arteriole. Both constricting the efferent arteriole and dilating the afferent arteriole are mechanisms for preserving renal blood flow in times of hypovolemia. NSAIDs and aspirin inhibit cyclooxygenase, the enzyme that helps convert arachidonic acid into PGs. With neither AII nor PGs, the glomerulus has lost both sources of protection from hypoperfusion. Consequently, GFR drops and BUN and creatinine climb as the kidney can no longer clear substances from the blood. If this situation persists, the renal parenchyma itself becomes ischemic and dies (i.e., ATN). The other category to consider is allergic interstitial nephritis, also associated with NSAID use, suggested by eosinophils in the urine or a convincing clinical presentation with fever and rash, less likely in this case.

Treatment for this patient involves discontinuing nephrotoxic drugs, appropriate volume regulation (diuretics, water restriction, IV fluids, as needed), and monitoring and correcting electrolyte abnormalities, including by emergent dialysis if needed.

Thumbnail: Renal Pathophysiology—Causes of Acute Renal Failure

Prerenal	Intrinsic renal	Postrenal

Hypovolemia
• Hemorrhage
• Dehydration
• Burns
• GI losses
• "Third space" sequestration (pancreatitis, burns, hypoalbuminemia)
	Acute tubular necrosis (ATN)
	• Ischemic (end point of prerenal ARF)
	  • Nephrotoxic
	    • Exogenous (radiocontrast, chemotherapy)
	    • Endogenous (rhabdomyolysis, hemolysis)
		Obstruction
		• Bilateral ureteric
		• Prostatic hyperplasia
		• Urethral stricture
		• Stones
		• Phimosis

Low effective renal plasma flow • Low cardiac output states • Increased systemic vasodilation (sepsis, antihypertensives) • Cirrhosis with ascites	Interstitial nephritis • Allergic (drugs: especially antibiotics, NSAIDs) • Infection (pyelonephritis) • Infiltration (sarcoidosis, leukemia, lymphoma)	Neurogenic bladder

Impaired renal autoregulation
• Cyclooxygenase inhibitors (NSAIDs, aspirin)
• ACE inhibitors
• Renal vasoconstriction (epinephrine, norepinephrine)
Renovascular obstruction renal artery stenosis
	Diseases of the glomeruli
	• Glomerulonephritis
	  • Nephritic
	  • Nephrotic
	  • Thrombotic microangiopathy
	    • HUS
	    • TTP
	    • DIC	

	Macrovascular diseases • Artery (atherosclerosis, vasculitis, malignant hypertension, scleroderma) • Vein (thrombosis, compression)	
	Acute renal transplant rejection	
$FE_{Na^+} < 1\%$	$FE_{Na^+} > 1\%$	
$U_{Na^+} < 10$ mg/dL	$U_{Na^+} > 20$ mg/dL	
Plasma BUN:Cr > 20	Plasma BUN:Cr < 10–15	

Key Points

▶ Acute renal failure may be divided into prerenal, intrinsic renal, and postrenal causes.

▶ The urinalysis and urine electrolytes provide clues to diagnosis:

  ▶ **Leukocyte esterase:** released by granulocytes. Evidence of pyuria.

  ▶ **Nitrites:** nitrates are converted to nitrites by (G⁻ rods). Indicates bacteriuria.

  ▶ **Ketones:** indicate metabolic acidosis (diabetic ketoacidosis, starvation).

▶ **Lipid:** Oval fat bodies   Nephrotic syndrome
     Maltese crosses
     (polarized light)

▶ **Casts:** Red cell casts   Glomerulonephritis (GN)
     White cell casts   Interstitial nephritis
     Muddy brown casts   Acute tubular necrosis

▶ **Cells:** Red cells   GN, tumors, trauma, UTI
     Dysmorphic red cells   GN
     (acanthocytes)
     White cells   Cystitis (lower UTI)

Questions

1. A 62-year-old woman is admitted to the hospital for ARF and a 24-hour urine collection is obtained. Urine volume is 600 cc/day. U_{Na+} is 5 mg/dL, U_{Cr} is 25 mg/dL, P_{Na+} is 140 mg/dL, and P_{Cr} is 3.5 mg/dL. What is the FE_{Na+}?

   A. < 1% suggesting prerenal failure
   B. > 2% suggesting intrinsic renal failure
   C. 1.5%, of limited use in this nonoliguric patient
   D. < 1%, of limited use in this nonoliguric patient
   E. 1.2%, making diagnosis difficult but prerenal unlikely

2. A 75-year-old man is referred to the ED after being seen in the clinic with an elevated BUN and creatinine on routine exam. The patient is not ill-appearing and has stable vital signs. A pelvic ultrasound from several years ago shows two normal-appearing kidneys. What is the most likely cause of renal failure in this patient?

   A. Kidney stone lodged in the right ureter → post-renal failure
   B. Diabetes mellitus → renal insufficiency
   C. Benign prostatic hypertrophy (BPH) → postrenal failure
   D. Sepsis → prerenal failure
   E. Goodpasture's syndrome → intrinsic renal failure

HPI: RL, an 82-year-old Asian American woman with long-standing diabetes, is brought from a local supermarket to the ED after complaining of shortness of breath and heart palpitations, with increasing confusion. Her granddaughter is present and is able to elucidate her recent history. She has been receiving hemodialysis three times per week for the past 3 years, but did not make her two most recent appointments this week. Her type 2 diabetes mellitus was diagnosed at age 49, and she currently takes insulin and captopril. She has several diabetic family members including her sister, mother, and both of her maternal grandparents. Her mother began dialysis at age 66 and died 10 years later of renal failure, and her maternal grandfather died at age 62 from a heart attack.

PE: T 40°C RR 23/min BP 155/91 Pulse 102 SaO$_2$ 92% at room air
The patient is an overweight woman who appears her stated age. Her breath has a faint fishy odor. Her cardiovascular exam is normal except for a faint rub, best heard at the left lower sternal border. She has diminished breath sounds in the right lung base and rales audible to one third of the way up her back. She has no cyanosis or clubbing of her extremities but she does have 3+ pitting edema extending to her knees bilaterally.

Labs: Glucose 280 mg/dL, Na$^+$ 148 mEq/L, K$^+$ 5.2 mEq/L, Cl$^-$ 90 mEq/L, HCO$_3^-$ 1mEq/L, BUN 110 mEq/L, creatinine 5.mg/dL, Hgb 8 g/dl, Hct 24%, platelets 150,000/μL, blood cultures × 2: *E. Coli*, sensitivities pending. Urinalysis: glucose 3+, ketones neg, protein 1+, nitrites 1+, leukocyte esterase 1+, blood 2+, broad waxy casts.

Thought Questions

- What are the causes of chronic renal failure (CRF)?
- What are the distinguishing characteristics of CRF?
- What is the treatment for ESRD and CRF?

Basic Science Review and Discussion

The kidney has many crucial functions. It produces hormones like erythropoietin; converts vitamin D to its active state; clears the blood of toxins; maintains electrolyte, fluid, and acid-base balance; and plays a crucial role in maintaining blood pressure. In **CRF**, the kidneys are unable to perform some or all of these functions. The central mechanism is loss of renal mass, secondary to damage from diabetes, hypertension, or glomerulonephritis. A vicious cycle of renal damage is established: loss of nephrons leads to hypertrophy and hyperfiltration of the remaining nephrons, creating "hypertension" in those nephrons, causing glomerular sclerosis and interstitial fibrosis. Kidneys have enormous functional reserve; up to 50% of nephrons may be lost without symptoms. Loss of 50% to 80% of nephrons leads to azotemia, and loss of more than 80% leads to uremia. **Azotemia** is an excess of urea or other nitrogenous compounds in the blood and presents with nonspecific symptomatology (e.g., malaise, fatigue). **Uremia** is the constellation of signs and symptoms that reflect the malfunctioning of all organ systems from untreated renal failure (see Thumbnail). These signs and symptoms result from the buildup of the toxic by-products of protein metabolism that are dependent on renal excretion and from the failure of crucial renal functions. Distinguishing features of chronic renal failure include the presence of **small kidneys on x-ray, renal osteodystrophy, peripheral neuropathy, and anemia.**

Renal osteodystrophy results from secondary hyperparathyroidism induced by the electrolyte imbalances wrought by a failing kidney. As the GFR drops, phosphorus excretion decreases. The resultant hyperphosphatemia leads to overproduction of PTH by the parathyroid glands. In CRF, there is also decreased activity of **1α-hydroxylase**, the renal enzyme responsible for converting vitamin D to its active form. Since active vitamin D normally increases Ca^{2+} uptake in the gut and Ca^{2+} and PO$_4^{3-}$ reabsorption in the DCT, decreased vitamin D activation leads to hypocalcemia and hyperphosphatemia, causing further up-regulation of PTH. A vicious cycle ensues. Renal osteodystrophy takes the form of either **osteitis fibrosa cystica** with increased osteoclast activity ($\uparrow$ PTH $\rightarrow$ $\uparrow$ osteoclast activity) or **osteomalacia** with a slowed rate of bone mineralization. Peripheral neuropathy tends to be more sensory than motor and includes paresthesias and the restless legs syndrome. The normochromic, normocytic anemia of CRF is due to decreased erythropoietin production, normally secreted by the peritubular capillary endothelium in response to hypoxia. Hypertension results from fluid overload and from decreased effective renal blood flow. The kidneys perceive the sluggish flow as they would hypovolemia, and the juxtaglomerular cells respond with renin production, activating the renin-angiotensin-aldosterone cascade further increasing blood pressure.

Laboratory results include elevated BUN and creatinine, hyperkalemia, broad waxy casts in the urinary sediment, and frequently decreased HCO_3^- from an anion gap metabolic acidosis (remember in the MUD PILES mnemonic, discussed in Acid–Base Physiology, Case 7, U stands for uremia). This is due to an impaired ability to produce the buffer ammonia. The hyperkalemia can lead to dangerous arrhythmias.

ESRD is the last stage of the progressive loss of renal function that occurs in chronic renal failure. At ESRD, patients have lost so much renal function that they are dependent on having that function replaced via transplantation or dialysis to minimize uremic symptoms. However, some uremic symptoms persist or progress despite optimal dialysis treatment. Ninety percent of ESRD is due to chronic renal disease.

Case Conclusion This patient with chronic renal failure is experiencing uremia secondary to missing two dialysis appointments and further exacerbated by a systemic infection (*E. coli* from a bladder infection). She is treated with IV antibiotics and is sent for emergent dialysis. She recovers although some of her symptoms linger. Given her age and overall health, she is not a good candidate for renal transplant surgery. Therefore, her doctors discuss with the family the importance of regular hemodialysis to avoid dangerous electrolyte disturbances. They explain that people with CRF have little renal reserve and that the urinary tract infection and subsequent bacteremia was enough of a metabolic stressor to overload the kidney's functional capacity.

Thumbnail: Uremia Head to Toe

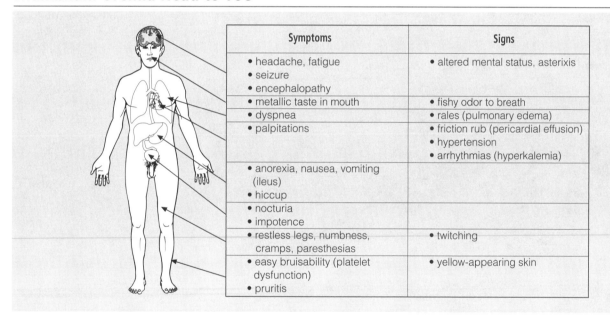

	Symptoms	Signs
	• headache, fatigue • seizure • encephalopathy	• altered mental status, asterixis
	• metallic taste in mouth	• fishy odor to breath
	• dyspnea	• rales (pulmonary edema)
	• palpitations	• friction rub (pericardial effusion) • hypertension • arrhythmias (hyperkalemia)
	• anorexia, nausea, vomiting (ileus) • hiccup	
	• nocturia • impotence	
	• restless legs, numbness, cramps, paresthesias	• twitching
	• easy bruisability (platelet dysfunction) • pruritis	• yellow-appearing skin

Key Points

▶ CRF is characterized by small kidneys, osteodystrophy, neuropathy, anemia, and uremia.

▶ Laboratory results include elevated BUN/Cr, hyperkalemia, and broad waxy casts in the urinary sediment.

▶ The "big three" causes of CRF are diabetes (30%), hypertension (25%), and glomerulonephritis (21%).

▶ Dialysis and transplantation are the treatments for CRF.

Questions

1. A 76-year-old woman has had progressive CRF for 10 years and has been receiving hemodialysis for the past 6 years. Complications of CRF include which of the following:
   A. Hyperkalemia
   B. Osteitis fibrosa cystica
   C. Anemia
   D. Pericarditis
   E. All of the above

2. A 68-year-old woman with CRF has persistent hypertension. She already takes lisinopril, an ACEI proven to reduce morbidity and mortality from CRF. Her doctor wants to prescribe an additional antihypertensive or diuretic but is not sure which one to use. This patient's CRF is severe enough that she will probably begin hemodialysis within the year. Which of the following medications would be the best choice and why?
   A. Triamterene because it is a potassium-sparing diuretic
   B. Spironolactone because it blocks the aldosterone receptor
   C. Furosemide because it is a potassium-wasting diuretic
   D. Acetazolamide because it inhibits carbonic anhydrase
   D. Mannitol because it is an osmotic diuretic

HPI: MK, a 63-year-old African-American man, presents to the Veterans Administration (VA) urgent care clinic complaining of blood in his urine for "a while" and a low-grade fever for at least a week or two (he only started taking his temperature when he discovered the blood). He admits to losing 30 pounds in the past 6 months. He states that he did not want to make the hour-long trek to the closest VA but realized he might not be able to "kick this thing" on his own. He also has hypertension and chronic bronchitis. He takes hydrochlorothiazide, captopril, and ipratropium. His mother, father, and younger sister have hypertension, his father and younger brother suffer from depression, and his oldest sister recently had a serious myocardial infarction (MI). He is a widower, lives alone, and works as a short-order cook. He drinks a pint of whiskey daily, admits to IVDU in the past but has not used IV drugs for 30 years. He has smoked one pack of cigarettes per day for the past 50 years.

PE: T 38.5°C RR 22/min BP 138/87 Pulse 69
The patient is an overweight man who appears fatigued and older than his stated age. He has distant breath sounds and scattered wheezes and an unremarkable cardiac exam. His abdominal exam is significant for a large left upper quadrant mass felt on deep palpation. It is otherwise soft, nontender with normoactive bowel sounds.

LABS: BUN 18 mEq/L, creatinine 1.1 mg/dL, WBC $10 \times 10^3/\mu L$, Hgb 18 g/dL, Hct 48%, platelets $280 \times 10^3/\mu L$. Urinalysis: glucose neg, ketones neg, protein neg, RBC 27/hpf, WBC 0–1.

Thought Questions

■ What are the most likely diagnoses and how can we narrow our list?

■ What is the pathophysiology of renal cell carcinoma?

■ What are the genetic associations with renal cell carcinoma?

■ What would our differential diagnosis be if this patient was 3 rather than 63?

Basic Science Review and Discussion

Renal cell carcinoma presents with hematuria (50%), flank pain or mass (40%), and systemic symptoms like fever (20%) and weight loss (33%). The "classic triad" of hematuria, flank pain, and abdominal mass occurs in only about 10% of patients. Thirty percent of patients have symptoms of metastatic disease at presentation (bone pain, cough). Patients can also present with secondary polycythemia (elevated hematocrit) due to increased production of erythropoietin, anemia due to bone marrow infiltration of tumor, or with paraneoplastic syndromes due to ectopic production of adrenocorticotropic hormone (ACTH), parathyroid hormone related peptide (PTHrP), and prolactin. Renal cell carcinoma can spread hematogenously, lymphatically, or via direct extension. The most common sites of metastases are the lungs and bones. Five-year survival decreases from 70% to 45% once metastases are present.

Renal cell carcinomas are adenocarcinomas. Eighty percent are clear cell (nonpapillary). The originating cell is the proximal tubule epithelium, and polygonal clear cells are seen on biopsy. Gross specimens reveal a solitary yellow mass, often located on the upper kidney pole and usually unilateral.

Smoking is the only clearly associated environmental factor. The immediate cause is unknown, with sporadic cases far outnumbering cases linked with dialysis or von Hippel-Lindau (VHL) syndrome. VHL syndrome is characterized by hemangiomas of the cerebellum and retina, and bilateral renal cysts that inevitably develop into multiple foci of renal cell carcinoma. VHL syndrome accounts for less than 5% of renal cancers. However, in *all* renal clear cell carcinomas, there is a deletion in the area of chromosome 3 containing the VHL gene, suggesting that the VHL gene acts as a tumor-suppressor gene.

In the setting of the patient's unintentional weight loss and gross hematuria, genitourinary (GU) malignancy, particularly renal cell carcinoma and transitional cell bladder carcinoma, should head our list of differential diagnoses. Both types of GU cancers present with hematuria and are found most commonly in the same patient population, namely older male smokers. Transitional cell carcinoma, however, is more frequently associated with irritative voiding symptoms (urgency, frequency), while renal cell carcinoma is more associated with an abdominal mass and systemic symptoms. Transitional cell carcinoma is the fourth most common cancer in men and the ninth most common in women, and can occur in the renal calyces or pelvis, the ureters, or, most commonly, the bladder. In addition to smoking, it is also associated with cyclophosphamide treatment or aniline dye exposure. Renal cell carcinoma accounts for 2.3% of all adult cancers. It is the most common of malignant renal neoplasms (95%). The other major primary malignant renal neoplasm is Wilms' tumor, an embryonal mixed tumor found in children, and thus not on our list of differential diagnoses in this patient.

In this case, given the presence of an abdominal mass, the initial evaluation would be an abdominal CT scan. In the absence of an abdominal mass, the diagnostic work-up for hematuria includes a urinalysis, urine culture, and cystoscopy (sensitive for bladder neoplasms). Further evaluation of masses and the search for metastases is typically performed with chest, abdominal, and pelvic CT scans.

Case Conclusion   Suspecting GU malignancy, we send the patient for an abdominal CT, which reveals a mass suspicious for renal cell carcinoma. A biopsy is obtained, which reveals polygonal clear cells. A chest CT reveals two small nodules in the right middle lobe of the lung suggestive of metastases. A bone scan reveals no bony metastases. The patient undergoes a lung lobectomy and a nephrectomy with lymph node dissection, and is discharged on chemotherapeutic agents. The gross specimen reveals a 4-cm solitary yellow mass located on the top pole of the left kidney. Our patient survives another 3 years before he arrives in the ED one day, complaining of left wrist pain. His wrist fractured when he attempted to lift a cast iron frying pan with only his left hand. An x-ray reveals a pathologic fracture (due to weakening of the bone structure by metastatic infiltration). A follow-up bone scan reveals multiple bony metastases. The patient is discharged to hospice and dies peacefully 4 months later.

Thumbnail: Renal Pathophysiology—Renal Cell Carcinoma

Frequency	2.3% of adult cancers
Age of onset	50–70 years old
High-risk group	Male (2:1), smokers
Clinical onset	**Flank tenderness, mass, fever, hematuria,** polycythemia ($\uparrow$ epo), paraneoplastic syndromes
Genetic association	**von Hippel–Lindau (VHL) gene** on chromosome 3
Gross appearance	Yellow mass located on upper pole of kidney solitary, unilateral, yellow
Cell type	Proximal convoluted tubule epithelium

Key Points

▶ Renal cell carcinoma is characterized by flank tenderness, abdominal mass, hematuria, and systemic symptoms (low-grade fever, weight loss).

▶ Transitional cell carcinoma is characterized by hematuria and frequency and urgency with urination.

▶ Wilms' tumor is a malignant embryonal mixed tumor found in children.

Questions

1. A 3-year-old patient presents with similar symptoms of fever, flank mass, and weight loss. Given this patient's different age and risk category, which two cancers would lead the diagnosis?

   A. Wilms' tumor and neuroblastoma
   B. Wilms' tumor and renal cell carcinoma
   C. Neuroblastoma and renal cell carcinoma
   D. Neuroblastoma and polycystic kidneys
   E. Renal cell carcinoma and polycystic kidneys

2. A 3-year-old boy presents to his pediatrician with developmental delay. Chromosome mapping reveals a rare mutation. Which of the following is not associated with Wilms' tumor?

   A. WAGR (**W**ilms' tumor, **a**niridia, **g**enital anomalies, mental **r**etardation) syndrome (autosomal dominant gene on chromosome 11p13)
   B. Denys-Drash syndrome (a missense point mutation mapped to chromosome 11p13)
   C. Prader-Willi syndrome (a deletion mapped to chromosome 15q12)
   D. Beckwith-Wiedemann syndrome (genomic imprinting at chromosome 11p15.5)
   E. Sporadic mutation of one copy of the *WT-1* gene

Case 1

1. D
2. B
3. D

Case 2

1. A
2. D

Case 3

1. B
2. B
3. C
4. C

Case 4

1. D
2. A

Case 5

1. B
2. B
3. E

Case 6

1. E
2. B
3. E

Case 7

1. C
2. C
3. C
4. D

Case 8

1. C
2. D
3. B

Case 9

1. E
2. C
3. E

Case 10

1. E
2. D
3. B
4. B

Case 11

1. B
2. E

Case 12

1. C
2. D
3. A
4. E

Case 13

1. E
2. C
3. E
4. B

Case 14

1. E
2. E

Case 15

1. D
2. C

Case 16

1. E
2. C

Case 17

1. A
2. C

Part II

Hematology

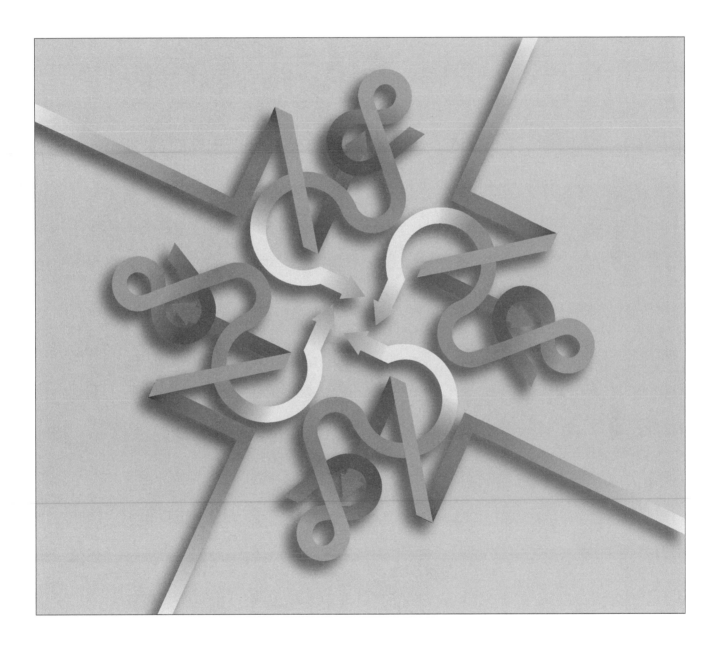

HPI: RC, a 25-year-old woman, comes to your office complaining of increasing fatigue and occasional heart palpitations for the last several weeks. She occasionally feels short of breath while having the palpitations, but denies any fever, chills or weight loss during this time. She does not have a history of asthma or any cardiac problems. She has never had symptoms like this before. PMH: Seasonal allergies. Last menstrual period was 1 week prior. Her periods are moderately heavy, lasting 5 to 7 days, cycling regularly every 30 days. She is not taking any medications.

PE: T 36.2°C HR 72 BP 125/72
Her conjunctiva look pale, and she has a soft systolic murmur heard best at the left second intercostal space. The rest of the exam is unremarkable.

Labs: Hgb 10 g/dL (low), Hct 30% (low), MCV 76 fL (low), serum iron 40 µg/dL (low), Transferrin 450 µg/dL (high), Ferritin 8 µg/dL (low).

Thought Questions

■ What is the general structure and function of red blood cells (RBCs) in the human body?

■ What is anemia and what are the general mechanisms for its development?

■ How are the different types of anemia usefully classified?

■ What is the pathophysiology of iron deficiency anemia, how does it present, and how is it treated?

Basic Science Review and Discussion

Red blood cells (RBCs or erythrocytes) are discoid shaped cells, roughly 8 µm in diameter, that function to transfer oxygen (O_2) from the lungs to other tissues and carry CO_2 from those tissues back to the lungs. The plasma membrane of a mature erythrocyte is made up of many transmembrane proteins that regulate the unique properties of deformability, tensile strength, and cell shape. An RBC must repeatedly deform through 2 to 3 µm capillaries during its 120-day life span and it must withstand the shear stresses of the circulation. The flattened shape of the erythrocyte maximizes surface area, allowing for faster diffusion and absorption of O_2 and CO_2.

Hemoglobin During erythropoiesis or RBC maturation, RBCs lose all cellular organelles and function anaerobically to preserve O_2 that is meant for other cells. The cytoplasm is filled with millions of oxygen-carrying proteins called **hemoglobin.** Each hemoglobin molecule has a tetramer of globin subunits and each subunit has a heme group with a central iron atom, which binds O_2 directly. Iron, therefore, plays an essential role in heme (and subsequently RBC) production.

Each of the four heme groups can carry an O_2 molecule; hemoglobin can carry a maximum of four oxygen molecules. When hemoglobin is saturated with oxygen, it has a bright red color; as it loses oxygen (deoxyhemoglobin), it becomes bluish (cyanosis). Hemoglobin's affinity for oxygen increases as successive molecules of oxygen bind. More molecules bind as the oxygen partial pressure increases until the maximum amount that can be bound is reached (100% saturation). As this limit is approached, very little additional binding occurs and the curve levels out, having a sigmoidal or S shape. The affinity of hemoglobin for oxygen is also affected by several other factors as seen in Figure 18-1.

Laboratory Assessment of Red Blood Cells In the lab, hemoglobin can be measured in a certain volume of blood and functions as a "direct" red blood cell measure. Other direct measures include the **mean corpuscular volume** (MCV), which is the average volume of an individual cell, and a red cell count (also called the RBC). A commonly reported measure, the **hematocrit** (Hct), is the proportion, by volume, of the blood that consists of red blood cells. The Hct is easily measured by placing a sample of blood in a tube and centrifuging down the red cell mass. The Hct is the proportion of the total length of the tube made up by RBCs. This can also be calculated by multiplying the red cell count by the MCV.

Various RBC disorders, such as anemia, can be identified by changes in RBC size or shape. This qualitative analysis of RBCs is done by microscopically examining a **peripheral blood smear.**

Anemia Anemia occurs when there is a decrease in red cell mass and is usually defined by a hemoglobin less than 12 g/dL in women and less than 14 g/dL in men. There are three general mechanisms for the development of anemia. The first is **decreased production** of RBCs (hypoproductive anemia), which can result from nutritional deficiencies (iron, vitamin B_{12}, or folate), low levels of erythropoietin (such as in chronic renal failure), bone marrow failure

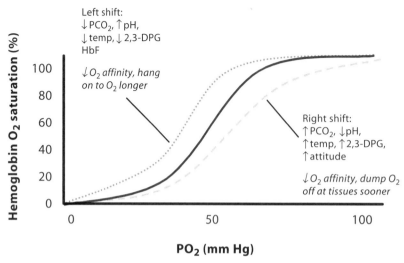

Figure 18-1 Hemoglobin-oxygen dissociation curve.

(aplastic anemia), or replacement of normal marrow by malignant cells (leukemias or metastatic bone disease). Another cause of anemia is **increased destruction** of circulating erythrocytes, as seen in hemolytic anemias, spherocytosis, and sickle cell disease. Finally, **blood loss** can be the cause of anemia. In the latter two mechanisms, a normal bone marrow compensates with an increase in red cell production, or erythropoiesis (hyperproductive anemia).

To determine whether a patient has a hypoproductive or hyperproductive anemia, one can measure the number of reticulocytes (immature blood cells) in the peripheral blood. An increased number of reticulocytes indicates hyperproduction of RBCs, while a normal or decreased number of reticulocytes means the bone marrow is not able to compensate. A useful classification of anemia is one based on the MCV (see Thumbnail).

Iron Deficiency Anemia RC is diagnosed with anemia since her hemoglobin is less than normal. Her MCV of 76 fL, indicates a microcytic anemia. Iron deficiency anemia, a microcytic type, is the most common form of anemia. Hence, when evaluating someone for a microcytic anemia, it is important to order iron studies. While the largest compartment of iron is found in hemoglobin (two-thirds total body iron), it is also found in a storage compound, ferritin, located in almost every tissue of the body. **Ferritin** synthesis is controlled by the amount of iron in the body. **Transferrin,** a transport molecule, binds much of the iron in the serum and is also an important indicator of iron status. Unbound serum iron, transferrin, and ferritin are all important iron studies. In iron-deficient states, serum iron is low and ferritin is low (not much iron to store), while transferrin is high (the body is mobilizing any stored iron because it is deficient). Our patient's lab values fit these parameters of iron deficiency. A peripheral smear would likely reveal small **hypochromic** (pale) erythrocytes.

Iron deficiency can be caused by **increased requirements** of iron, as seen in growing children and pregnant women; **decreased iron absorption,** sometimes seen in patients after gastrointestinal surgery; and, most commonly, **iron loss.** For premenopausal woman, menstrual blood loss is the most common cause. For men and postmenopausal women, blood loss from the GI tract is usually the cause.

Iron-deficient patients have the typical indications of anemia including dizziness, fatigue, heart palpitations, shortness of breath with activity, and skin/mucous membrane pallor. Other complaints or findings related more specifically to the low iron state include headache, paresthesias, glossitis (red, swollen, smooth tongue), stomatitis (inflammation of the oral mucosa), angular cheilitis (fissures at the mouth angle), and koilonychia (spooning of the nails). Standard treatment for iron deficiency anemia is oral iron, usually ferrous sulfate. Up to 20% of patients have significant side effects such as nausea, abdominal pain, constipation, or diarrhea; therefore, the supplements are often given with meals. Steps to stop or decrease any bleeding are advisable. Intramuscular or intravenous administration of iron is used in extreme cases or when severe malabsorption impairs iron absorption.

Anemia of Chronic Disease Anemia of chronic disease (ACD), the second most common type of anemia, is found in patients with chronic inflammatory, infectious, or neoplastic disorders. Systemic lupus erythematosus, rheumatoid arthritis, Crohn's disease, osteomyelitis, tuberculosis, lymphoma, and solid tumors are all examples. ACD can appear as micro- or normocytic. Impaired iron metabolism is a key feature of its etiology, namely impaired iron mobilization. Iron studies can distinguish it from iron deficiency. Hallmark findings of ACD are low serum iron despite normal to high ferritin (storage) levels. Treatment is directed at the underlying disease.

Case Conclusion   The patient is treated with oral iron supplements given three times a day with meals. Because the likely source of her iron deficiency anemia is her heavy periods (menorrhagia), she is also begun on oral contraceptive pills to decrease the monthly blood loss. Within 6 weeks, her Hgb has increased to 13.5 g/dL. She continues on iron supplementation once per day thereafter.

Thumbnail: Hematology—Breakdown of Anemias

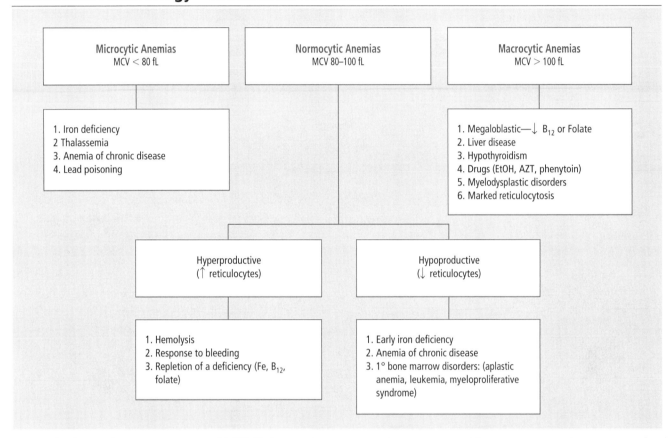

Key Points

- RBCs contain hemoglobin molecules, each with 4 O_2-binding iron groups.
- Hemoglobin-oxygen dissociation follows a sigmoidal curve.
- Three general mechanisms for anemia: ↓ production, ↑ destruction, blood loss.
- Iron deficiency is the most common type of anemia.

- Iron deficiency lab values: ↑ transferrin, ↓ serum iron, ↓ ferritin, ↓ MCV (microcytic), small hypochromic cells on peripheral smear.
- Blood loss is the most common cause of iron deficiency.
- Anemia of chronic disease: ↓ transferrin, ↓ serum iron, ↑ or normal ferritin.

Questions

1. A 78-year-old man comes to your office for a routine checkup. His medical history is significant for mild hypertension and hypercholesterolemia, for which he has been taking prescription medications for the last several years. He denies any alcohol or tobacco use, and describes his diet as "healthy." On physical exam you find an elderly, mildly cachectic ("wasted") man with pale conjunctiva. Lab tests reveal a Hct and iron studies consistent with iron deficiency anemia. His last Hct (1 year prior) was normal. What would you do next?

   A. A trial of iron and recheck Hct at next physical exam
   B. Repeat labs since the patient is asymptomatic
   C. Work-up for occult GI bleed
   D. Bone marrow biopsy
   E. Hb electrophoresis

2. A 58-year-old woman with a long history of iron deficiency anemia now presents with progressive dysphagia (difficulty swallowing), primarily with solid foods. On exam she has a swollen, painful, smooth-appearing tongue (glossitis) and spooning of her nails (koilonychia). Endoscopy reveals she has a large esophageal web, which has been obstructing food passage. Her most likely diagnosis is:

   A. Fanconi anemia
   B. Lead poisoning
   C. Esophageal cancer
   D. Plummer-Vinson syndrome
   E. Porphyria

> **HPI:** PT, a 75-year-old man, comes to your clinic for a routine physical exam. His medical history is significant for mild hypertension, coronary artery disease, degenerative lumbar disk disease and glaucoma. He denies alcohol or tobacco use and describes his diet as "good." (He cooks often with his wife and eats a variety of foods.)
>
> **PE:** The patient is slightly overweight and has pale conjunctiva. There is a loss of vibratory sense in the bilateral upper and lower distal extremities and loss of proprioception bilaterally in the toes. These findings are new since last year's exam.
>
> **Labs:** Hgb 11 g/dL, mean corpuscular volume (MCV) 111 fL, peripheral blood smear: megaloblasts and hypersegmented neutrophils noted.

Thought Questions

- What are the causes of macrocytic anemia?

- Why are folate and vitamin B_{12} important in the human diet?

- How are the clinical manifestations of folate and vitamin B_{12} deficiency similar? How are they different?

- What can you determine from a Shilling test?

Basic Science Review and Discussion

DNA synthesis is dependent on a derivative of folic acid, called tetrahydrofolate (H4 folate). The enzyme, **dihydrofolate reductase,** is responsible for converting folic acid to H4 folate (remember that the antibiotic, trimethoprim, and the chemotherapeutic agent methotrexate inhibit this enzyme). The "folate" contained in dietary supplements is folic acid, but the "folate" in the unsupplemented human diet is a methylated H4 folate. The methyl group is transferred to homocysteine via a reaction that requires vitamin B_{12} as a coenzyme. This reaction yields methionine and the utilizable H4 folate.

The tissues with the highest turnover of cells (such as the hematopoietic system) have the highest requirement for folate and therefore rely heavily on dietary intake of both folate and vitamin B_{12}. Deficiencies in either compound can result in a macrocytic anemia.

Folate Deficiency **Folate** is found in all tissues of the body, and most of the excess storage occurs in the liver. Stores are limited; serum levels fall after 3 weeks of insufficient intake and anemia begins to occur after 4 to 5 months. Folate is found naturally in many fruits and vegetables (asparagus, broccoli, spinach, bananas, melons, for example), and in the United States grains and cereals are often supplemented. Folate is absorbed in the proximal jejunum, and sometimes in the ileum after surgical resection of the jejunum.

Causes of folate deficiency include increased requirements (such as during pregnancy or after renal dialysis), decreased intake (often in alcoholics or those who have poor diets), and decreased absorption (in patients with celiac sprue or regional enteritis, or those who have undergone extensive resection of their small intestine).

Clinical manifestations are those of a slowly developing anemia. Patients often do not have symptoms of anemia until their hemoglobin is very low. Other symptoms include glossitis (painful tongue) and mucositis (mouth sores), because mucosal cells also have high turnover. Folate deficiency in pregnant women can result in **neural tube defects** in the fetus; therefore, it is important to have sufficient folate prior to the onset of pregnancy.

Vitamin B_{12} Deficiency Vitamin B_{12} (a derivative of **cobalamin**) is found only in foods of animal origin (meat, eggs, and dairy products). Similar to folate, vitamin B_{12} can also be found in cereals and grains due to supplementation. Unlike folate, the human body has plentiful stores of vitamin B_{12}; deficiency only manifests itself after years of deficit. Absorption of vitamin B_{12} requires several steps. In the stomach, vitamin B_{12} is released from food and binds to transport proteins, which protect it from the acidic environment. In the duodenum, vitamin B_{12} is released from the protein complex and is bound by **intrinsic factor** (IF). IF is synthesized by parietal cells located in the stomach. The vitamin B_{12}-IF complex is finally absorbed in the **distal ileum.**

Causes of vitamin B_{12} deficiency include increased requirements (occasionally in pregnancy), decreased intake (usually in strict vegetarians who exclude dairy products from their diet), and decreased absorption. Malabsorption of vitamin B_{12} can occur for several reasons. The most common cause of B_{12} deficiency is **pernicious anemia,** with a prevalence of 1% in the U.S. adult population. This is an autoimmune disease where antibodies destroy gastric parietal cells, resulting in little or no IF production. Patients with stomach resection or distal ileum resection or disease (Crohn's,

Whipple's) also have absorption difficulty. Infestation with the fish tapeworm *Diphyllobothrium latum* is a rare cause in the U.S.

Clinical manifestations of vitamin B_{12} deficiency, like folate, are of a slowly developing anemia. Unique to vitamin B_{12}, are **neurologic abnormalities,** which generally begin with paresthesias, loss of vibratory sense, and loss of proprioception (joint position sense). Findings can progress to gait ataxia, motor weakness, and altered mental state including dementia, depression, and even psychosis. Patients may present with neurologic deficits and no finding of anemia.

Lab Tests   Folate can be measured in the serum or in the red blood cells. Red cell levels correlate better with long-term tissue levels. Vitamin B_{12} levels are usually measured in the serum. Both folate and vitamin B_{12} deficiencies are "hypoproductive" and have a low reticulocyte count. **Macrocytosis** means a high MCV (greater than 100 fL). On the peripheral smear, red cells with large immature nuclei (called megaloblasts) can be seen. (Remember, normal RBCs do not have nuclei). Anemias secondary to folate and vitamin B_{12} deficiencies are sometimes called "**megaloblastic anemias.**" One diagnostic finding on the smear is **hypersegmented neutrophils** with five or more lobes (see Figure 19-1).

The **Shilling test** is a nuclear medicine study specific for detecting vitamin B_{12} deficiency and its cause. The first step is to give radiolabeled vitamin B_{12} orally and unlabeled vitamin B_{12} by intramuscular injection (the latter to saturate body stores). A 24-hour urine collection is then measured for radiolabeled vitamin B_{12} excretion. A less than normal excretion suggests that vitamin B_{12} is being malabsorbed. If this is the case, step 2 is performed. This is similar to step 1 with the addition of intrinsic factor given with the oral radi-

Megaloblast-RBC with large immature nucleus

Hypersegmented neutrophil

Figure 19-1 Peripheral blood smear findings in folate and vitamin B_{12} deficiencies.

olabeled vitamin B_{12}. If urinary excretion improves (meaning absorption improved), pernicious anemia is diagnosed. If excretion remains low, other causes of malabsorption are considered.

Treatment   Folate deficiency is treated with oral supplements. Vitamin B_{12} is best given by intramuscular injection, usually done monthly. It is important **not** to give folate to a patient with vitamin B_{12} deficiency. This may improve the anemia, but may actually worsen the neurologic problems. The early diagnosis of vitamin B_{12} deficiency is extremely important, as chronic neurologic deficits (e.g., more than 1 year) are often irreversible despite treatment. Vitamin B_{12} levels should be checked in every patient with a suspected macrocytic anemia, even if folate levels are low.

Other Causes of Macrocytic Anemias   **Liver disease** can cause macrocytosis due to altered cholesterol metabolism, which results in RBC membrane changes. Patients with **myelodysplastic syndromes** can have a macrocytic anemia, as well as abnormal white cell and platelet formation. **Drugs** [such as alcohol, phenytoin, or zidovudine (AZT)] can cause macrocytosis, through interference with folate metabolism. **Hypothyroidism** is an additional cause; the mechanism is unknown.

Case Conclusion   Additional labs: serum folate 7 ng/mL (normal 6–20); serum vitamin B_{12}, 97 pg/mL (normal 140–800). The patient was sent for a Shilling test, which revealed normal vitamin B_{12} absorption with the addition of intrinsic factor. The diagnosis of pernicious anemia was made. The patient was started on daily intramuscular injections of cyanocobalamin (vitamin B_{12}) for 1 week, then weekly injections for 1 month, and monthly injections for the remainder of life. At 2 months, the patient had a normal hemoglobin and improvement in his neurologic exam.

Thumbnail: Comparison of Folate and Vitamin B$_{12}$ Deficiencies

	Folate	Vitamin B$_{12}$
Biology	Involved directly in DNA synthesis (H4 folate) **Limited tissue stores**	Involved in reaction that converts natural dietary folate to a H4 folate **Plentiful tissue stores**
Clinical manifestations	Anemia symptoms, **neural tube defects** (in developing **fetus**)	Anemia symptoms, **neurologic deficits** (decreased vibratory and proprioceptive sense, ataxia, altered mental status)
Causes	• ↑ requirements (pregnancy , dialysis) • ↓ intake (alcoholism, poor diet) • ↓ absorption (jejunum—celiac sprue, regional enteritis)	• ↑ requirements (pregnancy) • ↓ intake (strict vegetarians) • ↓ absorption (gastric parietal cells produce **intrinsic factor** needed for transport to the distal ileum) Pernicious anemia—parietal cells/IF, Crohn's, Whipple's disease—ileum
Lab findings	Low serum or RBC folate level; macrocytic anemia, low reticulocyte count, megaloblasts, hypersegmented neutrophils	Low serum vitamin B$_{12}$ level; macrocytic anemia, low reticulocyte count, megaloblasts, hypersegmented neutrophils, **possible abnormal Shilling test**
Treatment	**Daily oral** folate supplement	**Monthly intramuscular** vitamin B$_{12}$ (cyanocobalamin) injection

H4 folate = tetrahydrofolate.

Key Points

▶ Folate and vitamin B$_{12}$ deficiency are both common causes of macrocytic anemia.

▶ Pernicious anemia (autoantibodies induce atrophy of parietal cells/↓ IF) is the most common cause of vitamin B$_{12}$ deficiency.

▶ It is important not to give folate to a patient with vitamin B$_{12}$ deficiency. This may worsen neurologic deficits, which may become irreversible.

▶ Liver disease, myelodysplastic syndromes, drugs (alcohol), and hypothyroidism can all cause macrocytic anemias.

Questions

1. A patient is referred to you for a Shilling test. Yesterday, an injection of nonradiolabeled B$_{12}$ and an oral dose of radiolabeled B$_{12}$ was administered. A 24-hour urine collection reveals abnormally low excretion of vitamin B$_{12}$ today. What do you do next?

   A. Call the referring physician and suggest that this patient likely has a decreased dietary intake of B$_{12}$ as the cause for his anemia.

   B. Call the referring physician and suggest that this patient likely has autoantibodies to his gastric cells as the cause for his anemia.

   C. Repeat the test and give radiolabeled B$_{12}$ by injection and nonlabeled B$_{12}$ orally.

   D. Repeat the test and give oral IF with the radiolabeled B$_{12}$.

   E. Treat the patient with both B$_{12}$ and folate.

2. An elderly woman is admitted to the hospital for pneumonia. On her admission labs it is noted that her Hgb is 9 g/dL and MCV is 106 fL. A serum folate level is ordered and is 2 ng/mL (normal 6–20). What do you do next to treat her anemia?

   A. Do nothing, her anemia will resolve with resolution of her pneumonia.

   B. Begin an oral folate supplement and continue with treatment of her pneumonia.

   C. Check a serum vitamin B$_{12}$ level before treating her anemia.

   D. Do not check iron studies before treating her anemia. You already have a diagnosis.

   E. Supplement her diet with iron.

HPI: A 10-year-old African American girl with sickle cell disease comes to the ED with severe back and leg pain, which began several hours earlier. She was feeling fine the day before, when she spent the entire day at an amusement park. Her father says this is a typical presentation of a "pain crisis," which his daughter experiences one or two times a year. Her last hospitalization was 7 months ago, during which she required intravenous narcotics and a blood transfusion to control the pain.

PE: T 38.1°C (100.6°F) HR 98 BP 115/75
The patient is thin and appears younger than her age. Her conjunctiva are pale. Her back is warm to the touch and is very tender.

Labs: Hb 9 g/dL (her baseline is 10 g/dL); blood cultures are pending.

Thought Questions

- What is the pathophysiology of sickle cell disease?

- What are the common clinical manifestations?

- How can the disease be detected and treated?

Basic Science Review and Discussion

While thalassemia is a *quantitative* abnormality of hemoglobin chain production, sickle cell disease (SCD) is a *qualitative* problem of structurally abnormal globin. SCD is caused by the formation of hemoglobin S (Hb S), which consists of two α chains and two mutant β chains. The mutation is the result of a single nucleotide substitution in the sixth codon of the β-globin gene (glutamine is replace by valine). In this country, **African Americans** are most at risk for carrying the gene mutation. One in 375 African American newborns has SCD, and 1 in 12 African Americans carry the gene. People from Spanish-speaking regions (South America, Cuba, Central America), Saudi Arabia, India, and Mediterranean countries, such as Turkey, Greece, and Italy, also have an increased prevalence.

In an oxygenated environment, Hb S is soluble, and the red blood cell maintains its normal discoid shape. Deoxy-Hb S has poor solubility, which results in polymerization of the protein, causing the red cell to become hard, sticky, and shaped like sickles used to cut wheat. This process is reversible and with oxygenation the sickle cells open up, leading to a repetitive cycle of sickling and unsickling. Eventually, the RBC becomes irreversibly sickled. These rigid, pointy sickle cells cause problems by occluding small blood vessels and prematurely hemolyzing, resulting in anemia.

Sickle Cell Disease A person who is homozygous for SCD inherits two copies of the mutation and produces no normal β-globin. **Chronic hemolytic anemia** is seen in SCD patients. Sickle cells circulate for only 10 to 20 days (as opposed to 120 days for normal RBCs). The spleen recognizes sickle cells as abnormal and traps them, causing painful enlargement of the spleen and usually infarction of the organ in the first few years of life (known as "**autosplenectomy**"). Functional asplenia early in life causes sickle cell patients to be more susceptible to infections from **encapsulated organisms** such as *Streptococcus pneumoniae, Haemophilus influenzae,* and *Neisseria meningitidis.* They are also at risk for **salmonella osteomyelitis.** These bacterial and viral infections (especially **parvovirus B19**) can precipitate acute exacerbations of anemia at the level of the bone marrow (**aplastic crisis**). Symptoms and signs of hemolytic anemia include jaundice, scleral icterus (yellow skin and eyes, respectively) and a high incidence of gallstones (all due to increased bilirubin). One of the most common reasons sickle cell patients seek medical attention is for an **acute pain crisis,** which results from the vaso-occlusion. Over time, sickle cell sufferers can experience damage to organs such as liver, kidney, lungs, and heart due to the anemia, vascular insufficiency, and eventually infarction of these organs. The mean life expectancy is around the fourth or fifth decade.

Sickle Cell Trait Individuals with **sickle cell trait** inherit one normal and one abnormal gene, producing roughly equal amounts of normal and mutant β-globin. Polymerization of deoxy-Hb S is concentration dependent, and dilution with normal hemoglobin reduces the extent of polymerization. Therefore, these individuals generally do not sickle, are asymptomatic, and have a normal life expectancy. One exception is the hyperosmolar, acidic, hypoxic renal environment, which may cause sickling in the kidney, with resulting difficulty in concentrating urine and possible renal damage in both SCD and sickle cell trait patients. Individuals heterozygous for sickle cell can also be heterozygous for β-thalassemia, causing little or no production of normal β globin and increasing the effects of Hb S.

Lab Tests Sickle cell anemia is generally normocytic. Sickled cells can be seen on the peripheral blood smear from individuals with SCD but not from those with sickle cell trait. Commercial tests are available that provide rapid results that determine whether Hb S precipitates when blood is mixed with a high ionic solution. Hb electrophoresis, a more lengthy process, provides a definitive diagnosis. The amino acid substitution in Hb S causes it to run apart from normal Hb (Hb A) on the gel.

Treatment   Agents such as **hydroxyurea,** erythropoietin, and 5-aracytidine have been shown to up-regulate γ-globin gene expression, producing more **Hb F.** Increased Hb F

diluties Hb S, reducing the amount of sickling that occurs. Studies have shown that hydroxyurea therapy can reduce that frequency of vaso-occlusive crises, improving the quality of life (and possibly decreasing end-organ damage) of sickle cell patients. Blood transfusions can treat acute episodes of anemia and pain crisis. Bone marrow transplantation is the only cure for sickle cell disease, but it carries a high risk of morbidity and mortality and is limited by a lack of available matching donors.

Case Conclusion   This case is a typical presentation of a vaso-occlusive pain crisis associated with sickle cell disease. The most likely precipitant of this girl's episode is dehydration due to running around at the amusement park the previous day. Dehydration increases the concentration of Hb S within RBCs, which increases sickle formation and vaso-occlusion. Mild fever and tenderness over the affected area are common. With intravenous hydration and moderate analgesics, the patient is nearly pain free. It is important to rule out infection in sickle cell patients, as they are more susceptible to certain organisms. Indeed, our patient's blood cultures came back negative. She will follow up in several weeks with her regular hematologist.

Thumbnail: Sickle Cell Disease

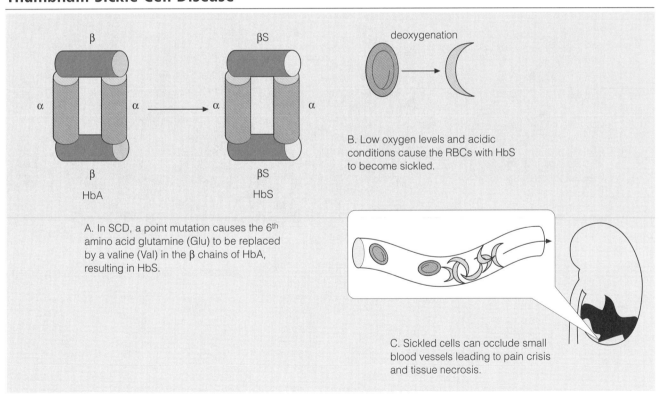

A. In SCD, a point mutation causes the 6th amino acid glutamine (Glu) to be replaced by a valine (Val) in the β chains of HbA, resulting in HbS.

B. Low oxygen levels and acidic conditions cause the RBCs with HbS to become sickled.

C. Sickled cells can occlude small blood vessels leading to pain crisis and tissue necrosis.

Key Points

▶ Sickle cell disease primarily affects African Americans.

▶ Sickle cell disease causes chronic hemolytic anemia, childhood autosplenectomy, increased risk of infection (salmonella osteomyelitis and encapsulated bugs), aplastic crisis (due to parvovirus B19 infection), acute pain crisis (vaso-occlusion) and ischemic organ damage.

▶ Treatment: Hydroxyurea → ↑ HbF → dilutes HbS and reduces amount of sickling.

Questions

1. An 8-year-old African American boy who has a chronic history of anemia is admitted to the hospital for a probable bone infection in his right thigh. An old electrophoresis result revealed 80% Hb S in his blood. What antimicrobial agent would you empirically start him on?

   A. Penicillin G
   B. Azithromycin
   C. Isoniazid
   D. Ceftriaxone
   E. Vancomycin

2. A 6-month-old African American girl is diagnosed with sickle cell disease. Besides sickled cells, what other abnormality might you see on the peripheral blood smear?

   A. Target cells
   B. Hypersegmented neutrophils
   C. Auer rods
   D. Spherocytes
   E. Schistocytes

HPI: NT is an 8-month-old boy of Italian parents who are recent immigrants from Sardinia. The baby has been crying frequently and often refuses to eat. He has not been febrile and has not had any symptoms of vomiting, diarrhea, or constipation. Upon questioning, the mother discloses she had mild anemia since she was a child. The father has no known medical problems, and the patient has no siblings. The patient's birth was full term and uneventful.

PE: This pale baby has a slightly enlarged spleen and appears small for his age. The rest of the exam is unremarkable.

Labs: Hb 5 g/dL (normal 10–13), the MCV is low. Peripheral blood smear reveals pale microcytic cells with variations in size and shape; a target cell is seen. Hb electrophoresis reveals elevated Hb F and Hb A_2 and no Hb A.

Thought Questions

■ What is the structure of hemoglobin?

■ What is the pathophysiology of thalassemia?

■ How do the syndromes of α- and β-thalassemia compare?

Basic Science Review and Discussion

In general, the Hb tetramer found in red blood cells is made up of two α-globin and two non–α-globin subunits. Normal adult hemoglobin (or Hb A) is made up of two α-globin subunits and two β-globin subunits. A less abundant adult hemoglobin, Hb A_2, is composed of two α-globin and two δ-globin chains, and fetal hemoglobin, Hb F, is made of two α-globin and two γ-globin chains. The α and β genes are expressed on different chromosomes, although their production in normal adults is balanced. A group of genetic disorders that lead to *quantitative* abnormalities of Hb subunit production are called **thalassemias,** which are causes of varying severities of anemia.

β-Thalassemia   β-Thalassemia is due to absent or diminished expression of β-globin genes. There is normally one β chain gene located on each chromosome 11, for a total of two gene copies. With little or no β chains to pair with, the α chains (produced in normal amounts) remain unpaired, precipitate, and cause premature red cell destruction. Excess α chains also precipitate in the bone marrow. The varying degree of disease severity depends on the number of abnormal genes inherited.

β-Thalassemia major (also known as "Cooley's anemia" or plain "thalassemia major") occurs when a person is homozygous for (or has inherited two copies of) the faulty β gene. The disease becomes apparent about 6 months after birth when Hb F production declines. At this time, a severe microcytic, hypochromic anemia begins requiring lifelong transfusions. Lack of oxygen delivery to the tissues sends signals to the bone marrow to increase production of erythrocytes. The bone marrow is teeming with abnormal erythrocyte production, a process called "ineffective erythropoiesis." With time, the marrow cavities (skull bones, facial bones, and ribs) expand, leading to the classic facial or skull bone distortions in an untreated patient due to excessive extramedullary hematopoiesis. Erythrocytes that do enter the circulation are identified as abnormal by the reticuloendothelial system (spleen and liver), and are taken up by these organs with ensuing enormous hepatosplenomegaly. Life expectancy in these patients is approximately 30 to 40 years.

A much milder syndrome, β-thalassemia minor, caused by the inheritance of only one faulty β gene (heterozygosity), is characterized by mild anemia (or no anemia), microcytosis, hypochromia, target cells, and basophilic stippling. This can often be mistaken as iron deficiency anemia, but it is important to avoid unnecessary iron therapy in these patients (see Treatment, on next page). There is generally no effect on the life span of β-thalassemia minor patients. An intermediate form of β-thalassemia, appropriately named β-thalassemia intermedia, is caused by inheritance of β genes with reduced (not absent) synthesis of β globin. β-thalassemia is most prevalent where malaria is endemic (especially in Mediterranean populations). It is proposed that thalassemia and/or the gene abnormalities that cause it provide a protective mechanism against the parasitic infection and has been naturally selected for in these areas.

α-Thalassemia   There are two α chain genes located on each chromosome 16, for a total of four gene copies. Deletion of one or more α-globin genes is the usual cause of α-thalassemia. In these syndromes, excess β chains can form β-4 tetramers (Hb H), which, similar to unpaired α chains, precipitate in the red cell. **Hydrops fetalis** is due to loss of all four α genes and results in γ-4 tetramers called **Hb Barts.** These infants are often stillborn due to congestive heart failure. Three missing genes result in **Hb H disease,** characterized by acute hemolysis when a patient is exposed to oxidant-forming medications or infections. Oxidative reactions increase the precipitation of Hb H and subsequent damage to red cells. Two missing α genes (and two normal α genes) cause **α-thalassemia trait,** characterized by mild or no anemia and mild microcytosis. This should be distinguished from iron deficiency anemia to avoid unnecessary iron therapy.

Individuals with one missing α gene are phenotypically normal (silent carriers), but can pass the gene to offspring. α-Thalassemia gene frequencies are highest among southern Chinese, Southeast Asians, and Pacific Island populations. African and Mediterranean descendants also have increased gene frequencies.

Lab Tests   Iron studies can rule out the much more common microcytic anemia, iron deficiency. Hb Barts (γ-4) can be quantified in umbilical cord blood and correlates with the amount of α-globin deficiency. β-Thalassemia can be detected by electrophoresis. Hb A_2 and Hb F are elevated since the excess α chains can pair with δ and γ chains, respectively.

Genetic Counseling   The inheritance of thalassemia is **autosomal recessive** and follows mendelian principles. Afflicted individuals and couples from endemic areas should seek counseling to determine the risk of passing thalassemia genes to their offspring.

Treatment   No therapy is indicated for mild forms of thalassemia (β-thalassemia minor, α-thalassemia trait, and α silent carrier). These patients should avoid iron therapy, which can cause toxic iron buildup (hemosiderosis) that can damage the heart, liver, and pancreas (in these patients the body has a sufficient iron supply and is being signaled to absorb excess iron due to the perceived anemia). β-Thalassemia major and Hb H disease require frequent transfusion therapy and iron chelation therapy to rid the body of excess iron. Bone marrow transplant has been successful in some β-thalassemia major patients.

Case Conclusion   NT was diagnosed with β-thalassemia major. Both his parents are carriers of the β-thalassemia gene (which is why his mother had anemia and father did not—both common presentations.) NT will continue regular blood transfusions and begin iron chelation therapy at around age 5, but will likely continue to have growth retardation and delayed sexual development. Unfortunately, it is unlikely he will make it past the fifth decade of his life.

Thumbnail: Thalassemia

β-Thalassemia	α-Thalassemia
β chain gene = 2 inherited copies	2 α chain genes = 4 inherited copies
Caused by absent or diminished expression of β-globin genes	Caused by deletion of one or more of the α-globin genes
2 main syndromes: β°/β°—β-thalassemia major (chronic anemia, splenomegaly, bone distortions, hemosiderosis, ↑ HbF) β/β°—β-thalassemia minor (mild or no microcytic anemia)	4 main syndromes: 4 missing genes—hydrops fetalis (incompatible with life) 3 missing genes—Hb H disease (acute hemolysis 2° to oxidative insult) 2 missing genes—α-thalassemia trait (mild or no microcytic anemia) 1 missing gene—α-thalassemia silent carrier (asymptomatic)

β, normal allele; β°, mutant allele.

Key Points

▶ Thalassemia is a heterogeneous group of genetic disorders that lead to *quantitative* abnormalities of Hb subunit production.

▶ β-Thalassemia is more common than α-thalassemia (especially in Mediterranean origins).

▶ Avoid iron therapy in thalassemia patients, which can cause toxic iron buildup.

Questions

1. An African American couple would like to have children. Both individuals are silent carriers of α-thalassemia ($-\alpha/\alpha\alpha$). You are asked to provide them with genetic counseling. What percent of offspring would you predict to also be silent carriers?

   A. 0%

   B. 25%

   C. 50%

   D. 67%

   E. 100%

2. If the frequency of the β-thalassemia major disease is 1/1600, what is the probability that a person in the general population (asymptomatic and no family history) is heterozygous for a mutant β-thalassemia allele?

   A. 1/1600

   B. 1/800

   C. 1/40

   D. 1/20

   E. 2/3

HPI: An 18-month-old girl is hospitalized for dehydration during an upper respiratory infection. On day 2, after the administration of IV fluids, her fever decreased from 102°F to 101°F. On day 3 it was noted that she was jaundiced (yellow skin) and had moderate scleral icterus (yellow conjunctiva).

PE: T 38.3°C (101°F) HR 101 BP 110/72
Well-developed baby girl, crying during entire exam. Moderate splenomegaly, also seen on x-ray.

Labs: Hb 8 g/dL, MCV 83 fL. Peripheral blood smear reveals normocytic cells and a few scattered spherocytes.

Thought Questions

■ What causes the production of spherocytes?

■ How do patients with hereditary spherocytosis present?

■ How can hereditary spherocytosis be detected in the laboratory?

■ What is the treatment of hereditary spherocytosis and possible complications of treatment?

Basic Science Review and Discussion

Interactions between red blood cell transmembrane and cytoskeleton proteins function to regulate the unique properties of RBC deformability, tensile strength, and discoid shape. Spectrin, ankyrin, band 3, and protein 4.2 are all such proteins. **Hereditary spherocytosis** (HS) is a **congenital disorder** that involves a genetic mutation that leads to decreased production in one of these proteins (most often cited, **spectrin**). Deficiencies in these proteins decrease RBC membrane strength and increase susceptibility to membrane fragmentation under physical stress (such as in the interendothelial slits in the splenic sinusoids). An uncoupling of the cytoskeleton and lipid bilayer can also occur, leading to the formation of microvesicles that can bleb off. The resulting loss of RBC surface area leads to the generation of spherical cells, called **spherocytes.** The spleen recognizes damaged cells and spherocytes and prematurely destroys them, causing a **hemolytic anemia.**

About 75% of patients with HS have an **autosomal-dominant** inheritance pattern. The remaining 25% are autorecessive forms or new mutations. In the United States, 1 in 5000 have the disorder, and it is most common among people of northern European descent. The clinical picture is highly variable, depending on the degree of hemolysis. Patients may have severe hemolytic anemia with significant growth and sexual retardation, or they may be asymptomatic with a normal life span if the hemolysis is mild or well compensated for by increased RBC production. A typical presentation of HS is a neonate or young child with **jaundice, splenomegaly, anemia, increased indirect bilirubin** (from RBC lysis), and spherocytes on a peripheral blood smear.

Lab Tests   A CBC will show evidence of anemia (decreased hemoglobin), but the MCV will usually be within normal limits (normocytic). The mean corpuscular hemoglobin concentration (MCHC), or the average concentration of hemoglobin in a volume of red cells, will be increased. A reticulocyte count is almost always high as the bone marrow tries to produce more red cells to compensate for the anemia. Other lab values indicate evidence of hemolysis: increased indirect bilirubin (an RBC breakdown product), increased lactate dehydrogenase (LDH) (an RBC component), and decreased free plasma haptoglobin (Hb binding product—more of it is complexed to free Hb released during hemolysis). The **osmotic fragility test,** a test specific for HS, will reveal cells with increased osmotic fragility. A peripheral blood smear can show spherocytes. It is important to perform a direct Coombs' test to rule out an immune-related cause of spherocytes and possible osmotic fragility.

Treatment   **Splenectomy** is the treatment for individuals with moderate to severe HS. Removal of the spleen nearly normalizes red cell survival. Splenectomy is often postponed until after age 4, when the mortality of postsplenectomy infection decreases significantly (remember, asplenic patients are at increased risk for infection by encapsulated bacteria). Postsplenectomy patients should be given prophylactic antibiotics and vaccinations for *Streptococcus pneumoniae, Neisseria meningitidis,* and *Haemophilus influenzae.*

Complications   Patients with HS, even those with mild or no symptoms, are at risk for exacerbations of their condition. Hemolytic crises can be precipitated by bodily stress, especially infections. In more severe cases, **aplastic crises** can occur (most often after parvovirus B19 infections) where RBC production is suppressed in the bone marrow. Chronic hemolysis raises the incidence of pigmented gallstones and its associated complications. Severe episodes can be treated with exchange blood transfusions.

Case Conclusion   This baby also had laboratory results suggesting hemolysis, including indirect hyperbilirubinemia and increased serum LDH. An osmotic fragility test was performed and it was noted that her red cells lysed sooner than normal red blood cells. A direct Coombs' test was also performed (which was negative) to rule out an immune-related hemolysis, which might also present with the same clinical scenario. On further questioning, it was revealed that when the patient's father was a child he had a splenectomy for an unknown reason (likely a positive family history of the disease). The baby was treated with supportive care, and her hemoglobin remained stable, avoiding the need for a blood transfusion. The likelihood for a future splenectomy at around age 5 was discussed with the family.

Thumbnail: Spherocytosis

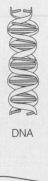

DNA

A. Hereditary spherocytosis is caused by a genetic mutation that leads to deficiency in RBC membrane proteins—spectrin, ankyrin, protein 4.2, or band 3.

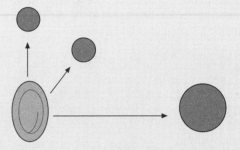

B. Uncoupling of membrane and cytoskeleton proteins leads to microvesicle blebbing, loss of surface area and spherocyte formation.

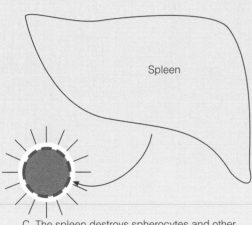

Spleen

C. The spleen destroys spherocytes and other weak fragmented cells resulting in a hemolytic anemia.

Key Points

▸ HS is a congenital disorder, most often with autosomal-dominant inheritance.

▸ HS is a disorder of the RBC membrane caused by a genetic mutation in RBC transmembrane or cytoskeleton proteins, often spectrin.

▸ Structural protein deficiencies result in decreased membrane strength, osmotic fragility, and the formation of spherocytes.

▸ Patients have varying degrees of hemolytic anemia and are prone to hemolytic and aplastic crises.

▸ Splenectomy is the treatment for HS.

Questions

1. Which of the following statements best describes a *positive* osmotic fragility test?

   A. The osmotically fragile RBCs will burst at a lower concentration of NaCl, because more water can go into the cell before it bursts.

   B. The osmotically fragile RBCs will burst at a lower concentration of NaCl, because less water can go into the cell before it bursts.

   C. The osmotically fragile RBCs will burst at a higher concentration of NaCl, because more water can go into the cell before it bursts.

   D. The osmotically fragile RBCs will burst at a higher concentration of NaCl, because less water can go into the cell before it bursts.

2. All of the following lab values are consistent with hemolysis EXCEPT:

   A. ↑ serum indirect bilirubin

   B. ↑ serum lactase dehydrogenase

   C. ↑ plasma haptoglobin

   D. ↑ urine hemosiderin

   E. ↑ urine hemoglobin

HPI: GP is a 67-year-old man who presented to his primary care physician after experiencing 2 months of continual headaches and dizziness. He gets occasional headaches but has never had one last this long. Past medical history includes mild hypertension, asthma, osteoarthritis, and gout. The patient is taking only a prescription NSAID (naproxen sodium). The patient smokes about half a pack of cigarettes a day, and occasionally drinks alcohol. On review of systems, the patient admitted to experiencing intense episodes of pruritus without any evidence of a skin rash.

PE: BP 140/78 HR 82 RR 18 T 97.9°F SaO$_2$ 97%
The patient is of normal weight, with ruddy skin and prominent veins. Funduscopic exam revealed prominent retinal veins. Lung and cardiovascular exams were unremarkable. Normal, active bowel sounds were heard; the abdomen was soft and nontender. The spleen was palpable to 5 cm below the costal margin. A thorough neurologic exam was nonfocal.

Labs: Hct 61% WBC 14,000 Platelets 529,000. The red cell count was elevated. Electrolytes and liver function tests were normal.

Thought Questions

- How does the body produce red blood cells?

- What diseases cause an increase in red blood cell production?

- What are the signs, symptoms, and treatments for polycythemia vera?

Basic Science Review and Discussion

Erythropoiesis The process of red blood cell (RBC) production is termed **erythropoiesis.** During early embryonic life, blood cells are produced in the **yolk sac** (which is extraembryonic tissue), and then in the **fetal liver** during the second trimester of pregnancy. In adult life, RBC production occurs in the **bone marrow.** The earliest precursor of RBC development is the pluripotent stem cell, which is capable of differentiating into any of the blood cell types. The earliest cell type committed to erythroid development is the **proerythroblast,** a large cell with basophilic cytoplasm (many ribosomes) and pale euchromatic (transcriptionally active) chromatin. The **basophilic erythroblast,** a large basophilic cell, begins to synthesize hemoglobin while the nucleus begins to condense and form a checkerboard appearance. As the nucleus is more condensed and the cell shrinks in size, it becomes a **polychromatophilic erythroblast.** This cell continues to synthesize hemoglobin, which gives it a grayish cytoplasm—a mixture of blue (ribosomes) and pink (hemoglobin) staining. Cell division ceases at this stage. As hemoglobin accumulates, the cell is called an **orthochromatophilic erythroblast.** The nucleus is pyknotic (dense), and the cell takes on a pink color. The last stages of erythroid development are characterized by the loss of the nucleus and nearly all of the cell's organelles. The orthochromatophilic erythroblasts encircle a macrophage, which phagocytoses their extruded nuclei. The enucleated nearly mature red cell is called a **reticulocyte.** It still contains some ribosomes and mitochondria, which causes it to stain and appear bluish as compared to a mature RBC.

The differentiation time from basophilic erythroblast to red cell is 1 week. The rate of erythropoiesis is regulated by the protein, **erythropoietin,** which is produced mainly by the kidneys in response to hypoxia (decreased oxygen). Erythropoietin acts by increasing the number of early committed erythroid stem cells that survive and by inducing the transformation of these cells into proerythroblasts. The protein also stimulates the early release of reticulocytes into the circulation. The gene for erythropoietin has been cloned and the protein can be produced in large quantities using recombinant DNA technology. It is frequently used for the treatment of anemias due to advanced kidney disease (where the kidney can no longer produce enough erythropoietin) or during cancer chemotherapy.

Polycythemia Vera **Polycythemia,** in general, is the presence of too many RBCs. Polycythemia vera (PV), or primary polycythemia, is an acquired myeloproliferative disorder that causes overproduction of predominantly erythrocytes, but also accompanying overproduction of white cells and platelets. The median age of onset is 60, and 60% of patients are men. PV is characterized by autonomous erythroid production that is independent of erythropoietin. Most patients present with symptoms related to **increased blood viscosity** and expanded blood volume including headache, dizziness, blurred vision, and fatigue. Pruritus (itching) is due to increased histamine levels released from increased basophils and mast cells, and usually is exacerbated by a warm bath or shower. The increased blood viscosity causes sludging of the RBCs, which can lead to abnormal platelet function and subsequent **thrombosis or hemorrhagic phenomena. Splenomegaly** is found in most patients. The hallmark of PV is a hematocrit above normal, especially above 60%, and an **elevated red cell mass.** RBC morphology is normal. **Serum erythropoietin levels are low,** which distinguish PV from other forms of polycythemia. The treatment of choice is regular phlebotomy to decrease the hematocrit. Occasionally, myelosuppressive therapy (chemotherapy) is used in refractory cases. Over time, approximately 5% of PV cases progress to acute myelogenous leukemia.

Other Causes of Polycythemia   PV must be distinguished from secondary causes of polycythemia. These include chronic hypoxia (smokers, high-altitude living, pulmonary disease), erythropoietin-secreting tumors (adult polycystic kidney disease, renal cell carcinoma, hepatocellular carcinoma), and endocrine abnormalities (pheochromocytoma, Cushing's syndrome). PV should also be differentiated from other myeloproliferative disorders such as essential thrombocytosis, myelofibrosis, and chronic myelogenous leukemia.

Case Conclusion   GP has polycythemia. A serum erythropoietin level was drawn and was lower than normal limits. This finding essentially rules out secondary causes of polycythemia, including erythropoietin-producing tumors (which would cause high serum levels). A carboxyhemoglobin level was drawn and was at the upper limits of normal. Given this finding and the normal oxygen saturation, there is no evidence of hypoxia as the cause of polycythemia. The patient is diagnosed with PV. The elevated white count and platelet levels are consistent with the diagnosis. The patient was started on weekly phlebotomy treatments.

Thumbnail: Polycythemia

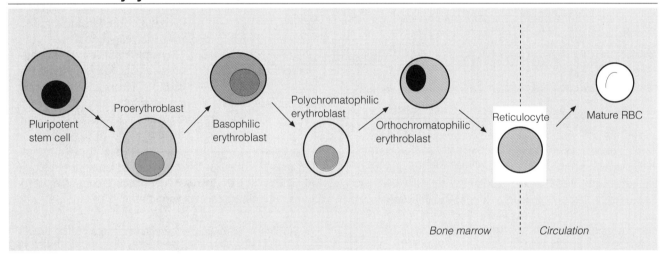

Key Points

▶ The rate of erythropoiesis is regulated by the protein erythropoietin, which is produced mainly by the kidneys in response to hypoxia.

▶ Polycythemia is the presence of too many RBCs.

▶ Primary polycythemia, or PV, is characterized by a high hematocrit, high red cell mass, and low serum erythropoietin level. White cells and platelets are also often increased. Symptoms include headaches, fatigue, pruritus, and thrombotic/hemorrhagic events. Regular phlebotomy is first-line treatment. Approximately 5% of PV cases progress to acute myelogenous leukemia.

▶ Secondary causes of polycythemia are distinguished from PV by a high serum erythropoietin level. These include hypoxia (heavy smokers, high altitude), erythropoietin-secreting tumors (adult polycystic kidney disease, renal cell carcinoma, hepatocellular carcinoma), and endocrine abnormalities (pheochromocytoma, Cushing's syndrome).

Questions

1. A 42-year-old woman with systemic lupus erythematosus has had progressive renal failure over the last year. She is not on dialysis. On examination she has pale conjunctiva and skin. Her hemoglobin is 8.0 g/dL, hematocrit 25%, MCV 88 fL. Total bilirubin is 0.9 mg/dL. The peripheral blood smear is normal. What is the cause of her anemia?

   A. Iron deficiency
   B. Microangiopathic hemolytic anemia
   C. Acute blood loss
   D. Hereditary spherocytosis
   E. Thalassemia
   F. Erythropoietin deficiency
   G. Vitamin B$_{12}$ deficiency

2. Polycythemia vera is associated with which correct combination of findings?

   A. Erythrocytosis, leukocytosis, thrombocytosis, splenomegaly, decreased erythropoietin
   B. Erythrocytosis, leukocytosis, thrombocytopenia, splenomegaly, decreased erythropoietin
   C. Erythrocytosis, leukopenia, thrombocytosis, splenomegaly, decreased erythropoietin
   D. Erythrocytosis, leukocytosis, thrombocytosis, splenomegaly, increased erythropoietin
   E. Erythrocytosis, leukocytosis, thrombocytopenia, splenomegaly, increased erythropoietin
   F. Erythrocytosis, leukopenia, thrombocytosis, splenomegaly, increased erythropoietin

HPI: A 61-year-old man with coronary artery disease and hypertension underwent a coronary artery bypass graft (CABG) procedure. Before the operation the surgeon ordered four units of packed RBCs to be cross-matched to the patient's type A, Rh negative blood. The patient required three units during the surgery. The patient had an uneventful recovery until the fifth postoperative day, at which time his Hb dropped from 15 to 8 g/dL. The patient appeared jaundice and spiked a temperature of 39.1°C; his urine appeared "tea-colored." As part of a work-up for a suspected hemolytic anemia, a direct Coombs' test was ordered.

Thought Questions

■ What are blood groups and why are they important in transfusion medicine?

■ What is an indirect Coombs' test and what other tests are used to match transfusion products?

■ What are some common transfusion reactions?

Basic Science Review and Discussion

Blood Groups   The major **blood types, A, B, O,** and **AB,** are based on the presence or absence of carbohydrate antigens on the RBC surface. Type A blood has the "A" antigen, type B blood has "B" antigen, type AB has both antigens, and individuals with type O blood have neither of these antigens. Individuals have "naturally" occurring antibodies in their serum (stimulated by the environment) directed against the AB antigen(s) that are *not* found on their red cells. For example, a person who is type B blood has anti-A in her plasma. These antibodies are usually IgM, which react at room temperature, bind complement, but do not cross the placenta. IgG forms of anti-A and anti-B are produced when individuals are exposed to red cells by pregnancy or transfusion.

The presence of the AB antigens on the surface of the red cell and the presence of AB antibodies in the plasma dictates what blood products can be safely transfused. Red cell products must be transfused only to recipients who lack the corresponding AB antibody in their plasma. Plasma products containing AB antibodies must be transfused only to recipients who lack the corresponding antigen on their red cell membranes. Since group O individuals lack any A or B antigens on their red cells, they are considered **universal blood donors.** Group AB individuals are **universal plasma donors** as they lack AB antibodies.

Another type of blood grouping is the **Rh** system. Of the numerous antigens in the Rh system, the D antigen is the most important. Rh(+) blood denotes the presence of the D antigen on the red cells of an individual's blood. The D antigen is strongly immunogenic and anti-D (anti-Rh) anti-

bodies are the leading cause of **hemolytic disease of the newborn.** When a Rh-negative pregnant woman carries a Rh-positive fetus, small amounts of D-positive red cells can enter her circulation. Her body can then produce anti-D IgG antibodies. If she becomes pregnant in the future with an Rh-negative fetus, the antibodies can cross the placenta and attack the red cells of the fetus. Rh-negative pregnant women are given a small amount of Rh immunoglobulin (anti-D), RhoGAM, which prevents their own formation of anti-D antibodies.

Over 600 red cell antigens are known, but only a small amount are considered clinically significant (capable of stimulating IgG antibodies), and may cause hemolytic transfusion reactions. Some examples are Kell, Duffy, or Kidd antigens.

Blood Testing   When a patient requires a blood transfusion, there are several tests that are done to find a compatible match in the blood bank. First, the patient's red cells are tested for the presence of A, B, and D antigens (blood typing). Next, an antibody screen (also known as an **indirect Coombs' test**) is performed by mixing a patient's serum with reagent red cells with known antigens (Figure 24-1). If the patient has serum antibodies directed against any of the red cell antigens, the specimen will agglutinate (clump) after antiglobulin is added. Another test is the **direct Coombs' test,** during which the patient's RBCs are mixed directly with antiglobulin (Figure 24-2). Patients with delayed hemolytic transfusion reactions or with autoimmune hemolytic anemias have red cells coated with antibodies that agglutinate, yielding a positive reaction.

Transfusion Reactions   Reactions to blood transfusions do occur and can even result in death. Reactions can be acute (immediate) or delayed, occurring days or weeks after transfusion. **Febrile nonhemolytic transfusion reactions (FNHTRs)** are one of the most common acute transfusion events. The patient often experiences chills, rigors, and a temperature increase of 1°C or more during or after the transfusion. This reaction is due to pyrogenic cytokines [interleukin-6 (IL-6) or tumor necrosis factor (TNF)] that are stimulated in the recipient by leukocytes in the transfused product or that have

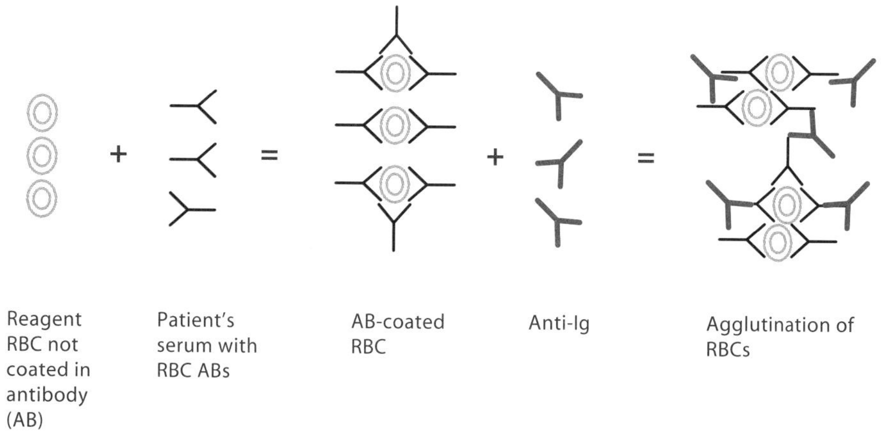

Figure 24-1 Indirect Coombs' test.

already been produced in the transfusion product during storage. Most patients are pretreated with an antipyretic (e.g., acetaminophen) to avoid this reaction.

A **hemolytic transfusion reaction,** a less common but more serious transfusion reaction, also causes fever. These reactions can be acute or delayed. Acute hemolytic transfusion reactions occur most commonly when ABO incompatible blood is transfused. The most common cause is human error in matching identification of the patient and appropriate blood product! Antibodies in the patient's serum react with

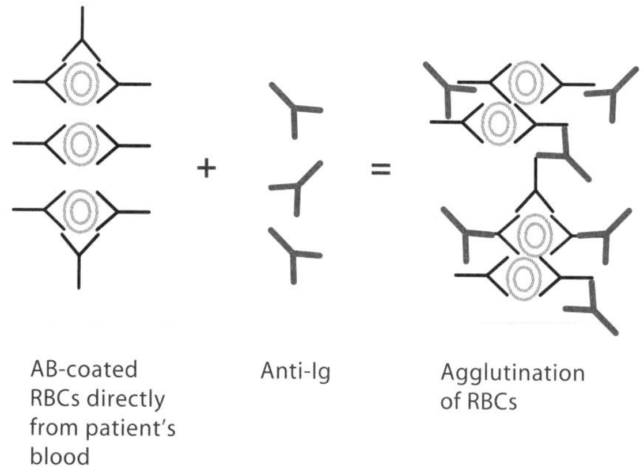

Figure 24-2 Direct Coombs' test.

antigens on the transfused cells and complement-medicated **intravascular hemolysis** occurs. Along with fever, patients may have chills, chest pain, hypotension, and diffuse bleeding. Renal failure, shock, and DIC can follow. This is an extremely serious reaction, as death occurs in 10% to 40% of cases. Delayed reactions occur when a person is sensitized during a previous transfusion but has undetectable antibodies on pretransfusion testing. Several days to weeks after the second transfusion, the patient produces more antibodies, which coat the surface of the transfused cells. Presenting symptoms are fever, anemia, and jaundice due to **extravascular hemolysis** as the antibody-coated RBCs are removed in the spleen. A direct Coombs' test is often positive. These reactions may go undetected due to their delayed nature. Treatment includes a procedure, called *elution,* that removes antibodies from the surface of the red cells.

Another common reaction is an **allergic transfusion reaction,** occurring in 1% to 3% of all transfusion recipients. These are mediated by preformed IgE in the recipient to some transfused allergen. Hives and pruritus are common, but reactions can progress to bronchospasm, hypotension, and anaphylaxis. Treatment is with antihistamines, which are often given to all patients before a transfusion to prevent this event.

Case Conclusion The direct Coombs' test was positive. According to the patient's records, he had been transfused two units of red cells the previous year for his first CABG procedure. A formal investigation of a suspected transfusion reaction was performed. There was no evidence of clerical or laboratory error. The pretest direct Coombs' test of the transfused blood was negative. As a part of the patient's treatment, an elution was performed and the antibodies were then identified in the laboratory as JKb, a Kidd antigen. It was determined that the patient underwent a delayed hemolytic transfusion reaction. He was sensitized to the Kidd antigen during the previous transfusion, but his antibody titer was too low to be detected on pretransfusion testing. The patient was given further supportive care and was discharged from the hospital on day 9. It was noted in his records that all future transfusion products be screened for this antigen and avoided.

Thumbnail: ABO Blood Group Antigens, Antibodies, and Compatibility

Group	ABO antigens of red cells	Compatibility of red cells	Antibodies in plasma	Compatibility of plasma
O	None	Transfuse to all patients (universal donor)	Anti-A, Anti-B	O patients only
A	A	A and AB only	Anti-B	A or O
B	B	B and AB only	Anti-A	B or O
AB	A and B	AB only	None	Transfuse to all patients (universal donor)

Key Points

▸ ABO blood types are based on red cell antigens. Patients receiving blood products from another person must have a compatible blood type.

▸ An antibody screen (also known as an indirect Coombs' test) is performed by mixing a patient's serum with reagent red cells with known antigens to determine which RBC antibodies are present in the patient's serum.

▸ A direct Coombs' test detects the presence of pre-formed antibody-coated RBCs in the patient's blood and can be positive in autoimmune hemolysis and delayed transfusion reaction.

▸ Hemolytic disease of the newborn occurs when Rh-negative mothers are sensitized by Rh-positive babies. If pregnant with a subsequent Rh-positive child, anti-D (Rh) antibodies can cross the placenta and attack the newborn's RBCs. RhoGAM is given early to prevent this occurrence.

▸ Acute hemolytic transfusion reaction is caused by direct ABO incompatibility. Delayed hemolytic transfusion reactions can be caused by antibody sensitization during pregnancy or prior transfusions.

▸ Allergic transfusion reactions, mediated by IgE, can cause hives and, in severe cases, shock and anaphylaxis.

Questions

1. Which of the following correctly describes how a direct Coombs' test is performed?

   A. The patient's serum is mixed with test RBCs and agglutination is measured.

   B. The patient's serum is mixed with mouse RBCs and agglutination is measured.

   C. The patient's RBCs are mixed with anti-human immunoglobulin/complement mouse antibodies and agglutination is measured.

   D. The patient's RBCs are mixed with anti-mouse immunoglobulin/complement human antibodies and agglutination is measured.

2. Which of the following statements is correct regarding Rh immunoglobulin (RhoGAM)?

   A. It prevents the production of anti-D antibodies.

   B. It is given to all Rh-positive pregnant women at the time of delivery.

   C. It blocks IgM antibodies from crossing the placenta.

   D. It can trigger hemolytic disease of the newborn in some patients.

HPI: HK is an 18-month-old boy who presents with a painful left knee. His father relates that the child had large bruises following the immunizations at 15 months. He also states that someone in his wife's family, possibly the wife's father, had a similar history of "easy bruising," as a child. PMH: Increased bleeding postcircumcision.

PE: Warm, tender, and swollen left knee with decreased muscle size in left quadriceps in comparison to right quadriceps. Remainder of physical exam is normal.

Labs: Platelets 330,000/dL, PTT 80 seconds, PT 12 seconds.

Thought Questions

- What diagnostic considerations are most likely based on the patient's presentation and bleeding times?

- What is the inheritance pattern and variable expression of this disorder?

- How should this patient be treated and managed to prevent recurrent episodes?

- What infectious organisms are possible complications of treatment?

Basic Science Review and Discussion

Patients with coagulation disorders may present with one of two general symptom profiles. Patients who have a **platelet disorder** present with **mucosal bleeding** (e.g., gums, nosebleeds), **ecchymoses,** as well as **purpural and petechial rashes.** Those with **deficient clotting factors** present more commonly with **hemarthroses, bleeding into soft tissue or muscle, or increased bleeding after trauma or surgery** (Table 25-1).

Coagulation Cascade   For proper blood coagulation to occur, soluble plasma fibrinogen must be converted to fibrin. A deficiency in fibrin or more commonly an inability to convert fibrinogen to fibrin prevents normal fibrin function. Therefore, the primary platelet plug is not encapsulated and will not form a stable hemostatic clot. The process of activating fibrin requires a functional coagulation cascade. Each factor, except factor XIII, is a **serine protease,** which activates the following reaction in the cascade. The activated form of the factor is represented with a lowercase *a*. In the classical view, the intrinsic and extrinsic pathways converge in the common pathway (Figure 25-1).

Modeling the extrinsic and intrinsic pathways allows the use of prothrombin time (PT), partial thromboplastin time (PTT), and thrombin time (TT) in diagnosing coagulation disorders; however, in vivo the model is not accurate. The modified view is currently most representative of the clotting pathway within the human body.

The modified pathway links the extrinsic and intrinsic through VIIa's activation of IX. This allows two means of activating X. This is necessary due to an in vivo inhibitor of VIIa and tissue factor—tissue factor pathway inhibitor (TFPI). Increased thrombin is then dependent on IXa activating X. This explains the bleeding seen in patients with hemophilia A despite a normal PT. This model also accounts for the bleeding seen in a small number of patients deficient in factor XI (Figure 25-2).

Hemophilia   A diagnosis of moderate or severe **hemophilia** is the most likely consideration in this case due to the patient's labs (increased PTT with normal PT and normal platelet count) the clinical presentation (bleeding postcircumcision and recurrent joint bleeds with increased activity), and the described inheritance pattern (**X-linked recessive**). Hemophilia A is five times more common than hemophilia B; however, both are inherited in the same pattern.

Table 25-1 Comparison of bleeding disorders

Patient presentation	Category	Most common diagnoses
Spontaneous mucosal bleeding; nonpalpable purpuric rash and ecchymoses	Platelet disorder	Qualitative platelet disorder—*von Willebrand disease, Bernard-Soulier syndrome, Glanzmann thrombasthenia, storage pool diseases* Reduced platelet count—*thrombocytopenias*
Hemarthrosis with muscle and joint involvement, spontaneous or post minor trauma; prolonged bleeding following surgery	Clotting factor deficiency	*Hemophilia A* (factor VIII deficiency), *hemophilia B* (factor IX deficiency)

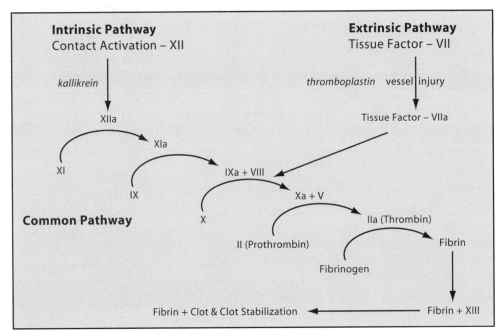

Figure 25-1 Coagulation cascade.

Hemophilia A is the most common form of a factor deficiency. While the majority of patients inherit the disease, 33% of cases result from random mutation of the *FVIII* gene on the long arm of the X-chromosome. Variable amounts of viable protein are produced in affected individuals, which are grouped as mild, moderate, or severe. Mild hemophiliacs (5% to 20% coagulation factor activity compared to normal expression) present with bleeding posttrauma. Moderate hemophiliacs (1% to 5%) bleed posttrauma, and occasionally spontaneously. Severe hemophiliacs (less than 1%) present with frequent spontaneous bleeding episodes and are likely to develop joint deformities, which can be crippling if not properly treated. While it is unusual for females to develop the disease due to its pattern of expression, carrier females may present with bleeding following severe trauma. Most carriers express 50% to 70% normal FVIII levels.

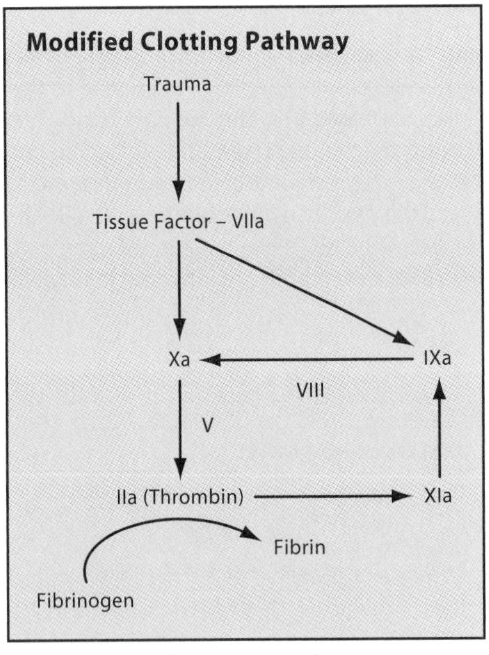

Treatment of hemophilia A or B is determined by the level of factor that is functionally produced by the patient. Patients are advised on limiting physical activity and contact sports. Families are also routinely screened to determine if the mother is a carrier and if future children should be tested during pregnancy. Severe hemophiliacs require a prophylactic regimen of FVIII transfusions to prevent spontaneous bleeding, yet mild hemophiliacs require replacement therapy only for surgeries or following trauma. Mild hemophiliacs may also show benefit with **deamino-8-D-arginine vasopressin (DDAVP)** (desmopressin) treatment. DDAVP causes a transient rise in FVIII levels by triggering its release from endothelial cells. Currently, FVIII replacement therapy uses recombinant FVIII and immunopurified FVIII, which has greatly reduced the degree of infectious diseases spread by blood products. During the 1980s, over 50% of hemophiliacs contracted **HIV** through blood transfusions. Prior to the surge in HIV among hemophiliacs, the incidence of hepatitis C was on the rise as well. Both of these have caused AIDS, chronic hepatitis, and cirrhosis to be among the leading causes of death among severe hemophiliacs.

Modified Clotting Pathway

Trauma

Tissue Factor – VIIa

Xa ← IXa

VIII

V

IIa (Thrombin) → XIa

Fibrin

Fibrinogen

Figure 25-2 Modified clotting pathway.

Case Conclusion   HK was admitted to the hematology day clinic and transfused with recombinant FVIII to 30% correction. The hemarthroses of the left knee were treated symptomatically with elevation and ice. Additional labs showed a 0% production of FVIII protein and HK was diagnosed with severe hemophilia A. A follow-up visit was scheduled to discuss prophylactic treatment and to screen HK's mother and sisters by restriction fragment length polymorphism (RFLP) analysis to determine their carrier status.

Thumbnail: Hematology—Lab Tests of Coagulation

PT and **PTT** are common laboratory measures of a patient's intrinsic and extrinsic clotting pathways. PT may be expressed as international normalized ratio (INR), which is the ratio of a patient's PT over the normal PT. **TT (thrombin time)** is a third less commonly used measure of the coagulation cascade.

Laboratory value	Potential deficiency	Most common diagnoses
Thrombin time (TT) nl 14–16 seconds	Fibrinogen—deficient or abnormal Inhibition of thrombin	*Disseminated intravascular coagulation (DIC)* Heparin therapy
Prothrombin time (PT) nl 10–14 seconds, a measure of extrinsic pathway function	Deficiency or abnormality in one or multiple of factors II, V, **VII**, X, and fibrinogen	*Liver disease* *Warfarin therapy* DIC
Partial thromboplastin time (PTT) nl 30–40 seconds, a measure of intrinsic pathway function	Deficiency or abnormality in one or multiple of factors II, V, **VIII, IX**, X, XII, and fibrinogen	*Hemophilia A* (VIII) *Hemophilia B* (Christmas disease, IX) *Heparin therapy* Warfarin therapy DIC

Factor XIII is not assessed by either PT or PTT. For this reason a patient with nl PT and PTT yet recurrent bleeding episodes is suspect for a factor XIII deficiency. **Factor XII** and in most cases **factor XI** deficiencies show increased PTT but no increased bleeding clinically.

Key Points

▶ The most common factor deficiency leading to increased bleeding is hemophilia A, FVIII.

▶ Both *FVIII* and *FIX* genes are located on the long arm of the X-chromosome with an X-linked recessive inheritance pattern.

▶ PT and PTT provide an in vitro assessment of the factors involved in the extrinsic and intrinsic pathways, respectively.

▶ Platelet disorders present clinically as mucosal bleeding, ecchymoses, and purpural and petechial rashes.

▶ Clotting factor deficiencies present clinically as hemarthroses, bleeding into soft tissue or muscle, and bleeding posttrauma or surgery.

Questions

1. Elective surgery is scheduled for a 14-year-old boy with no history of bleeding problems. During routine labs an elevated PTT is found and determined to be a deficiency in FXII. The patient's PT, platelet count, and all other labs are normal. The family consults you to determine if the surgery should be performed. The most appropriate action is?

   A. Cancel the surgery and determine if replacement therapy is needed.

   B. Reassure the family and proceed as planned.

   C. Perform the surgery only after infusing purified FXII.

   D. Cancel the surgery and reorder labs including PTT, PT, and TT.

   E. Perform the surgery after vitamin K supplements and fibrinogen IV.

2. Which of the following regarding FVIII deficiency is true?

   A. PT is prolonged.

   B. Vitamin K administration is adequate treatment to prevent bleeding.

   C. It is less common than FIX deficiency.

   D. Girls are affected more commonly than boys.

   E. Severe hemophiliacs should be placed on prophylactic therapy despite the risk of HIV transmission.

3. A 22-year-old man is brought to the ED following a gang fight. Two deep lacerations are observed in the lower right quadrant of his abdomen. The lacerations are bleeding profusely despite applied pressure for 20 minutes. Diffuse swelling, erythema, and rubor are noted in his right ankle and left knee. The patient is unresponsive. An astute medical student notices a medical alert bracelet among the pile of the patient's belongings. It indicates the patient has mild hemophilia A. The expected labs and treatment plan are which of the following?

   A. Normal PT, prolonged PTT; treatment with recombinant FVIII

   B. Normal PT, prolonged PTT; treatment with recombinant FIX

   C. Prolonged PT, normal PTT; treatment with recombinant FVIII

   D. Prolonged PT, normal PTT; treatment with recombinant FIX

   E. Prolonged PT, prolonged PTT; treatment with recombinant FVIII

4. A 4-year-old boy presents with recurrent bleeding into soft tissue and muscle. Some rib fractures are noted in the child's chart. At the prior visits, PT, PTT, and TT were tested. All normal results were reported consistently, except for a transient period as an infant during which PT and PTT were slightly elevated. During this visit the father is concerned since the child's bruising has continued. The physician identifies symmetric bruising along the child's midaxillary line. X-ray of the ribs indicates new rib fractures overlaid on healing fractures. His PT, PTT, and TT are currently normal. The next step in working up this child's case is which of the following?

   A. Reorder PT, PTT, and TT.

   B. Order a von Willebrand's factor (vWF) count including multimers and ristocetin.

   C. Check the platelet count.

   D. Check vitamin K levels.

   E. Contact child protective services and the team's social worker on call.

HPI: JK is a 24-year-old woman with recurrent bleeding following wisdom tooth extraction. PMH: Recurrent nose-bleeds began in her early teens and are still present. The patient bled excessively following a tonsillectomy at age 9. She also mentions that episodically her menstrual bleeding has been longer than normal.

Labs: Bleeding time 23 minutes (nl less than 8 minutes) PTT 44 seconds (nl 25–35 seconds) PT 12 seconds (nl 12–14 seconds) FVIII coagulant activity 25% of nl Platelets 250,000 μL (nl 150,000–350,000/μL)
JK's physician suspects a platelet disorder based on the clinical presentation. However, her counts are within normal limits. Due to the combination of clinical presentation and lowered FVIII activity, her physician suspects von Willebrand's disease.

Thought Questions

- What is the mechanism of platelet adhesion and aggregation?

- What are the common hereditary platelet disorders?

- What are the three types of von Willebrand's disease?

- How does treatment with DDAVP increase vWF and FVIII levels?

Basic Science Review and Discussion

Platelets are responsible for the formation of the initial hemostatic plug, which initially adheres to the subendothelial connective tissue following vessel insult. Vessel damage exposes subendothelial microfibrils, which bind to multimers of **vWF. Glycoprotein Ib** on the surface membrane of platelets complexes with the bound vWF; this complex formation exposes **glycoprotein IIb/IIIa** on the platelet membrane. Circulating **fibrinogen** binds to this glycoprotein at both ends, forming a matrix and allowing platelet aggregates to form. An additional glycoprotein, Ia, forms a direct adhesion to collagen (Figure 26-1).

Platelet exposure to **thrombin** and **collagen** cues its granule release. The release of arachidonate from granules leads to increased thromboxane A_2 levels and decreased cAMP concentration. Increased thromboxane A_2 levels augment platelet aggregation and cause local vasoconstriction. Medications that prevent the drop in cAMP are able to inhibit platelet function. Platelet granules also release adenosine diphosphate (ADP), serotonin, fibrinogen, lysosomal enzymes, thromboglobulin, and platelet factor 4 (heparin neutralizing factor). Increasing ADP and thromboxane A_2 levels positively feed back and further the platelet plug.

Inherited Platelet Disorders Deficiencies in the key glycoproteins found on the platelet membrane account for the inherited platelet disorders such as **Glanzmann's thrombasthenia** and **Bernard-Soulier syndrome. Glanzmann's**

thrombasthenia is a deficiency in GPIIb/IIIa, which prevents proper aggregation of platelets through fibrinogen. Lab values indicative of GPIIb/IIIa deficiency detail a normal platelet count with poor aggregation to most agonists. Bleeding as a result of this defect in primary platelet plug formation occurs within the first few months of life. Glanzmann's thrombasthenia is inherited in an autosomal-recessive pattern. Likewise, **Bernard-Soulier disease is an inherited autosomal-recessive deficiency. Depleted GPIb prevents platelet adhesion to vWF,** which is the primary means of platelet attachment to the vessel wall via subendothelial connective tissue. Bleeding in Bernard-Soulier disease is severe and improves gradually with age. Diagnostic tests indicate **poor aggregation to ristocetin and thrombin, abnormally large platelets, and variably deficient platelet counts.** Replacement therapy with functional platelets provides treatment for both disorders. Rarely, deficiencies in platelet granule contents may be inherited (storage pool diseases), leading to excessive bleeding.

Von Willebrand's Disease Glanzmann's thrombasthenia, Bernard-Soulier disease, and storage pool diseases increase bleeding time, yet PT and PTT remain unchanged. In **von Willebrand's disease** (deficient vWF), **PTT may be elevated in addition to an increased bleeding time. vWF, previously known as FVIII related antigen, actually acts as a carrier molecule for FVIII.** vWF is released by endothelial cells and platelets, in which vWF is found within α granules. Molecularly, vWF forms large multimers and leads to von Willebrand's disease following point mutations or large deletions in the vWF gene. This disease is inherited in an **autosomal-dominant** pattern.

Von Willebrand's disease is the most common inherited bleeding disorder and has three subtypes. **Quantitative reductions in the levels of vWF occur in types 1 and 3. Type 2 von Willebrand's disease is a functional deficiency with 4 etiologies.** Treatment of von Willebrand's disease may include FVIII replacement therapy if its activity in the patient is decreased, as well as DDAVP to boost vWF levels. DDAVP increases vWF and therefore also FVIII levels by triggering its release from endothelial cells.

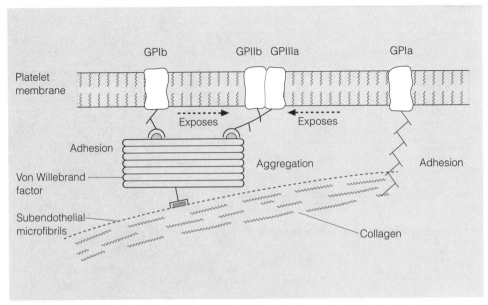

Figure 26-1 Platelet adhesion. (Adapted from Hoffbrand AV, Pettit JE, Moss PAH. Essential haematology, 4th ed. Osney Mead, Oxford: Blackwell Science, 2001.)

Case Conclusion JK's physician ordered vWF levels and platelet aggregation studies. The results indicated low vWF, defective aggregation to ristocetin, and normal aggregation to ADP, collagen, and thrombin. JK was diagnosed with von Willebrand's disease and transfused with FVIII to raise her above 30% activity. DDAVP was given to raise her von Willebrand factor. She was discharged after a full recovery.

Thumbnail: Hematology—von Willebrand's disease vs Hereditary Platelet Disorders

	Hereditary platelet defects		
Disease	**Bernard-Soulier disease**	**Glanzmann's thrombasthenia**	**von Willebrand's disease (vWD)**
Inheritance pattern	Autosomal recessive	Autosomal recessive	Autosomal dominant
Deficiency of	Membrane glycoprotein Ib	Membrane glycoprotein IIb-IIIa	von Willebrand factor (vWF)
Protein function	vWF receptor	Fibrinogen receptor	Bind subendothelial connective tissue to platelet
Defect in	Platelet adhesion vWF and therefore subendothelium	Primary platelet aggregation	Platelet adhesion to subendothelial connective tissue
Clinical presentation	• More severe bleeding than vWF deficiency • Improves with age	• Severe bleeding disorder • First presentation as neonate	• Mild bleeding with variable presentation in heterozygous • Severe bleeding with early onset in homozygous
Poor aggregation test to	Ristocetin and thrombin	All agonists except ristocetin	Ristocetin
Treatment	• Replacement therapy with purified platelets	• Replacement therapy with purified platelets • Monoclonal anti-GPIIb-IIIa antibodies	• Replacement therapy with purified FVIII or fresh frozen plasma • DDAVP—vasopressin derivative which causes vWF release from endothelial cells
Notes	Large platelet size and low platelet count	Normal platelet count	• Most common inherited bleeding disorder • vWF acts as a carrier molecule of FVIII (in some cases of vWD reduced FVIII levels are present)

Questions

1. What percent of the population is affected by von Willebrand's disease?

   A. 0.2%
   B. 0.5%
   C. 1.0%
   D. 2.0%
   E. 5.0%

2. Platelets contain vWF within which granules and which clotting factor does vWF carry?

   A. α Granules, FV
   B. α Granules, FVIII
   C. α Granules, FIX
   D. δ Granules, FV
   E. δ Granules, FVIII

3. A 19-year-old woman presents with menorrhagia to her family physician. Her chart indicates a family history of excessive bleeding. The patient also complains of a red and swollen left knee with reduced mobility. Her labs include a normal PT, slightly elevated PTT, prolonged bleeding time, moderately reduced FVIII activity levels, and decreased ristocetin cofactor activity. A quantitative loss in vWF is found, and no decrease in large weight vWF multimers. The most likely diagnosis is which of the following?

   A. Type 1 von Willebrand's disease
   B. Type 2A von Willebrand's disease
   C. Type 2M von Willebrand's disease
   D. Type 2N von Willebrand's disease
   E. Type 3 von Willebrand's disease

4. A 7-year-old girl with recurrent mucosal bleeding, petechiae, and ecchymoses is seen for a consult. The patient's labs indicate mild thrombocytopenia and large platelets on smear. Decreased aggregation to ristocetin and thrombin is also noted. PT and PTT are normal. A detailed family history reveals an autosomal-recessive pattern of inheritance. The most likely diagnosis is which of the following?

   A. Glanzmann's thrombasthenia
   B. Bernard-Soulier disease
   C. von Willebrand's disease
   D. Hemophilia A
   E. Hemophilia B

HPI: AN is a 15-year-old girl with a seizure disorder brought by ambulance to the ED with 3 days of **fever** and **cough,** and now with **altered mental status.** According to her mother, she was recently diagnosed with a grand mal seizure disorder and started **antiepileptic therapy** with **phenytoin** 3 weeks ago. Three days ago she developed a mild fever, malaise, sore throat and cough. The fever resolved eventually, but her cough and **pharyngitis** persisted. Two days ago, she began to develop oral lesions consistent with **thrush,** and has since quickly deteriorated with declining mental status without evidence of prior seizure activity as she normally has.

PE: T 37.6°C HR **105** BP **95/50** RR **30** SaO$_2$ **95%** at room air. On exam, the patient was **somnolent** but arousable, and in mild respiratory distress. Her exam was significant for **diffuse oral thrush; diffuse rhonchi** in all lung fields, and **multiple erythematous papules** on her upper and lower extremities. She had no focal neurologic deficits.

Labs: A scraping of the oral thrush was observed under microscope with KOH preparation and revealed **budding yeast** and **pseudohyphae** consistent with a *Candida* sp. Her CBC with differential revealed an **absolute neutrophils count of 315/μL.**

Thought Questions

- What is the normal function of neutrophils, and what are the molecular and cellular events that mediate inflammation?

- What is the definition of neutropenia, and what pathophysiology underlies this phenomenon?

- What are the clinical manifestations of neutropenia?

- How is neutropenia diagnosed and treated?

Basic Science Review and Discussion

Neutrophils and Inflammation The above case demonstrates the importance of neutrophils as the first-line defense against mucocutaneous and systemic infection. **Neutrophils** or **polymorphonuclear (PMN) cells** develop from myeloid precursors in the bone marrow under the influence of granulocyte-colony-stimulating factor (G-CSF) and granulocyte macrophage-colony-stimulating factor (GM-CSF). They progress through several stages of differentiation, from myeloblast to mature neutrophil with its characteristic multilobed nucleus and cytoplasmic granules. These granules contain bactericidal enzymes and other components required for pathogen killing. Neutrophils are then released into circulation in response to the cytokines IL-1, TNF-α, and C3e. Neutrophils are in one of two states while in the intravascular space, either free floating or in contact with the endothelium. The latter population of neutrophils is said to be "marginated." **Margination** is a low-affinity adherence of PMNs to endothelial cells via **selectins,** resulting in "rolling" of these cells on endothelial surfaces. If a pathogen-like bacteria breaches the skin or mucosal barrier,

the products released from bacteria and damaged tissue (e.g., cytokines) up-regulate expression of **integrins** in leukocytes and **intercellular adhesion molecules-1** and **-2** in endothelial cells. These receptors cause increased "stickiness" or **tight adhesion** of neutrophils to the endothelial surface. Neutrophils then undergo **diapedesis** (i.e., transmigration through the endothelial cell layer), and migrate toward the site of injury by following a molecular gradient of **chemokines** (*chemo*attractant *cyto*kines) such as IL-8, complement component C5a, and kallikrein, released from that site (see Figure 27-1).

Alternatively, neutrophils resident in the tissue may recognize new invading bacteria by their **pathogen-associated molecular patterns,** structures commonly expressed by microorganisms. Such pathogens may also be **opsonized,** or bound by complement fragment C3b, to increase the efficiency of phagocytosis and killing by neutrophils. If the body has been previously exposed and has developed humoral immunity to a pathogen, that pathogen may be opsonized by immunoglobulin, a more specific binding interaction that similarly promotes phagocytosis. Microbial killing proceeds via an **"oxidative burst"** representing the formation of toxic oxygen products like hypochlorous acid, hypochlorite, and chlorine that oxidize phagocytosed microorganisms. Proteins and enzymes like defensins, lysozyme, and proteases also aid in killing. Neutrophils then release multiple cytokines that recruit other leukocytes of the innate and adaptive immune systems to promote the rest of the inflammatory immune response.

Neutropenia Neutropenia is defined as a decrease in neutrophil count below that of normal standard limits (normal range 1800–10,000/μL). However, African Americans and other populations may have normal counts of 500 to

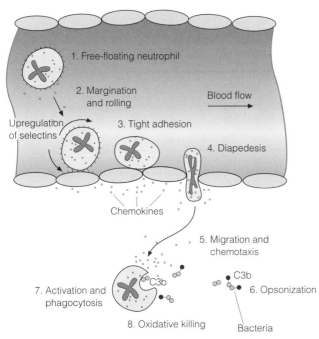

Figure 27-1 Schematic of neutrophil recruitment, activation, and inflammation. Free-floating neutrophils are recruited by cytokines released from damaged tissue. Several receptors are up-regulated to facilitate endothelial cell adhesion and diapedesis. This is followed by migration to the site of damage through the influence of chemokines.

1000/µL with no adverse consequences. Clinically relevant neutropenia is associated with an **absolute neutrophils count of < 500/µL,** which increases risk of serious bacterial and fungal infection. Neutropenia may exist as part of a

pancytopenia or aplastic anemia. The most common form of neutropenia is iatrogenic as an incidental reaction to drugs. Neutropenia can result from myelosuppression due to cytotoxic and immunosuppressive drugs, as neutrophils have a short half-life of 6 to 7 hours in circulation and may be the first to be depleted of all blood cells. Alternatively, drugs may serve as **haptens,** or agents that by themselves are not immunogenic but when bound to a carrier protein, such as a self-protein, can elicit an immune response. This can lead to autoimmune recognition of self-protein from previous sensitization to the hapten-protein complex. In the case of neutropenia, this phenomenon targets neutrophils and leads to increased peripheral destruction. Neutropenia is an ominous sign in bacterial sepsis, which can increase neutrophil demand beyond the body's capacity to regenerate. Other causes include HIV infection, congenital disorders (Felty's syndrome with the triad of isolated neutropenia, rheumatoid arthritis, and splenomegaly), and other autoimmune disease [large granular lymphocytosis, a clonal abnormality of T cells or natural killer (NK) cells that attack neutrophils] (Table 27-1).

Patients may be asymptomatic or may present with infections from gram-positive or gram-negative aerobic bacteria or fungi, such as *Candida* or *Aspergillus*. Common sites include the upper respiratory tract, lungs, and the perirectal area. Mucosal infections can progress to systemic infection. In severely neutropenic patients, signs of infection may be absent due to blunted inflammatory response from the neutropenia. Bone marrow biopsy may aid in determining whether neutropenia is caused by decreased production or increased peripheral destruction.

Table 27-1 Causes of neutropenia

Decreased production	Peripheral destruction
• Drugs: *Note all drugs begin with "c" or "p" (at least on this list). Think "causes of poor production"* • Cytotoxic agents (cyclophosphamide) • Antibiotics (chloramphenicol, penicillin,) • Anticonvulsants (carbamazepine, phenytoin) • Antipsychotics (clozapine, phenothiazines) • Hematologic disease: idiopathic, cyclic neutropenia, aplastic anemia • Myelofibrosis/bone metastases • Nutritional deficiency: B$_{12}$/folate deficiency • Infection: tuberculosis, measles, viral hepatitis, EBV, HIV/AIDS	• Antineutrophil antibodies and/or splenic/lung trapping → phagocytosis by macrophages • Autoimmune disorders: Felty's syndrome, RA, SLE • Drugs as haptens: α-methyl dopa, phenothiazine • Wegener's granulomatosis

RA, rheumatoid arthritis; SLE, systemic lupus erythematosus.

Case Conclusion With the suspicion that her isolated neutropenia was caused by recent initiation of phenytoin therapy, her regimen was changed. Her blood cultures grew *Candida albicans*. A bone marrow biopsy was performed, which revealed an isolated depletion of myeloid precursors, with all other cell lines intact. She was in critical condition for several weeks supported with the broad-spectrum antibiotic amphotericin B and G-CSF. Her neutropenia resolved after 7 days. Despite her critical condition, she recovered, and her antiepileptic therapy was switched to oral phenobarbital. She had no subsequent episodes of neutropenia or candidal infections.

Table 27-2 Diagnostic work-up for neutropenia

Diagnostic test	Indications	Results/implications
CBC with differential	Signs of infection	Identifies isolated neutropenia, absolute neutrophils counts less than 500/μL, or pancytopenia
Blood culture and sensitivity	Signs of infection	Confirms systemic bacterial or fungal infection, species, and antibiotic sensitivity
Serum B$_{12}$ and folate	All neutropenic patients, esp. alcoholics	Suggests megaloblastic anemia and hypoproliferative state from malnutrition
Bone marrow biopsy	1. Unexplained neutropenia lasting greater than a few weeks 2. Pancytopenia 3. Neutropenia with serious infection	*Isolated absence of myeloid precursors* → agranulocytosis likely due to a drug reaction *Absence of all precursors* → work-up for aplastic anemia *Normal bone marrow* → suggests peripheral destruction (autoimmune, sepsis, hypersplenism)
Antineutrophil antibody	Neutropenia with signs of CVD	Suggests autoimmune etiology
Cytogenetic testing and chromosomal analysis	Younger patients Suspicion of congenital anomaly	Identifies hereditary neutropenias, e.g., Felty's syndrome

CBC, complete blood count; BM, bone marrow; CVD, collagen vascular disease.

Thumbnail: Hematology—Neutropenia

Definition	Absolute neutrophil count < 500/μL, or below normal laboratory range

Pathophysiology and etiologies	1. Drug-induced—chemotherapy, antibiotics, antiepileptics, antipsychotics
	  a. Cytotoxic and immunosuppressive drugs—myelosuppression
	  b. Immune haptens—autoimmunity to drug–self-antigen complex
	2. Autoimmune disease—rheumatoid arthritis, systemic lupus erythematosus
	3. Infection—HIV, tuberculosis, Epstein-Barr virus (EBV), measles, viral hepatitis
	4. Congenital disease—Felty's syndrome

Clinical manifestations	Mucosal infection with bacteria or fungus → systemic infection
Diagnosis	CBC with differential [absolute neutrophil count (ANC) < 500/μL]; blood culture and sensitivity; serum B$_{12}$ and folate, bone marrow biopsy; antineutrophil antibody
Prognosis	Most patients with drug-induced agranulocytosis recover with supportive care Prognosis dependent on etiology and level of neutropenia

Key Points

▶ Neutrophils are the first-line defense against mucocutaneous and systemic infection and are the first to proliferate after a new infection.

▶ Clinically relevant neutropenia is associated with an absolute neutrophils count of less than 500/μL, which increases risk of serious bacterial and fungal infection.

▶ Neutropenia arises from several conditions that fall into two main categories: (1) insufficient production, and (2) accelerated destruction. The most common etiology is drug reaction.

▶ Neutropenia manifests in increased risk of mucosal infection with bacteria or fungus that easily transforms into a systemic infection.

Questions

1. A 10-year-old boy has a congenital deficiency in leukocyte adhesion molecules, namely the common integrins required for "tight adhesion" of leukocytes to endothelium. He is at play in the yard when he is scraped, and the wound becomes infected with bacteria. What laboratory abnormality would you expect to find several hours after this event and what effect would this disease have on the boy?

   A. Elevated WBC with neutrophilia (elevated neutrophils) → normal wound healing
   B. Elevated WBC but with neutropenia → abnormal wound healing
   C. Elevated WBC with neutrophilia → abnormal wound healing
   D. Decreased WBC but with neutrophilia → normal wound healing
   E. Decreased WBC with neutropenia → abnormal wound healing
   F. Decreased WBC with neutrophilia → normal wound healing

2. SR, a 19-year-old woman with rheumatoid arthritis, is diagnosed with her second episode of bacterial pneumonia in the past month and is discovered to have a low white blood cell count with an isolated neutropenia confirmed on blood smear. On exam, she is noted to have splenomegaly. What is most likely in the differential diagnosis of her neutropenia?

   A. Acute leukemia
   B. Felty's syndrome
   C. Large granular lymphocytosis
   D. Chronic myeloid leukemia
   E. Myelofibrosis with myeloid metaplasia

HPI: AA is a 68-year-old African-American man who presents with 3 weeks of gradually worsening **fatigue, epistaxis,** and **nonhealing oral lesions.** He noticed increasing **dyspnea on exertion** with his daily 1 mile walks and now can, at most, walk around the house. His epistaxis has occurred daily and is now becoming increasingly difficult to stop. He also notes **increased bruising** to minor trauma. He developed multiple oral ulcers 1 week ago, which have not improved since. Prior to this, he had had an upper respiratory infection after visiting his granddaughter, who was sick with a fever and rash. His past medical history is significant for a recent history of **hepatitis with negative serologies,** and thus presumed to be due to alcohol, although he denies heavy alcohol use. His family history is significant for **sickle cell anemia,** although he has never had symptoms suggestive of this disease nor has he been evaluated for it. He worked for a **petroleum** company for 40 years, and is now retired.

PE: T 37.6°C HR **109** BP 135/65 RR **36** SaO$_2$ 99% at room air.
The patient is a thin, ill-appearing man in mild respiratory distress during exertion. His physical exam is significant for **scleral pallor,** dried blood in his nares, **mucosal petechiae,** multiple buccal and labial **aphthous ulcers,** and **diffuse ecchymoses** on his upper and lower extremities with no evidence of bone tenderness. His cardiovascular and abdominal exams are benign; he has no organomegaly.

Labs: WBC **3500/μL,** absolute neutrophil count **358/μL,** monocytes **1%,** lymphocytes 25%, Hct **26%,** MCV **105 fL,** platelets **85,000/μL.** *Peripheral blood smear* revealed **large RBCs, few platelets and granulocytes,** with **rare hyperlobulated neutrophils. Bone marrow biopsy** produced a **pale and dilute aspirate,** which microscopically appeared **fatty** with **less than 20% cellularity,** consisting of a few red cells, lymphocytes, and scant megakaryocytes. Blood cultures were negative for bacteria.

Thought Questions

- What are the basic functions of white blood cells?

- What are the causes of pancytopenia? How are these diagnosed?

- What are the clinical features of pancytopenia? How is pancytopenia treated?

Basic Science Review and Discussion

The leukocytes of the **innate immune system** rely on the nonspecific recognition of **pathogen-associated molecular patterns (PAMPs),** molecular structures commonly expressed by many microorganisms in order to carry out their multiple functions. This recognition activates various mechanisms of pathogen elimination including phagocytosis, cell killing, and recruitment of other leukocytes that have their own roles in amplifying, refining, or suppressing the immune response (Table 28-1).

Pancytopenia is defined as a decrease in circulating mature blood cells, leading to the characteristic *leukopenia, anemia,* and *thrombocytopenia.* In the simplest terms, it results from some insult leading to a dynamic abnormality in blood cell production, distribution, usage, and survival. Such abnormalities may occur in two compartments, either within the bone marrow or in peripheral circulation. An insult may cause enough damage to hematopoietic stem cells that their numbers no longer adequately support the

body's requirements. In **aplastic anemia,** pancytopenia is accompanied by a marked reduction of all hematopoietic precursors in the bone marrow. Alternatively, damage may result in cytogenetic abnormalities that simply *impair* cell proliferation and differentiation, and thus prevent adequate replenishment of circulating blood cells, as found in **myelodysplastic syndromes (MDS).** Normal bone marrow cell replacement may also occur with **myelophthisic diseases,** wherein fibroblasts are stimulated to lay down collagenous material in the bone marrow, thereby crowding out normal hematopoietic cells and causing abnormal release of immature cells. There are three possible categories of bone marrow histopathology that may result (Table 28-2).

The main clinical features of pancytopenia are those associated with anemia, thrombocytopenia, and neutropenia. Physical exam findings include petechiae, ecchymoses, retinal hemorrhage, skin, and mucosal pallor. Pelvic and rectal exams may reveal cervical bleeding or blood in the stool. Hepatosplenomegaly may also be present as a sign of extramedullary hematopoiesis when the bone marrow is unable to meet the body's requirements. Often, the etiology of pancytopenia is suggested by history. In **aplastic anemia,** where pancytopenia arises from the destruction of hematopoietic precursors, a blood smear reveals *normal-appearing cells but in markedly reduced numbers,* with evidence of compensatory RBC production. In **MDS** where there is abnormal cell proliferation and differentiation, a blood smear would reveal a distinct population of large RBCs along with *abnormal-appearing and hypofunctioning*

Table 28-1 Review of white blood cells of the innate immune system

Cell type	Characteristics and functions
Neutrophils (PMNs)	• **Primary phagocyte of the innate immune system;** recognizes PAMPs; have no class II MHC proteins for antigen presentation • Can better recognize and phagocytose pathogens opsonized with immunoglobulin and complement component C3b via Fc surface receptors.
Eosinophils	• **Parasite recognition**—leukocyte with *red-staining cytoplasmic granules* that recognize and *attack large extracellular pathogens* (e.g., parasites) • Recognize parasites opsonized with IgE via the Fcε-receptor, which activates degranulation of vesicles containing lytic enzymes • **Parasite killing**—lytic enzymes, including *major basic protein,* are released extracellularly to attack pathogen membranes; may also cause local tissue damage • **Immediate hypersensitivity reactions** (e.g., asthma)—eosinophil granules contain *histaminase,* which degrades histamine, a mediator of allergic reactions • Recruited and activated by T$_H$2 **helper cells** via cytokines **IL-4** and **IL-5**
Basophils and mast cells	• **Basophils,** leukocytes with *blue-staining cytoplasmic granules* • **Mast cells** are functionally similar to basophils but *reside in tissue,* e.g., skin, mucosa, and have *receptors with bound IgE* that recognize certain allergens • **Immediate hypersensitivity reaction**—releases histamine (which increases vascular permeability, smooth muscle contraction, and glandular secretion), adenosine (activates masts cells, inhibits platelet aggregation), SRS-A, ECF-A, etc. • Both have **Fcε-receptor,** which binds IgE-opsonized allergens → induces degranulation of cells, which initiates inflammatory reaction • Massive degranulation can lead to severe reaction such as **anaphylaxis** • Late-phase response involves recruitment of other leukocytes
Macrophages/monocytes	• Monocytes are circulating leukocytes, while macrophages are monocytes that have migrated to an extravascular site like lymph nodes, spleen, bone marrow, etc. • **Phagocytosis** of bacteria, viruses, and other *small* foreign particles via Fc receptors that recognize immunoglobulins opsonizing foreign antigen; eliminates tumor cells • **Antigen presentation**—ingested foreign particles are processed and fragments are bound to class II MHC on macrophages for antigen presentation to T-cells, activating the adaptive immune response • **Cytokine production**—released **IL-1, IL-6, IL-10,** and **TNF-α** mediate several aspects of the inflammatory reaction
Dendritic cell or Langerhans cells *(when associated with skin or mucosa)*	• Lymphoid/myeloid-derived cells important in both innate and adaptive immunity • **Innate immunity**—recognize bacterial PAMPs, which bind dendritic cell TLR → up-regulate class II MHC and co-receptor expression → enhance antigen presentation and cytokine production → promote adaptive immune response • **Antigen presentation**—most important function; has both class I and II MHC • **Cytokine production**—produces **IFN-α** in response to viral infections → *activates NK cells* to kill virally infected cells; *recruits T- and B-cells*
Natural killer (NK) cells	• **Nonimmune cytotoxic killing**—recognize reduced expression of class I MHC and stress-induced protein expression on the cell surface of virally infected cells, cancer cells, as well as foreign cells; *does not require prior exposure to target* • Kills via **perforins** and **granzymes,** inducing *apoptosis* of targeted cell

PMN, polymorphonuclear cell; PAMP, pathogen-associated molecular patterns; LPS, lipopolysaccharide (component of endotoxin of gram-negative bacteria); Fc, constant fragment of antibody; IL, interleukin; SRS-A, slow-reacting substance of anaphylaxis; ECF-A, eosinophil chemotactic factor of anaphylaxis; TNF, tumor necrosis factor; MHC, major histocompatibility complex; TLR, toll-like receptor; IFN, interferon; NK, natural killer; APC, antigen-presenting cell.

platelets and neutrophils. Other causes of pancytopenia with cellular bone marrow must be ruled out, such as severe malnutrition, B$_{12}$ or folate deficiency, drug reaction, and infection wherein aplasia is transient or reversible. In **myelophthisic disease,** the peripheral smear reveals cell morphologies consistent with **disturbances in the blood–bone marrow barrier** where mature and immature WBCs, RBCs, and platelets are abnormally released into circulation. Circulating red cells are nucleated or **tear-drop–shaped;** WBCs include myeloid precursors; platelets are elevated and giant in size.

Bone marrow studies provide definitive diagnosis. In aplastic anemia, bone marrow destruction results in a dilute, fatty, and grossly pale aspirate that is **hypocellular with < 20% cellularity.** In MDS, the bone marrow is normal or hypercellular with **dysplastic morphologies,** including RBCs with **ringed sideroblasts,** hypogranulated and hyposegmented myeloblasts, and poorly nucleated megakaryocytes. Lastly, myelophthisic disease is characterized by a "dry tap," where no aspirate can be produced. The presence of granulomas suggests an infectious etiology. Treatable causes such as tuberculosis and fungus must be ruled out.

Table 28-2 Causes of pancytopenia by bone marrow histopathology

Hypocellular bone marrow	Cellular bone marrow	Bone marrow fibrosis
Acquired aplastic anemia:	*Myelodysplastic syndromes*	*Primary myelofibrosis*
• Idiopathic (> 80% of cases)	• Radiation, benzene	• Myelofibrosis with myeloid metaplasia (MMM)
• Toxic exposure—radiation, chemotherapy, benzene (in petroleum)	• Late toxicity of chemo/radiation therapy	*Secondary myelofibrosis* (Myelophthisis)
• Drugs—chloramphenicol, carbamazepine, cimetidine	*Substrate deficiencies:* • Megaloblastic anemia	• Mycobacterial infection
• Viruses—EBV, non-A/B/C hepatitis, CMV, B19	• Anorexia nervosa, starvation	• Fungal infection
Inherited aplastic anemia:	*Other bone marrow disease*	• HIV
• Fanconi's anemia	• Chronic leukemia/lymphoma	• Sarcoidosis
Immune diseases:	• Metastatic bony Infiltration usage:	• Radiation therapy
• Transfusion—GVHD	*Overwhelming infection*	• Gaucher's disease
• PNH	*Hypersplenism* (sequestration)	• Chronic leukemia/lymphoma
Pregnancy	*Nonspecific toxicity:* alcohol	
	Immune disease: PNH, SLE	

EBV, Epstein-Barr virus; CMV, cytomegalovirus; B19, parvovirus B19; GVHD, graft-versus-host disease; PNH, paroxysmal nocturnal hemoglobinuria; CML, chronic myeloid leukemia; MM, multiple myeloma; HCL, hairy cell leukemia; SLE, systemic lupus erythematosus; HIV, human immunodeficiency virus.

Case Conclusion AA is diagnosed with a pancytopenia with apparent hypocellular bone marrow suggestive of bone marrow failure. He is thus treated with supportive care, prophylactic antibiotics, fluids, packed red blood cells, and platelet transfusions. This is followed up with GM-CSF therapy to support bone marrow regrowth.

Thumbnail: Hematology—Pancytopenia

	Aplastic anemia	Myelodysplastic syndrome	Myelophthisic anemias
Pathophysiology	*Destruction* of bone marrow stem cells, causing insufficient production of circulating blood cells	*Damage* to stem cells causing *abnormal* proliferation and differentiation → release of hypofunctioning blood cells	Bone marrow fibrosis → replacement of normal cells and disturbance of blood–bone marrow barrier → release of premature and abnormally shaped cells
Etiology	Idiopathic (80%) Viruses Environmental exposures Chemotherapy/radiation Drugs Congenital disease Autoimmune disease Pregnancy	Environmental exposures Chemotherapy/radiation *Rule Out:* Nutritional deficiencies Overwhelming infection Hypersplenism Myeloproliferative Disease	Primary hematologic disease Metastatic tumor in bone marrow Infection Infiltrative disease Radiation therapy
Epidemiology	Biphasic age distribution: young and elderly	Elderly, mean age 68 years Male > female	Adults > 50 years old
History	Abrupt or insidious onset of bleeding, bruising, fatigue, palpitations, frequent mucosal infection	Insidious onset of anemia, thrombocytopenia, neutropenia	Insidious onset of anemia S/Sx, thrombocytopenia, neutropenia, Abdominal fullness
Physical exam	Petechiae, ecchymoses, bleeding, Pallor, ↑RR, ↑HR Signs of infection (mucosa)	Pallor, tachycardia, tachypnea Signs of bleeding, diathesis Signs of infection	Massive splenomegaly Signs of anemia, thrombocytopenia Signs of infection

Laboratory findings	Pancytopenia
	 < 20% bone marrow cellularity
	 Severe aplastic anemia: includes 2 of 3 criteria:
	   1. ANC < 500/μL
	   2. Platelets < 20,000/μL
	   3. Reticulocytes < 1%
		Pancytopenia
		 Normal or hypercellular bone marrow
		 Morphologically and functionally abnormal blood cells with elevated blasts in blood and bone marrow
			Pancytopenia
			 Tear-dropped shaped RBCs
			 ↑ WBC, RBC blasts
			 Giant abnormal platelets

Key Points

▶ White blood cells provide basic functions of immune defense through phagocytosis, cell killing, and leukocyte recruitment for the amplification, refinement, and even suppression of the immune response.

▶ Pancytopenia is the combined presence of *leukopenia, anemia,* and *thrombocytopenia* that results from an insult causing a dynamic abnormality in blood cell production, distribution, usage, and survival.

▶ Most etiologies of pancytopenia can be diagnosed by peripheral blood smear and bone marrow biopsy, which will reveal a hypocellular bone marrow, a normal or hypercellular bone marrow, or bone marrow fibrosis.

Questions

1. What is the least likely etiology of AA's pancytopenia from the history?
   A. Parvovirus B19 infection
   B. Post-hepatitis aplasia
   C. Benzene exposure during years in petroleum plant
   D. Fanconi's anemia
   E. Undiagnosed sickle cell trait with new overlying cytomegalovirus (CMV) infection compromising already compromised hematopoietic capacity

2. PR is a 59-year-old woman who presents with respiratory distress and is eventually diagnosed with *Streptococcus* pneumonia. Her recent medical history includes recent initiation of the antiseizure drug carbamazepine after a recent stroke. She has a long history of alcohol abuse and is noted by her caseworker to have poor appetite and food intake. Her exam is significant for rhonchi in the right upper lobe. Her labs reveal a pancytopenia with hypersegmented neutrophils. Subsequent bone marrow biopsy reveals a normal-appearing cellular bone marrow. What is the least likely cause of her pancytopenia?
   A. Drug reaction
   B. Vitamin B_{12} deficiency
   C. Parvovirus B19 infection
   D. Alcohol toxicity
   E. Pernicious anemia

HPI: CR is a 38-year-old man admitted with bacterial sepsis. He is currently in a sedated state, and his history is unknown. It is suspected that the sepsis was caused by the patient's IV drug use.

PE: CR is febrile (39.8°C), tachycardic (pulse 110), and tachypneic (RR 38). Track marks are located on his left ankle and right arm. Multiple petechiae and bruises are located on his chest and abdomen as well as over his IV sites. Indurated and confluent purpura are present on his right arm. Swelling and discoloration of the feet are noted.

Labs: Hgb is low (8.7 g/dL), WBC is high (18,500/μL), platelets are low (16,000/μL), and both PT and PTT elevated (23 seconds and 95 seconds, respectively). CR's physician believes the sepsis may be linked to the thrombocytopenia and elevated PT and PTT.

Thought Questions

- What is the typical clinical presentation of thrombocytopenia?

- What are the common causes of thrombocytopenia?

- What is the role of the immune system in the pathogenesis of idiopathic (autoimmune) thrombocytopenic purpura (ITP)?

- What is the clinical difference between thrombotic thrombocytopenic purpura (TTP) and hemolytic uremic syndrome (HUS)?

- What are the common causes of disseminated intravascular coagulation (DIC)?

Basic Science Review and Discussion

Platelet abnormalities in either **quantity (thrombocytopenia) or function** result in incompetent primary hemostasis. The clinical presentation is characterized by **spontaneous skin purpura (palpable or nonpalpable), ecchymoses, mucosal hemorrhages, and hematomas.** Normal platelet counts range from 150,000 to 450,000/μL; however, symptoms of thrombocytopenia develop when patients' counts fall below 50,000/μL. Under conditions of platelet destruction, the numbers of megakaryocytes within the bone marrow increase in order to compensate. The produced platelets in the peripheral bloodstream may appear **larger than normal** due to premature release from the bone marrow. If bone marrow depletion is involved, examination of the bone marrow shows depleted numbers of megakaryocytes and normal-sized, circulating platelets.

Thrombocytopenia may arise due to a variety of etiologies: **(1) failures of platelet production, (2) increased consumption of platelets including sequestration, and (3) drug or toxin interaction with platelet function.** Platelet production is decreased as a selective depletion of megakaryocytes or during general bone marrow failure. The latter, bone marrow failure, is the most common cause of thrombocytopenia. Bone marrow failure occurs due to radiotherapy, aplastic anemia, leukemia, myelofibrotic and myelodysplastic syndromes, multiple myeloma, and HIV infection. Platelet counts drop as they are sequestered in hypersplenism, cirrhosis, and some malignancies. Consumption of platelets is commonly due to an immune process, either directly against the platelets themselves (such as ITP), or as a result of infections, drug-induced, post-transfusion, or fetomaternal blood mixing. **TTP in familial or acquired form and the related HUS dramatically deplete platelet counts by consumption. In DIC, consumption is not limited to platelets, and affects clotting factors as well.** The last category, drugs and toxins, includes ionizing radiation, ethanol, chloramphenicol, idoxuridine, penicillamine, benzene, organic arsenic, rifampicin, sulfonamides, trimethoprim, diazepam, carbamazepine, acetazolamide, tolbutamide, chlorpropamide, heparin, and quinidine.

Idiopathic (Autoimmune) Thrombocytopenic Purpura ITP is considered for the majority of cases only as a diagnosis of exclusion. ITP occurs as chronic and acute forms. In both forms the bone marrow increases platelet production five times normal, due to shortened life span of the circulating platelets. Adults typically develop chronic ITP with a 3:1 greater incidence in women ages 15 to 50. While it is termed idiopathic, chronic ITP is associated with other autoimmune disorders such as SLE, malignancies such as chronic lymphocytic leukemia (CLL), Hodgkin's, and HIV infection. Clinically, patients present without splenomegaly, and less severe symptoms than expected based on platelet counts. This is possibly attributed to younger platelets that have superior function in circulation. The course of the disease is insidious and relapsing over time. **The patient's own immune system causes the platelet destruction through IgG autoantibodies to platelet proteins such as glycoproteins IIb-IIIa or Ib complex.** Antibody covered platelets are then destroyed in the spleen by macrophages, decreasing the life span from 7 days to a few hours. Treatment of chronic ITP includes steroids, splenectomy, high-dose intravenous immunoglobulin, and immunosuppressive medications.

Acute ITP presents in children following a viral infection such as chicken pox or infectious mononucleosis. An immune complex formation is formed similar to that in chronic ITP, causing platelet consumption. The majority of cases are self-limited and resolve in 4 to 6 weeks. However, 20% go on to develop chronic ITP. In severe cases, steroids are used as treatment.

Thrombotic Thrombocytopenic Purpura   TTP results from **excessive platelet aggregation due to the lack of an inhibitory protein, metalloprotease (caspase).** Caspases are responsible for the inhibition and degradation of high molecular weight multimers of vWF. Aggregates of vWF multimers trigger platelet adhesion and collection as microthrombi in small vessels. While this process does not also trigger the clotting cascade, the presence of **microthrombi leads to fever, jaundice, thrombocytopenia, traumatic hemolytic anemia, acute renal failure, CNS changes, seizures, and, potentially, coma.** Patient's laboratory values indicate low platelets, increased megakaryocytes, normal PT and PTT, low Hct and Hgb, RBC fragments on smear, and bilirubinemia. In familial TTP an inherited deficiency of caspase is present. Acquired forms occur postinfection, due to the production of an inhibitory antibody that interferes with caspase function. **Plasmapheresis to remove antibodies and the vWF multimers is the initial treatment of TTP.** A 90% mortality rate is reported for untreated cases.

Hemolytic uremic syndrome (HUS) shares a similar, yet limited, presentation to TTP. HUS commonly occurs among **children, and end-organ involvement is limited to the kidneys.** There are **no neurologic symptoms in HUS, while they are present in TTP.** *Escherichia coli* and *Shigella* infections are associated with HUS. Caspase levels are normal, and treatment focuses on controlling hypertensive symptoms and dialysis.

Disseminated Intravascular Coagulation   Platelet destruction occurs in DIC as in ITP, TTP, and HUS. DIC is considered a broad-spectrum disease following the release of numerous procoagulants causing **widespread activation and subsequent depletion of both platelets and the clotting factors.** Procoagulants in two forms contribute to the pathogenesis of DIC. Infectious agents (gram-negative and meningococcal septicemia, HIV, CMV, hepatitis infections, and septic abortions) and severe hypothermia or burns damage the endothelium and create excessive collagen exposure, triggering the cascade. DIC is also triggered by particles traveling in the bloodstream that act as procoagulants themselves, such as in mucin-secreting adenocarcinomas, acute myelogenous leukemia (AML), liver disease, transfusion reactions, premature separation of the placenta (placental abruption), and emboli of amniotic fluid. The result of abnormal excesses of thrombi in the microvasculature is the production of fibrin split products that interfere with the normal coagulation pathway. Thrombin and plasmin degrade circulating fibrinogen, prothrombin, and factors V and VIII. In compensated DIC, the liver is still capable of clearing the fibrin split products and producing ample coagulation factors to replace those being used. As the liver becomes unable to meet this function (known as decompensated DIC), the loss of clotting factors and platelets results, and bleeding is the number one clinical concern.

Clinical presentation in the acute setting includes bleeding, purpura, traumatic hemolytic anemia (due to shearing of the RBCs as they pass through vasculature containing thrombi and fibrin strands), **and bilateral necrosis of the renal cortex.** Chronic DIC presents with increased thrombosis and decreased bleeding. Laboratory values in DIC indicate thrombocytopenia, markedly **elevated PT, PTT, and TT, and high levels of D-dimers (fibrin degradation products) in both the serum and urine.** Schistocytes, broken RBCs, are present on smear. Treatment of DIC focuses on resolving the underlying cause. To prevent additional bleeding, patients are transfused with **fresh frozen plasma and concentrates of platelets.**

Case Conclusion   CR is found to have acute DIC, and his condition worsens before intravenous antibiotics and fresh frozen plasma can be effective. He develops acute renal failure and diffuse hemorrhage into his abdomen and GI system. He dies 24 hours after being admitted to the hospital.

Thumbnail: Hematology—Thrombocytopenia

Common Causes of Thrombocytopenia

Decreased production	Consumption/sequestration	Drugs/toxins	
Selective megakaryocyte depletion	Idiopathic thrombocytopenic purpura	Ionizing radiation	Cytotoxic drugs
Megaloblastic anemia	Thrombotic thrombocytopenic purpura	Ethanol	Chloramphenicol
Myelodysplastic syndrome	Hemolytic uremic syndrome	Idoxuridine	Penicillamine
Myelofibrosis	Disseminated intravascular coagulation	Benzene	Organic arsenic
Radiotherapy	Post-transfusion	Gold salts	Rifampicin
Leukemia	Thrombocytopenia	Penicillins	Sulfonamides
Multiple myeloma	Pregnancy associated	Trimethoprim	Chlorpropamide
Aplastic anemia		Tolbutamide	Heparin
		Quinidine	

ITP vs. TTP: Autoantibodies in ITP are to glycoprotein IIb-IIIa or Ib complex. Antibodies in acquired TTP are to metalloproteases (caspase).

TTP vs. HUS: TTP involves neurologic symptoms in addition to systemic symptoms. HUS is limited to renal involvement with no neuro symptoms.

DIC vs. ITP, TTP, and HUS: DIC leads to diffuse hemorrhage due to depletion of both platelets and clotting factors. Thrombocytopenias (ITP, TTP, and HUS) deplete only platelets and clinically manifest with mucosal bleeding, purpura, ecchymoses, and hematomas.

Key Points

▶ Thrombocytopenia is most commonly caused by inadequate production of platelets that is due to nonselective bone marrow failure.

▶ Platelet morphology on smear provides diagnostic findings in differentiating decreased platelet production from increased consumption of platelet sequestration. In the latter presentation, platelets appear immature and abnormally large. In contrast, smears representative of decreased platelet production depict platelets of normal morphology.

▶ Hemolytic uremic syndrome presents acutely in children postinfection and in the majority of cases is self-resolving with symptomatic treatment.

▶ Diagnosis of disseminated intravascular coagulation relies heavily on the finding of markedly elevated d-dimers in circulation.

Questions

1. A 32-year old patient presents with a history of gingival bleeding, lethargy, pallor, and recurrent infection. Petechiae are noted on exam over the buccal mucosa as well as over the ankles and perirectal area. Aspiration of bone marrow was difficult. The physician suspects a common cause of this patient's thrombocytopenia following microscopic examination of the bone marrow. The physician most likely saw which of the following?

   A. Normal granulocyte development, decreased number of megakaryocytes, normal erythroid development

   B. Normal granulocyte development, decreased number of megakaryocytes, decreased erythroid development

   C. Decreased granulocyte development, decreased number of megakaryocytes, decreased erythroid development

   D. Normal granulocyte development, increased megakaryocyte size, normal erythroid development

   E. Decreased granulocyte development, decreased number of megakaryocytes, normal erythroid development

2. The most common cause of acute DIC is?

   A. Gram-negative septicemia

   B. CMV infection

   C. Mucin-secreting adenocarcinoma

   D. Obstetric complications

   E. Severe hypothermia

3. A 12-year-old girl complains to her mother of new bruises over her shins and forearms. Upon examination by her pediatrician, petechiae in her oropharynx are noted in addition to the excessive bruising. Her labs indicate a normal hemoglobin and normal WBC count with a normal differential. However, her platelet count is $4000/\mu L$. Smear depicts larger than normal platelet size. She is otherwise normal with no systemic symptoms of renal failure, no pallor, abnormal connective tissue findings, or neurologic symptoms. The most likely diagnosis is?

   A. Hemolytic uremic syndrome

   B. Systemic lupus erythematosus

   C. Aplastic anemia

   D. Thrombotic thrombocytopenic purpura

   E. Idiopathic thrombocytopenic purpura

4. The pathogenesis of the patient presentation in question 3 is most likely due to?

   A. Circulating malignant cells

   B. Autoimmune production of antibodies to glycoprotein IIb/IIIa or Ib

   C. Depletion of platelet stem cells in the bone marrow

   D. A drug reaction

   E. Platelet sequestration within the liver

> **HPI:** PS is a 19-year-old woman coming in for a follow-up visit for an episode of deep venous thrombosis (DVT) 2 weeks ago. At that time she had presented with painful leg swelling, and following serial compression ultrasound the diagnosis was made. She is currently not taking oral contraceptives and does not smoke.
>
> **PE:** The patient is in good health currently and scans reveal no evidence of malignancy. Her prior medical history is unremarkable, except for three prior episodes of DVT over the past 7 years.
> Her physician is puzzled by the multiple episodes of DVT without an obvious risk factor in her history. The physician decides to work up the most likely hereditary causes of DVTs in the hope of isolating the etiology.

Thought Questions

- What is Virchow's triad and how does it explain the pathogenesis of DVT?

- What are the common acquired risk factors for DVT?

- What are the common hereditary risk factors for DVT?

- What course of treatment is recommended for a patient with recurrent DVT?

Basic Science Review and Discussion

As the balance between thrombosis and thrombolysis is disturbed, arterial and venous thrombi form. Arterial thrombi form under high shear conditions and are characterized as white, platelet-rich, fibrin-poor thrombi containing few to no RBCs. Venous thrombi form under low shear conditions and are characterized as red, platelet-poor, fibrin-rich clots containing RBCs. Abnormal blood flow, endothelial injury, and procoagulant and anticoagulant factors are the main determinants of thrombus formation. Virchow's triad summarizes the three factors predisposing a patient to thrombi as (1) stasis of blood flow, (2) hypercoagulability of blood, and (3) vessel wall damage. Vessel wall damage is significant in arterial thrombi, while the hypercoagulability of blood is the main component of venous clot formation. Stasis of blood flow applies equally to both.

Acquired risk factors for DVT affect stasis of blood flow and to a lesser degree, hypercoagulability. **DIC is the most common acquired hypercoagulable state encountered in the hospital setting.** Factors that lead to increased stasis include nephritic syndrome, dehydration, pelvic obstruction, pregnancy, varicose veins, hyperviscosity, polycythemia, prolonged immobility, stroke, and cardiac failure. For patients with considerable risk factors (obese, elderly, or previous family history) the incidence of postoperative venous thrombosis is markedly increased. Carcinoma of the breast, lung, prostate, pancreas, and bowel have also been linked to venous thrombosis. Blood disorders such as PV, essential thrombocythemia, paroxysmal nocturnal hemoglobinuria, and SCD are associated with increased viscosity or thrombo-cytosis and thus increased thrombi. An acquired risk factor applicable to the majority of women within the United States is estrogen therapy either as contraception or postmenopause. High-dose estrogen therapy is correlated with increased FII, FVII, FVIII, FIX, and FX production. In women on such medication, postoperative thrombi are a significant risk. Women who experience multiple miscarriages may be predisposed to thrombi due to a different risk factor, known as antiphospholipid antibody syndrome. This syndrome occurs in patients with **SLE. These patients develop an antibody (lupus anticoagulant) to a specific phospholipid, which paradoxically causes an increased PTT, while clinically leading to increased thromboembolic events and recurrent miscarriages.** Other autoimmune diseases are associated with a similar phenomenon; however, the antibodies are developed to cardiolipin and β_2-glycoprotein. Complications of antiphospholipid antibody syndrome include peripheral limb ischemia, myocardial infarction and stroke.

Inheritable Coagulopathies The acquired risk factors become highly significant in patients who are predisposed to coagulopathy due to an inherited condition. Hereditary disorders of thrombosis (factor V Leiden mutation, antithrombin III deficiency, protein C deficiency, protein S deficiency, prothrombin allele G20210A, hyperhomocystinemia, and abnormal fibrinogen) are geographically heterogeneous throughout the world, with increased incidence in North America and Europe.

Approximately **40% of patients with familial thrombophilia are resistant to activated protein C (aPC). Known as factor V Leiden, a point mutation changing amino acid 506 from arginine to glutamine is present in the FV gene that prevents cleavage by activated protein C.** Cleavage by protein C inactivates FV, which decreases the conversion of prothrombin to thrombin. Patients heterozygous at the factor V Leiden allele are five to 10 times more likely to develop thrombosis, and **homozygous patients are 50 to 100 times more likely.** Diagnosis of factor V Leiden is based on molecular testing of the gene itself. Following polymerase chain reaction (PCR) and amplification of a patient's sample of WBCs, restriction enzyme digests are used to determine if the patient is normal, heterozygous, or homozygous at the allele. **Three to five percent of Caucasians carry the mutant allele.**

An **autosomal-dominant deficiency of antithrombin III** contributes to venous thrombosis in a small percentage, 1% to 2%, of patients with hereditary thrombophilia. **Antithrombin III is responsible for inactivating factors II (thrombin), IXa, Xa, and XIa.** Diagnosis is based on a functional assay of antithrombin III levels. Heterozygotes with 30% to 60% of normal antithrombin III levels are symptomatic, typically with a first thrombosis in the second or third decade of life.

Four percent to ten percent of patients with hereditary thrombophilia have a deficiency in either protein C or protein S. Protein C deficiency is inherited in an autosomal-dominant pattern with variable penetrance. Homozygous infants develop DIC and/or infantile purpura fulminans. **Protein S is a necessary cofactor for protein C, allowing it to cleave factor V.** A deficiency in protein S presents similarly to protein C deficiency and follows an autosomal-dominant inheritance as well.

A mutation in **prothrombin allele G20210A causes approximately 20% of hereditary thrombophilia.** The mutation, present in 3% of the population, **doubles the risk of thrombosis by increasing the plasma level of prothrombin.** The elevated prothrombin concentration leads to increased active thrombin and down-regulation of the fibrinolytic system.

New research **shows hyperhomocystinemia either acquired or as hereditary homocystinuria (autosomal recessive) to be linked with vascular disease and increased risk for both arterial and venous thrombosis.** There is no current data to show if lowering the levels of homocystine in these patients is effective in lowering this risk. Acquired factors, which increase the risk of hyperhomocystinemia, include vitamin B_{12} or B_6 deficiencies, cyclosporin, smoking, renal damage, as well as increased age and male gender.

Treatment of Coagulopathies Treatment of acquired and hereditary states of episodic thrombosis involves **heparin therapy initially and in some cases lifelong warfarin (Coumadin) treatment.** Heparin catalyzes the rate of antithrombin III activity. This reduces the level of active clotting factors, specifically thrombin, IX, X, and XI. Heparin is administered in the acute setting by intravenous infusion, and low molecular weight heparin with a longer half-life is given by subcutaneous injection. Oral anticoagulants, such as warfarin, for chronic treatment are vitamin K antagonists. **Vitamin K is required for the activity of factors II, VII, IX, and X, due to its ability to γ-carboxylate the glutamic acid residues of these serine proteases.** Warfarin requires 5 days to be fully effective due to varying half-lives of the clotting factors. For this reason therapy should be overlapped for 5 days when moving a patient from heparin to warfarin.

Case Conclusion PCR and restriction enzyme digest of PS's factor V gene indicates a mutation at amino acid 506 (arginine to glutamine). Her physician informs her of the diagnosis of factor V Leiden and discusses long-term therapy options including warfarin.

Thumbnail: Hematology—Inhibition of Clotting Cascade

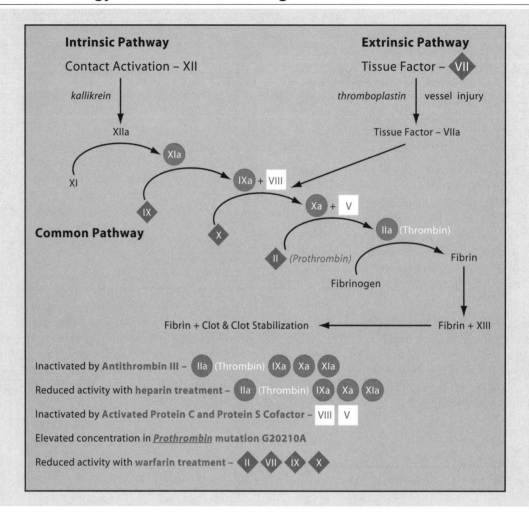

Key Points

▶ Arterial thrombi—high shear conditions—white, platelet rich, fibrin poor, few to no RBCs

▶ Venous thrombi—low shear conditions—red, platelet poor, fibrin rich clots containing RBCs

▶ Virchow's triad—stasis of blood flow, hypercoagulability of blood, and vessel wall damage

▶ Hereditary homocystinuria unlike the other common coagulopathies is inherited as an autosomal-recessive trait.

▶ Antiphospholipid antibody syndrome may present clinically as recurrent miscarriages due to placental thrombi.

Questions

1. The most common inherited cause of increased risk of venous thrombosis is?

   A. Factor V Leiden mutation

   B. Protein S deficiency

   C. Protein C deficiency

   D. Antithrombin deficiency

   E. Prothrombin allele G20210A

2. The clotting factor with a half-life of almost 5 days is?

   A. FII

   B. FV

   C. FVIII

   D. FIX

   E. FX

3. A 13-year-old boy accidentally ingests his grandfather's warfarin. His mother brings him to the ED 72 hours after ingestion. On physical exam the physician notes bruising of the child's trunk. Labs are ordered and indicate which of the following?

   A. Prolonged PT, prolonged PTT, decreased platelet count

   B. Prolonged PT, prolonged PTT, normal platelet count

   C. Prolonged PT, normal PTT, normal platelet count

   D. Normal PT, normal PTT, decreased platelet count

   E. Prolonged PT, normal PTT, decreased platelet count

4. A 31-year-old woman presents to the hospital clinic following three miscarriages with her most recent pregnancy terminating at 6 weeks. She has a history of DVT and has undergone chronic therapy for SLE. Her only abnormal laboratory finding is an elevated PTT. Her most likely diagnosis is which of the following?

   A. Antithrombin deficiency

   B. Prothrombin allele G20210A

   C. Factor V Leiden mutation

   D. Lupus anticoagulant

   E. Protein C deficiency

HPI: LS is a 50-year-old man admitted for elective surgery. A left internal jugular line was placed prior to surgery for administration of medications. Just prior to surgery, the patient complained of pain in his left arm, and swelling was noticed in his left arm and neck. His physician suspected thrombosis, and Doppler images noted clots within the left internal jugular and left subclavian veins. Surgery was postponed, and LS was treated with intravenous heparin. The clot was well controlled with heparin therapy in the initial 24 hours. Five days following the initial heparin treatment, LS complained of pain and swelling in his right thigh. Doppler noted a femoral clot.

PE: Multiple petechiae were observed on the ankles and mucosa.

Labs: Hgb 14.2 g/dL (nl 13.5–17.5 g/dL) WBC 5000/μL (nl 4–11,000/μL) Platelets 7500/μL (nl 150–400,000/μL)

LS's physician is concerned due to the recurrent thrombosis and consults with a fellow physician on what changes in this patient's treatment are needed.

Thought Questions

■ What are the indications for heparin therapy?

■ What are the complications of heparin therapy and alternative treatments?

■ What are the important drug interactions for patients on warfarin (Coumadin)?

■ What are the common fibrinolytic agents and their mechanisms of action?

■ What are the common antiplatelet medications?

Basic Science Review and Discussion

While much of modern medicine, surgery, and obstetrics have been devoted to decrease bleeding and combat bleeding disorders, there are a variety of agents used in medicine for their anticoagulant effects. In the setting of patients with pathologic embolic or thrombotic events such as DVT, pulmonary embolism (PE), MI, or stroke, these drugs can save lives. The most commonly used and clinically relevant of these medications are discussed below.

Heparin   Heparin has multiple indications due to its ability to effectively inhibit venous thrombi formation. In clinical cases of **PE, unstable angina pectoris,** and **DVT,** heparin is a primary treatment. It also is used prophylactically in cardiopulmonary bypass surgery and in pregnant women predisposed to DVT. Heparin's mechanism of action is its catalytic activity on antithrombin III. **Up-regulating antithrombin III leads to irreversibly deactivated thrombin, IIa, FIXa, FXa, and FXIa. PTT can be used to monitor heparin therapy.** The PTT typically is maintained between 1.5 and 2.5 times normal. In addition, heparin prolongs TT and slightly increases PT, while bleeding time is normal. Heparin is administered **intravenously.**

Three complications of heparin therapy are possible. First, heparin inhibits both the clotting cascade and secondary interaction with platelet function. In some cases excessive bleeding results and the heparin must be discontinued. **Protamine** is the recommended antagonist, which **inactivates heparin.** Second, following 2 months of therapy, heparin has been shown to complex to essential minerals within the bone structure, **inducing osteoporosis.** Third, **heparin-induced thrombocytopenia** (HIT) occurs in roughly 5% of patients on heparin therapy. Typically 5 days following the onset of treatment, patients paradoxically experience **thrombosis and a concomitant fall of greater than 60% in platelets.** If this occurs, heparin must be stopped and the patient switched to a direct thrombin inhibitor such as hirudin or lepirudin. HIT results from an IgG antibody that is produced to the heparin-platelet factor 4 complex. The complex is initially created when platelet factor 4 is released from within platelet granules. This complex forms on the surface membrane of platelets, and the **binding of IgG antibody induces platelet activation and aggregation.** Increased consumption leads to subsequent decreases in quantity.

Due to these complications of intravenous unfractionated heparin therapy, **low molecular weight (LMW) heparin** has been developed, which has a lower frequency of inducing HIT and rarely leads to osteoporosis. LMW heparin is similar in mechanism to traditional heparin since it binds to antithrombin III; however, it only **inhibits factors IXa, Xa, and XIa with no inhibition of thrombin.** Patients on LMW heparin are monitored by FXa activity rather than PTT. Other benefits of LMW heparin are its extended half-life (allowing once-a-day dosing) and subcutaneous rather than intravenous administration.

Warfarin   An advantage of warfarin (Coumadin) therapy over heparin is its oral dosing. Warfarin prevents coagulation by **blocking postribosomal γ-carboxylation of the glutamic acid within clotting factors II, VII, IX, and X.** Postribosomal γ-carboxylation is the function of vitamin K within the liver as the serine proteases are synthesized. Treatment with this or other vitamin K antagonists depletes the clotting factors and is effective therapy once each factor has dropped significantly below its half-life. For FVII this takes less than 24 hours. However, FX requires 3 to 5 days to drop to levels ensuring proper anticoagulant therapy. For this reason, when patients are transferred to warfarin from other anticoagulants, **therapy is overlapped for 5 days.** Warfarin therapy can be monitored by PT or **INR** (the international normalized ratio, which is the ratio of the patient's PT to a normal PT), with a target INR of 2.5.

There are toxicities associated with warfarin. It readily crosses the placenta and is a potent teratogen. Since the majority of warfarin circulates bound to albumin with the body, and its metabolism involves the P-450 reactions within the liver, drug interactions are numerous. Interactions that potentiate warfarin's anticoagulant activity include inhibitors of cytochrome P-450 (chloramphenicol, allopurinol, cimetidine, fluoroquinolones, and metronidazole), displacers of warfarin from albumin (sulfonamides, phenylbutazone, phenytoin, and aspirin), and medications that reduce the vitamin K uptake or production within the GI tract (neomycin). Inducers of cytochrome P-450 decrease warfarin's anticoagulant activity (barbiturates, rifampin, glutethimide). Overdose of warfarin is treated with removal of warfarin therapy, and start of intravenous **fresh frozen plasma** or factor concentrates with **vitamin K supplement.**

Fibrinolytics Treatment with fibrinolytic agents within 24 hours (ideally within 6 hours) has shown benefit following MI, cerebral strokes, PE, and arterial thrombosis. The originally isolated fibrinolytic agent, streptokinase, from streptococci combines with plasminogen, forming a protein complex. **This complex functions as a protease and cleaves free plasminogen into plasmin. Plasmin digests fibrin, fi-** brinogen, FV, and FVIII, producing fibrin split products and lysing the thrombus. Urokinase is also a protease, which works by the same mechanism. Activation of plasminogen to plasmin by urokinase and streptokinase is systemic and in cases of cerebral strokes with hemorrhage are not recommended. Tissue plasminogen activator (tPA) has a higher affinity for fibrin and creates fibrinolysis localized to the thrombus rather than systemically. Other fibrinolytic agents include single-chain urokinase type plasminogen activator (SCU-PA), and acylated plasminogen streptokinase activator complex (APSAC).

Antiplatelet Medications Acetylsalicylic acid (ASA), aspirin, is the most commonly used antiplatelet medication. It is currently recommended for patients with coronary artery disease and potentially those with thrombocytosis. **Aspirin inhibits synthesis of thromboxane A_2 by irreversibly inhibiting cyclooxygenase. Aspirin's ability to cause irreversible inhibition allows it to target platelet's enzymatic activity over endothelial cells, which use the same enzyme.** The activation of platelets is dependent on a decrease in cAMP concentration. Drugs such as dipyridamole prevent this drop by inhibiting phosphodiesterase. Treatment with dipyridamole creates resistant platelets with markedly decreased activation rates. Ticlopidine and clopidogrel prevent reduced cAMP by blocking ADP receptor-dependent signal transduction, which normally cues the reduction in cAMP and increases platelet binding to fibrinogen. Ticlopidine toxicities include neutropenia and thrombocytopenia. Abciximab, tirofiban, and eptifibatide are monoclonal antibodies that bind to and inhibit the GPIIb/IIIa receptor on the platelet membrane. While other medications may be used for extended treatment, abciximab can be used once only and has been prescribed to prevent complications for high-risk patients undergoing percutaneous transluminal coronary angioplasty.

Case Conclusion LS is diagnosed with HIT, which is causing the thrombi 5 days after the onset of heparin therapy. Due to cross-reactivity of the antibody inducing HIT, LS cannot be treated with LMW heparin. Instead, the heparin is discontinued and LS is treated with lepirudin, a thrombin inhibitor. His clotting is controlled, and he is discharged with a full recovery.

Thumbnail: Hematology—Anticoagulant Medications

Antithrombotic agents			Fibrinolytic agents	Antiplatelet agents
IV	Sub-Q	Oral	Streptokinase	Aspirin
Heparin	Low molecular	Coumadin	Urokinase	Dipyridamole
Hirudin	weight heparin	(warfarin)	Tissue plasminogen activator	Ticlopidine
Lepirudin			Acylated plasminogen- streptokinase	Clopidogrel
			Activator complex	Abciximab
			Single-chain urokinase plasminogen activator	Tirofiban
				Eptifibatide

Clotting cascade

↓

Clot formation—fibrin

Streptokinase, urokinase, tPA

+

Plasmin ← Plasminogen

+

Factor XIIa, kallikrein

+ ← Plasmin

↓

Fibrin split products
D-dimers

Key Points

▶ Heparin complications include thrombotic thrombocytopenia, which develops in up to 5% of patients 5 days following the initial heparin therapy.

▶ Heparin is the antithrombotic agent preferred for prophylactic or treatment in pregnant mothers.

▶ Warfarin's anticoagulant potency is affected by drugs that up-regulate or down-regulate cytochrome P-450, decrease vitamin K update or production, and displace warfarin from albumin.

▶ tPA in some clinical cases may be preferred over urokinase or streptokinase due to its greater affinity for fibrin and therefore greater localization to thrombi.

▶ Aspirin is the most commonly used antiplatelet agent. It effectively inhibits platelets as an irreversible inhibitor of cyclooxygenase. This prevents synthesis of thromboxane A_2, a vasoconstrictor and platelet activator.

Questions

1. A 46-year-old woman presents with left lower extremity swelling and pain. She exhibits Homans' sign, and a Doppler ultrasound shows a DVT in the popliteal fossa. She is begun on IV heparin therapy, but after several days develops thrombocytopenia. Which alternate treatment would be contraindicated?

   A. Aspirin
   B. Warfarin
   C. Hirudin
   D. Enoxaparin
   E. Argatroban

2. A 55-year-old man is on warfarin for chronic anticoagulation in the setting of atrial fibrillation. He presents to his primary care physician complaining of nosebleeds and bleeding gums, and has severely elevated indices. How should he be treated?

   A. Protamine
   B. Vitamin K and protamine
   C. Fresh frozen plasma and vitamin K
   D. Aminocaproic acid
   E. Flumazenil

3. A 62-year-old man presents to the ED with right-sided hemiparesis and slurred speech. His daughter reports that the symptoms began less than 1 hour ago. The attending physician suspects a stroke and orders imaging studies. These indicate a left hemisphere cerebral thrombus with potential secondary hemorrhage. Of the possible anticoagulants, the most recommended in this clinical situation is?

   A. Urokinase
   B. Streptokinase
   C. Hirudin
   D. Warfarin
   E. tPA

HPI: A 68-year-old man is admitted to the hospital for pneumonia. PMH: Significant for diabetes mellitus, cardiovascular disease, and severe aortic stenosis.

PE: The patient has significant scleral icterus (yellow sclera) and appreciable jaundice.

Labs: Hgb 10 g/dL HCT 30% MCV 85 fL Reticulocytes 6% (nl 0.5–1.5%). Total bilirubin 2.5 mg/dL (normal 0.2–1.0). A direct Coombs' test was done.

Thought Questions

- What are the signs and symptoms of a hemolytic anemia?

- What are schistocytes and in what type of anemia are they found?

- What underlying diseases are associated with autoimmune hemolytic anemias?

- Why does glucose-6-phosphate dehydrogenase (G6PD) deficiency lead to hemolysis?

Basic Science Review and Discussion

In general, hemolytic anemias are **normocytic** (normal MCV) and **hyperproductive** (increased reticulocytes). Symptoms and signs of hemolytic anemia include those of anemia (headache, fatigue, shortness of breath, heart palpitations) and those of hemolysis: **jaundice, scleral icterus** (yellow skin and eyes, respectively), and a high incidence of gallstones (all due to increased bilirubin). Laboratory findings of hemolysis include an **increased serum LDH** (released from RBC during hemolysis), **increased serum bilirubin** (a breakdown product of hemoglobin), and **decreased free plasma haptoglobin** (a hemoglobin-binding protein that gets quickly cleared when bound).

Microangiopathic Hemolytic Anemia   Microangiopathic **hemolytic anemia** (MAHA) is an acquired anemia in which erythrocytes undergo lysis in the circulation. This intravascular red cell fragmentation is caused by **mechanical damage** to the RBC membrane. The damage can be caused by either shear stress force such as when RBCs pass through damaged (e.g., in aortic stenosis) or faulty prosthetic cardiac valves. Damage can also occur when RBCs come into contact with abnormal vascular endothelial surfaces such as in patients with aortic aneurysms, TTP, malignant hypertension, vasculitis, and DIC. Patients present with typical signs of a hemolytic anemia and features of their underlying cardiac or vascular disease. The hallmark of MAHA is the presence of **schistocytes (**cells with two or more membrane projec-

tions or pointy ends) and RBC fragments on the peripheral blood smear caused by the direct damage of the RBC membrane. Treatment is targeted at correcting the underlying disease such as resection of the aortic aneurysm or replacement of a damaged cardiac valve. While the hemolysis continues, patients should be supported with iron and folate so that the bone marrow can continue to be hyperproductive. In extreme cases, red cell transfusions may be necessary.

Autoimmune Hemolytic Anemia   Autoimmune **hemolytic anemia** (AIHA) is an acquired anemia caused by the presence of circulating autoantibodies that bind to RBCs and cause their premature destruction. The complement system plays a role in the lysis of targeted RBCs. The majority of AIHA cases (80% to 90%) are mediated by **warm-reacting autoantibodies** (antibodies that bind to red cells at 37°C). **IgG** antibodies and/or complement bind to the red cell membrane and target it for macrophage phagocytosis. Part of the red cell membrane is internalized by the macrophage, and when the red cell is released it reseals and forms a sphere (due to lost surface area). These rigid **spherocytes** get trapped in the spleen and are prematurely removed by phagocytosis (extravascular hemolysis). A smaller portion of AIHA cases are mediated **cold-reacting autoantibodies** (antibodies that bind to red cells at less than 37°C). These antibodies are typically **IgM** and they activate and bind complement optimally at 20° to 25°C. They can also directly agglutinate red cells at temperatures at 0° to 5°C. The formation of spherocytes and extravascular hemolysis occur as described above.

AIHAs can occur in otherwise healthy individuals or in patients with underlying diseases. Warm-reacting antibodies are associated with lymphoproliferative malignancies (lymphoma, chronic lymphocytic leukemia), and rheumatic disorders (SLE). Cold-reacting antibodies can be associated with infectious mononucleosis and *Mycoplasma pneumoniae* infections. The clinical manifestation of AIHA can be rapid in onset or insidious, developing over months. The symptoms are that of anemia (headache, dizziness, shortness of breath) and jaundice. Individuals with cold-reacting antibodies experience cold-induced acrocyanosis (blue fingers, toes) because of cold-mediated vaso-occlusion at these peripheral sites where the body temperature is lower.

Common laboratory test findings are those for general hemolysis, and the presence of spherocytes on the blood smear. A more definitive test for AIHA is a **positive direct Coombs' test** in which the patient's red cells are reacted with specific reagents to determine the presence of immunoglobulin or complement bound to the red cells. In warm antibody autoimmune hemolysis, one would expect the presence of any of the following: (1) IgG alone, (2) IgG plus complement components (C3 and C4), or (3) C3 or C4 alone. In cold antibody disease the direct Coombs' test is positive only for the presence of C3 or C4 because IgM falls off during the washing procedures. The initial treatment for AIHA is systemic **steroids** (e.g., prednisone), although only two thirds of patients respond. Additional treatment includes **splenectomy.** Occasionally cytotoxic drugs or plasmapheresis is used. The most effective treatment for cold-reacting antibody disease is to keep the patient warm, which sometimes requires the patient's moving to locations with warm weather year round.

G6PD Deficiency   **G6PD** is an enzyme in the pentose phosphate pathway. G6PD deficiency is a **sex-linked** genetic disorder that causes episodic hemolysis in response to infection, to exposure to oxidant drugs (sulfas, quinine), or to eating fava beans. Infection, certain drugs, and fava beans cause the formation of free radicals that can oxidize glutathione and complex it with hemoglobin. This results in oxidized hemoglobin, which precipitates inside red cells as **Heinz bodies.** Normal cells protect themselves against oxidant damage by reducing glutathione with reduced nicotinamide adenine dinucleotide phosphate (NADPH). Individuals deficient in the enzyme G6PD are unable to regenerate NADPH. Red cells with Heinz bodies are identified as abnormal and undergo premature phagocytosis. Sometimes **bite cells** are seen on a peripheral blood smear. Eleven percent of African-American males have a mutant form of the enzyme, and enzyme activity is reduced to 5% to 15% of normal. A Mediterranean variant causes a more severe disease as individuals have less than 1% normal enzyme activity. Individuals with G6PD deficiency are instructed to avoid drugs known to precipitate hemolysis (the list is very long), and they are supported with transfusions through episodes of hemolysis.

Case Conclusion   The patient's direct Coombs' test came back negative. Review of the peripheral blood smear showed schistocytes and RBC fragments. The patient's findings are consistent with microangiopathic hemolytic anemia. (If the direct Coombs' test was positive and blood smear showed spherocytes, one might suspect an autoimmune hemolytic anemia.) Severe aortic stenosis can cause shear stress on RBC membranes while they pass over the calcified valve. Treatment for the anemia is surgical replacement of the diseased valve. In the meantime, the patient was started on folate and iron supplements to maintain his active reticulocytosis. There was not an indication for transfusion at this time, but the patient will be monitored regularly.

Thumbnail: Comparison of Select Hemolytic Anemias

	Microangiopathic hemolytic anemia	Autoimmune hemolytic anemia		G6PD deficiency
		Warm-reacting	Cold-reacting	
Etiology	Mechanical damage → RBC fragmentation • Aortic stenosis • Aortic aneurysm • Prosthetic cardiac valves • TTP • Malignant HTN • DIC Vasculitis	IgG +/− Complement binds RBC → partial phagocytosis → RBC reseals → spherocyte → trapped/lysed in spleen • Idiopathic • Lymphoproliferative disease • Rheumatic disease	IgM autoantibody agglutinates RBCs (at low temp) and binds complement → phagocytosis → spherocyte → lysed in spleen • Idiopathic • Lymphoproliferative disease • Mononucleosis infection Mycoplasma infection	Free oxygen radicals → oxidizes Hb → Hb precipitates (Heinz body) → phagocytosis/lysis of RBCs • Oxidant drugs • Infection Fava beans
Clinical picture	Underlying cardiac or valvular disease	Previously healthy or underlying disease	Acrocyanosis	• Sex linked genetics • ↑ in African Americans Episodic hemolysis
Laboratory	• Schistocytes C • RBC fragments	• Spherocytes ● • (+) Direct Coombs' • IgG +/− C3/C4 or C alone	• Spherocytes ● • (+) Direct Coombs' • C3, C4 only	• Bite cells ➷ • ↓ G-6-PD enzyme activity
Treatment	• Treat primary disease • Folate/iron supplement	• Steroids • Splenectomy • Cytotoxic drugs Plasmapheresis	• Warmth • Steroids • Splenectomy	• Avoid precipitating drugs • Red cell transfusion during severe episodes

Key Points

▶ Hemolytic anemias are normocytic and hyperproductive.

▶ Specific signs of hemolysis include jaundice and scleral icterus.

▶ Laboratory findings include an increased serum LDH, increased serum bilirubin, and decreased free plasma haptoglobin.

Questions

1. An African American college student is planning a trip to South America. A week prior to departure he begins a course of antimalarial pills (Mefloquine) that you have given him while working at the university travel clinic. Several days later he begins feeling ill and comes back to see you. His labs are as follows: Hgb 10 g/dL, HCT 30%, MCV 87 fL, and reticulocytes are 8%. The peripheral smear shows bite cells. His blood is direct Coombs' negative. What is the pathophysiology of his illness?

   A. IgG autoantibodies bind RBCs and cause partial phagocytosis by macrophages.

   B. IgM-drug complexes bind RBCs and cause complement-mediated lysis.

   C. Mechanical vascular damage causes RBC fragmentation.

   D. Cold-mediated vaso-occlusion of peripheral veins.

   E. Oxidized Hb precipitates in the RBC and causes phagocytosis by macrophages.

2. A 33-year-old woman presents to the ED with a fever and appears confused. She is alert and oriented only to person. Her exam is unremarkable except for some moderate scleral icterus. Laboratory results: Hgb 9 g/dL, HCT 27%, MCV 88 fL, reticulocytes 5%, platelets 50,000, total bilirubin 2.2 mg/dL, and creatinine 2.4 mg/dL. What do you expect to see on the peripheral blood smear?

   A. Bite cells

   B. Schistocytes

   C. Target cells

   D. Spherocytes

   E. Hypersegmented PMNs

Case 18

1. C
2. D

Case 19

1. D
2. C

Case 20

1. D
2. A

Case 21

1. C
2. D

Case 22

1. D
2. C

Case 23

1. F
2. A

Case 24

1. C
2. A

Case 25

1. B
2. E
3. A
4. E

Case 26

1. C
2. B
3. E
4. B

Case 27

1. C
2. B

Case 28

1. D
2. C

Case 29

1. C
2. D
3. E
4. B

Case 30

1. A
2. A
3. B
4. D

Case 31

1. D
2. C
3. E

Case 32

1. E
2. B

Part III

Oncology

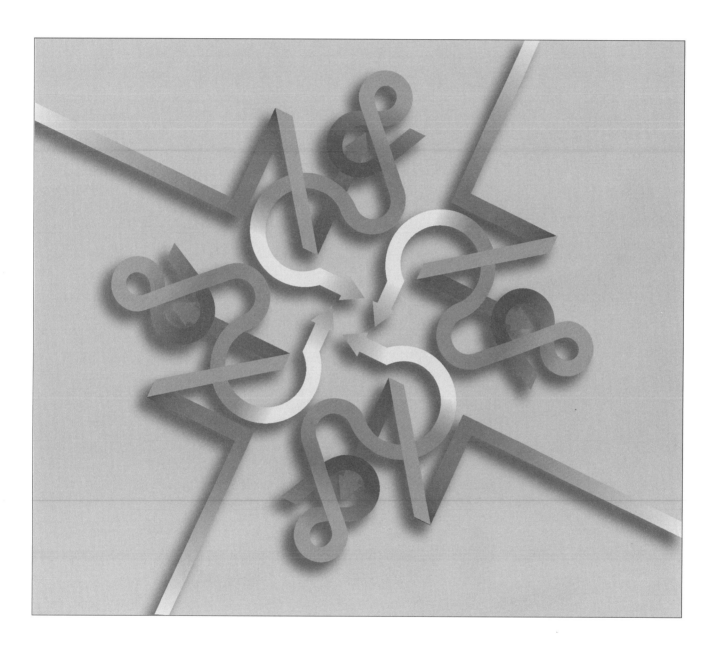

HPI: TL, a 59-year-old woman, presents with 5 days of **fever and night sweats.** She also noted a 20-pound **unexplained weight loss** in the last 3 months from her previous weight of 150 pounds. She has also had an intermittent cough with mild wheezing when lying on her right side. She has had no sick contacts nor symptoms suggesting infection. She had a negative purified protein derivative (PPD) 1 year ago and has no risk factors for tuberculosis exposure. PMH: Hashimoto's thyroiditis during her 20s; now hypothyroid taking L-thyroxine. No history of smoking or drinking.

PE: T 38.6°C BP 135/75 HR 85 RR 20 SaO$_2$ 98%
The patient is thin and ill-appearing. Her exam is significant for **positional wheezing** audible anteriorly on the right middle chest when lying on the right side and **nontender lymphadenopathy** consisting of two 2.5-cm rubbery nodules in the left axillary and right inguinal regions.

Labs/Studies: CBC and other routine labs are normal.
Chest x-ray reveals a 3-cm **mediastinal mass** protruding into the right pleural cavity.

Thought Questions

- What are the neoplasms of lymphoid origin and how do they arise?

- What are the histologic subtypes of these neoplasms and what are their characteristics?

- What are the clinical manifestations of lymphoid neoplasms?

- How are lymphoid neoplasms diagnosed, staged, graded, and treated?

Basic Science Discussion and Review

Lymphomas are solid tumors of lymphoid origin that arise from the malignant transformation of a lymphoid cell leading to its clonal proliferation. They are related to leukemias and are different only in that they do not arise in the bone marrow and are not characterized first by their presence in circulation. Figures 33-1 and 33-2 are diagrams of B-cell and T-cell differentiation and the leukemias and lymphomas associated with different stages of maturation.

Hodgkin's disease (HD) is a lymphoma characterized by the presence of **Reed-Sternberg cells** (or "owl's eye cells"), which are the true neoplastic components of the tumor. These cells are thought to secrete cytokines and thereby recruit reactive infiltrates, which make up the bulk of the tumor. All other lymphomas are categorized as **non-Hodgkin's lymphomas** (Table 33-1).

HD presents as singular nontender lymphadenopathy along the **central axis** of the body with *contiguous spread* to other nodal groups. In contrast, non-Hodgkin's lymphomas present at *multiple sites* in *peripheral nodal groups* with *noncontiguous spread*. Both diseases may present with **"B-symptoms,"** namely fever, night sweats, and weight loss, associated with cytokine release of lymphocytes.

Diagnosis of lymphoma is established by examination of a tissue biopsy. For non-Hodgkin's lymphoma, prognosis

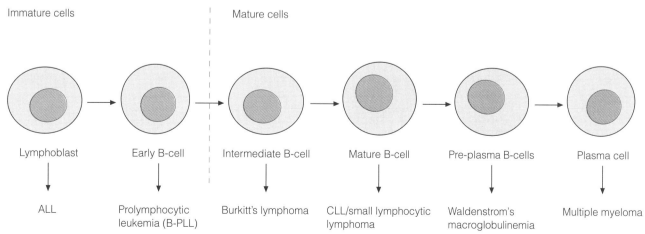

Figure 33-1 B-cell differentiation and malignant transformation into lymphomas and leukemias.

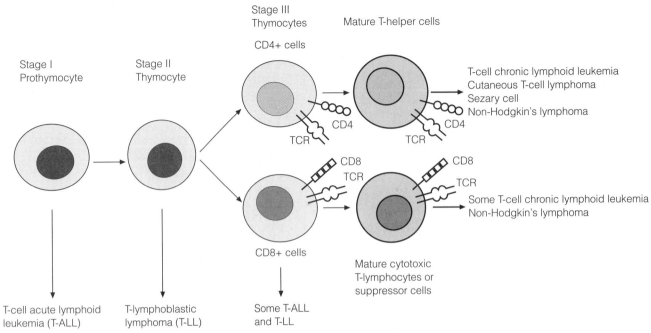

Figure 33-2 T-cell differentiation and malignant transformation into lymphomas and leukemias.

Table 33-1 Common non-Hodgkin's lymphoma subtypes

Common adult subtypes	
Follicular lymphoma*	**Germinal center B-cell lymphoma** (*mature and follicular*) *Most common form of NHL*, Age > 40 years; indolent course **t(14,18)** linking proto-oncogene, *bcl-2*, to Ig-heavy chain locus → *bcl-2* prevents apoptosis of lymphocyte
Small lymphocytic lymphoma	**Solid tumor counterpart to chronic lymphoid leukemia**, *mature B-cells in diffuse pattern* are slow-growing and migratory; indolent course; age 50–60 years Asymptomatic LAD, bone marrow/organ involvement; evolves into CLL
Diffuse large B-cell lymphoma*	**Aggressive tumor**, usually *intermediate- or high-grade cells, diffuse pattern* 20% of NHL; mean age = 60 years old; associated with immunodeficiency Presents with localized solid tumor then later dissemination; rapidly fatal
Mycosis fungoides	**Cutaneous T-cell lymphoma infiltrating dermal/epidermal junction** Mid-50s; common in males, blacks; indolent progressive course; incurable
Sézary syndrome	**Cutaneous T-cell lymphoma infiltrating skin and peripheral circulation** Sézary cells have "cerebriform" nuclei; median survival 8–9 years
Adult T-cell leukemia/lymphoma	**T-cell neoplasm of HTLV-1 infected patients** → skin lesions, LAD, HSM, lymphocytosis, hypercalcemia, CD4+ "flower cells" in blood; rapidly progressive, fatal within 1 year
Common childhood/adolescent subtypes	
Lymphoblastic lymphoma	**Solid tumor counterpart to** *immature* **B-cell acute lymphoblastic leukemia** Leukocytosis LAD, HSM, bone marrow failure, CNS/skin infiltration
Burkitt's lymphoma*	**Peripheral B-cell lymphoma/leukemia** of *mature* B-lymphocytes, *diffuse* pattern, *high grade* → most rapidly proliferating of any cancer Endemic in Africa and South America, associated with HIV EBV infection is thought to mediate malignant transformation Peripheral LAD, intra-abdominal mass, CNS infiltration **"Starry sky"**-appearance of lymphoid tissue

*Most tested lymphomas on USMLE Step 1.
LAD, lymphadenopathy; HSM, hepatosplenomegaly.

Table 33-2 Rye classification system for Hodgkin's disease (HD) histologic subtypes

Subtypes	Epidemiology	Pathology	Prognosis
Lymphocyte predominant	Least common	Mostly lymphocytes, L+H cells, rare RS cells	Best
Nodular sclerosing	Most common esp. in women	Nodular fibrosis with lymphocytes, lacunar cells, eosinophils, histiocytes, RS cells	Intermediate
Mixed cellularity	Older and HIV+ patients	No nodular fibrosis, irregular scarring, necrosis, many RS cells	Intermediate
Lymphocyte depleted	Rare; common in HIV+ patients	Few lymphocytes, RS cells, more atypical cells	Worst

RS, Reed-Sternberg; L+H, lymphohistiocytic ("popcorn cells").

depends on *grade* (degree of differentiation). Cells are either *mature* or *immature, B-cell* or *T-cell* in origin. Growth patterns either adhere to the normal *follicular* structure or grow in *diffuse* sheets. In general, the more mature the malignant cells are, the less aggressive and slower growing the neoplasm, and vice versa. Paradoxically, more mature cells of low-grade lymphomas disseminate earlier and wider as normal lymphocytes do, while less mature, high-grade lymphomas disseminate later, often presenting as a localized mass. Untreated, low-grade lymphomas can develop into high-grade lymphomas.

HD is classified by histologic subtype (Table 33-2). Prognosis for HD is most dependent on *stage* (size and nodal involvement) and is poorer among those with "B-symptoms" (Table 33-3). Generally, localized disease is treated with **radiation therapy.** More disseminated disease is treated with **chemotherapy.** Hodgkin's disease has among the most successful rates of cure.

Multiple myeloma and **Waldenström's macroglobulinemia** are both neoplasms of *immunoglobulin-secreting B-lymphocytes* (Table 33-4). They occur among older adults (mean age 60 years) and present with anemia and serum hyperviscosity (blurry vision, priapism, headaches, altered mental status, peripheral blood smear showing **Rouleaux formation** of red blood cells) due to massive overproduction of immunoglobulin proteins. These diseases can be distinguished by identifying monoclonal IgG or IgM via serum protein electrophoresis (**SPEP**), as well as **Bence-Jones proteins** consisting of κ and λ light chains via urine protein electrophoresis (**UPEP**), the radiographic presence or absence of lytic bone lesions, or via bone marrow examination. They are both incurable and have a mean survival of 3 to 4 years.

Table 33-3 Ann Arbor staging system for Hodgkin's disease

Stage 1	*Single* lymph node region or single extralymphatic organ involvement
Stage 2	Involvement of two or more lymphoid tissues on the *same side of the diaphragm*
Stage 3	Involvement of lymph node regions on *both sides of the diaphragm*
Stage 4	*Disseminated involvement* of organs, tissues, bone marrow, lymph nodes
Category A: Patients are **A**symptomatic	
Category B: "B-symptoms"—fever, night sweats, and weight loss > 10% original body weight	

Table 33-4 Plasma cell disorders/monoclonal gammopathies

	Multiple myeloma	Waldenström's macroglobulinemia
Pathophysiology	Monoclonal IgG- and κ or λ light chain-secreting B-lymphocyte neoplasm—bone marrow infiltration	IgM-secreting plasma cell neoplasm—variant of diffuse small lymphocytic lymphoma—no bony infiltration
Clinical presentation	Anemia, hyperviscosity syndrome, **bone pain**, bone fractures, recurrent infection, renal failure, proteinuria	Anemia, hyperviscosity syndrome, **no bone pain**, HSM, LAD, peripheral neuropathy, proteinuria
Diagnosis	SPEP, UPEP, blood smear, x-ray	SPEP, UPEP, blood smear, x-ray
SPEP	Monoclonal **IgG** spike	Monoclonal **IgM** spike
X-ray	**Lytic bone lesions diffusely**	**No lytic bone lesions**

Case Conclusion   Biopsies of the left axillary and right inguinal nodes reveal follicular lymphoma. Given that the patient presented with fever, night sweats, and weight loss, she was thought to have more advanced disease, and combination chemotherapy was initiated with chlorambucil, vincristine, and prednisone. She achieved complete remission, but relapsed 2 years later presenting with repeated B-symptoms and lymphadenopathy. She was found to have histologic transformation of follicular lymphoma to diffuse large B-cell lymphoma. She is now undergoing aggressive chemotherapy for her relapse.

Thumbnail: Non-Hodgkin's Lymphoma vs. Hodgkin's Lymphoma

	Non-Hodgkin's lymphoma	Hodgkin's disease
Epidemiology	**75%** of all lymphomas Mean age of onset = 42 years Risk factors: ionizing radiation exposure, viral infection (EBV, HTLV-1), autoimmune disease, immunosuppression	**25%** of all lymphomas **Bimodal distribution:** 20s and > 50s Men > Women Increased in HIV+ with more aggressive disease
Pathophysiology	Varied translocations affect cellular proliferation of lymphoid cells	Malignant Reed-Sternberg cells recruit inflammatory cells
Clinical presentation	Nontender enlargement of **multiple nodes** in **peripheral nodal groups** with **noncontiguous spread** to other nodes; extranodal lymphoid tissue involvement; generalized pruritus; B-symptoms	Nontender enlargement of a **single node or nodal group** with **contiguous spread** to adjacent nodes along the **central axis;** mediastinal or abdominal lymphadenopathy (LAD); generalized pruritus; B-symptoms; clinical anergy
Diagnosis	Lymph node/tissue biopsy; histologic examination	**Reed-Sternberg cells** on lymph node biopsy
Staging/grading	Prognosis **depends on** *grade:* follicular vs. diffuse; small vs. large B-cell vs. T-cell vs. mixed	Prognosis **depends on** *stage* (spread and pattern of nodal involvement): Ann Arbor stage 1–4, category A/B
Common histologic subtypes	Follicular lymphoma Diffuse large B-cell lymphoma Burkitt's lymphoma	Lymphocyte predominant Nodular sclerosing Mixed cellularity Lymphocyte-depleted
Therapy	Radiation therapy, chemotherapy, immunotherapy, autologous, allogeneic stem cell transplantation	Radiation therapy for stages I and II Combination chemotherapy for stages III and IV

Key Points

▶ Lymphomas are solid tumors of lymphoid origin; HD is defined by the presence of Reed-Sternberg cells, while all other lymphomas are designated as non-Hodgkin's lymphomas.

▶ HD manifests with central axis lymphadenopathy with contiguous spread to other lymph nodes, while non-Hodgkin's lymphoma manifests as a peripheral lymphadenopathy with noncontiguous spread.

▶ Plasma cell neoplasms hypersecrete monoclonal IgM, IgG, or immunoglobulin light chains (κ or λ) and produce disease related to serum hyperviscosity.

Questions

1. A 62-year-old man presents with anemia, bone pain, and blurry vision. Which lymphoma does he most likely have, what would be the most useful diagnostic test or procedure one would order, and what would be the characteristic finding?

   A. Waldenström's macroglobulinemia, serum protein electrophoresis, IgM spike
   B. Multiple myeloma, serum protein electrophoresis, IgG spike
   C. Follicular lymphoma, lymph node biopsy, small-cleaved cells in follicular pattern
   D. HD, lymph node biopsy, lymphocyte-predominant morphology
   E. Burkitt's lymphoma, lymph node biopsy, mature B-lymphocytes in diffuse pattern

2. A 40-year-old woman presents with isolated cervical lymphadenopathy with no fever, night sweats, or weight loss. A lymph node biopsy is performed and histopathology reveals small lymphocytes and rare Reed-Sternberg cells. Staging is done with MRI and she is found to have disease limited to one cervical nodal group. How would one classify her disease and what would be her prognosis?

   A. Follicular lymphoma with a prognosis of 5 to 10 years without treatment and 50% to 75% response to chemotherapy and radiation with complete remission
   B. HD stage IA with 85% to 95% 5-year survival and high potential for cure
   C. HD stage IIA with 85% to 95% 5-year survival and high potential for cure
   D. HD stage IB with poorer prognosis than stage IA
   E. Diffuse large B-cell lymphoma, which is rapidly fatal without treatment but highly responsive to chemotherapy

3. A 55-year-old HIV+ man with a CD4 count of 180 and viral load of 25,000 on highly active retroviral therapy presents with 4 days of fever and night sweats and 4 weeks of nonproductive cough. He has a history of a positive PPD with negative chest x-ray. On exam, he has multiple enlarged cervical, axillary, and inguinal lymph nodes, which he had noted to be slowly growing over the last several months. Subsequent chest and abdominal x-rays reveal a mediastinal mass and a single pulmonary nodule and abdominal mass. A repeat PPD is done and is found to be negative. Which of the following is the least likely explanation for his presentation?

   A. HD with anergy due to T-cell dysfunction associated with the lymphoma.
   B. Diffuse large B-cell lymphoma with mediastinal involvement causing nonproductive cough.
   C. Multiple myeloma causing T-cell dysfunction and recrudescence of tuberculosis.
   D. Burkitt's lymphoma with several rapidly growing lymph nodes and anergy caused by advanced AIDS.
   E. All answers above can explain his presentation.

HPI: A 63-year-old man comes to your primary care clinic for a refill of his allergy medication. You notice a **lesion on his nose** and question him about it. He recalls the lesion has been present for about 5 years and seems to be **gradually enlarging.** It is intermittently **itchy** and occasionally **bleeds** and scabs if he scratches vigorously. The patient adds that he worked as a **lifeguard** for 15 years and has always enjoyed swimming at the beach. With the exception of mild seasonal allergies, he is otherwise in good health.

PE: The patient is a **light-skinned** man. He has a 3 × 4 cm erythematous papule on the left side of his nose. It has a **pearly, translucent appearance** with visible telangiectatic vessels. The center is **ulcerated** and covered with a crust. He has no other lesions on his skin. The remainder of his exam is within normal limits.

Thought Questions

- What is the differential diagnosis of this lesion?
- What are major risk factors for malignancy?
- How do basal cell carcinoma and squamous cell carcinoma differ?
- What type of treatment do you recommend? Does this patient need to be seen in follow-up?

Basic Science Review and Discussion: Premalignant and Malignant Epidermal Tumors

Nonmelanoma Skin Cancers Nonmelanoma skin cancers are divided into two categories: basal cell carcinoma and cutaneous squamous cell carcinoma. Despite the fact that there are over a million cases of nonmelanoma skin cancers diagnosed each year, only 2000 patients die from the disease annually. This low mortality rate is primarily due to the low rate of metastasis in either of these malignancies. However, it is important that physicians be able to recognize and treat these epithelial malignancies because they may progress to metastasis if neglected over the years.

Basal Cell Carcinoma Basal cell carcinoma (BCC) is the **most common type of skin cancer.** In the United States alone, there are between 750,000 and 950,000 cases diagnosed annually; 85% of cases involve head and neck structures, especially the nose. The risk of developing BCC is directly proportional to cumulative ultraviolet (UV) exposure and inversely proportional to degree of skin pigmentation. Other risk factors include sites of chronic inflammation or injury, such as with scars or burns.

Technically, the name basal cell carcinoma is a misnomer, as the cells more closely resemble follicular cells than basal layer cells. Nevertheless, BCC cells do appear histologically "basaloid," with palisading nuclei. Basal cell carcinoma **grows slowly,** approximately 1 to 2 cm per year. Thus, the morbidity of BCC is largely due to local damage caused by relentless growth with invasion of adjacent structures. Nonetheless, there is almost no risk of metastasis. The extremely rare event of metastasis has occurred only in large, long-standing lesions that have been neglected for decades.

The classic presentation of BCC is as a **pink pearly white papule** with prominent telangiectatic vessels. However, the morphology of individual cases is diverse enough that BCC is often confused with actinic keratosis, squamous cell carcinoma, melanoma, chronic inflammation, or psoriasis. Definitive diagnosis is made by biopsy. Primary treatment is by Mohs surgical excision, a technique that involves removal of the lesion followed by immediate inspection of frozen pathology sections and reexcision if positive margins are found. Reconstructive surgery is often required after removal of large lesions. Close follow-up is also necessary because BCC has a high rate of recurrence, and the larger the tumor, the more likely it is to recur. Lesions greater than 2 cm have a recurrence rate of 25% even after full surgical treatment of the primary lesion.

Actinic Keratoses Actinic keratoses are dysplastic **precursors of squamous cell carcinoma.** Also known as solar keratoses, these lesions are extremely common; as many as 50% of fair-skinned adults develop actinic keratosis. This dysplasia is caused by prolonged exposure to the sunlight with a resultant buildup of keratin. Some lesions produce so much keratin that a "**cutaneous horn**" develops. While most lesions may regress or remain stable over a lifetime, the risk of malignant transformation is sufficient to warrant the removal of these potential precursor lesions. Removal can be accomplished in the same manner as for a common wart: by gentle curettage or by freezing.

Cutaneous Squamous Cell Carcinoma Cutaneous squamous cell carcinoma (SCC) is the second most common type of skin cancer and occurs primarily in the elderly. The underlying cause of SCC is DNA mutagenicity. Accordingly, factors that predispose or cause epithelial damage have been found to be risk factors. These include fair skin, **excessive sunlight UV rays,** industrial carcinogens, chronic ulcers, old burn scars, and ionizing radiation. Early-onset SCC is observed in xeroderma pigmentosum, which arises from a defect in DNA repair mechanisms of the skin. In addition, immunosuppressed individuals (such as organ transplant recipients) are also at increased risk for developing SCC.

Clinically, preinvasive carcinoma in situ (also known as **Bowen's disease**) appears as sharply defined, red scaling plaques. More advanced invasive lesions are nodular with evidence of hyperkeratosis and ulceration. Note that SCC

can occur anywhere on the skin, including even the lip, mouth, and genitalia. On microscopic inspection, there is full-thickness atypia of the epidermis, with sheets of squamous epithelium and central foci of keratinization ("**keratin pearls**").

SCCs are usually recognized early while they are still easily treatable with Mohs excision. The incidence of metastasis is greater than that for BCC, but is still low. Indeed, the risk of metastasis is lower if the malignancy occurs de novo than if the cancer arises from a precursor lesion. However if metastasis does occur, mortality is high (5-year survival of 35%).

Case Conclusion   Punch biopsy demonstrated irregular clusters of darkly staining basaloid cells with peripheral palisading nuclei. A diagnosis of infiltrative BCC was made. The patient successfully underwent **Mohs surgical excision** of the lesion, followed by reconstructive surgery. He was scheduled for regular follow-up visits every 6 months. Three years later, a recurrent lesion was noticed at the site of the initial lesion. The patient underwent repeat excision of the entire lesion. Postoperative radiation therapy was delivered to the surgical site. The patient has been disease-free since then.

Thumbnail: Basal Cell Carcinoma and Squamous Cell Cancer

Name	Epidemiology	Appearance	Risk factors	Prognosis
Basal cell carcinoma	Most common skin tumor	Morphology: pearly, translucent nodule with telangiectasias Histology: "basaloid" cells with palisading nuclei	UV light, fair skin, age, chronic skin inflammation	High recurrence rate, almost never metastasizes
Squamous cell carcinoma	2nd most common skin malignancy	Morphology: red, scaly plaque Histology: sheets of epithelial cells, "keratin pearls"	UV light, fair skin, age, actinic keratosis, Bowen's disease, chronic skin inflammation, xeroderma pigmentosum	Rarely metastasizes

---

Key Points

▶ BCC is the most common skin cancer; SCC is the 2nd most common skin cancer.

▶ Both BCC and SCC have low overall mortality rates.

▶ Definitive diagnosis of skin cancer is by biopsy and treatment is by surgical excision.

Questions

1. Both SCC and BCC share many of the same risk factors. Which of the following is a major risk factor for SCC but not for BCC?

   A. Excessive sunlight exposure
   B. Actinic keratosis
   C. Chronic decubitus ulcer
   D. Tanning salons
   E. Dysplastic nevus

2. JR is a 38-year-old recipient of a kidney transplant. She has been on immunosuppressive medication for 6 years to ensure that her body does not reject the transplant. She now comes to you with a suspicious skin lesion on her left forearm and you are concerned about malignancy. What histologic feature on her biopsy would confirm your suspicions of SCC?

   A. Palisading nuclei
   B. Acanthosis
   C. Keratin pearls
   D. Basaloid cells
   E. Follicular cells

3. It is important to know where to look for skin malignancies in order to diagnose them. Among the following sites, where is BCC most likely to be located?

   A. Ears
   B. Hands and feet
   C. Chest
   D. Genitalia
   E. Shoulders

HPI: DB is a 28-year-old Caucasian man who presents to your office for removal of a "mole" on his right shoulder. He does not remember whether the lesion was present at birth, but he believes he has had it since early childhood. In the past few months, he reports that it has become itchy, and he has noticed that it has grown in size. He also notes that the lesion has changed in color from light brown to **dark purple.** Upon further questioning, he states that he enjoys the outdoors, but does get **sunburned** frequently. Otherwise, the patient reports no health problems and is taking no medications.

PE: DB has blue eyes, red hair, and a **fair complexion.** There is a 1.7 × 2.1 cm variably pigmented plaque on the back of his right shoulder. It has an **ill-defined border** and contains small irregular nodules that have a darker color and a "pebble-like" indurated surface. The lesion does not demonstrate bleeding or ulceration. No other cutaneous lesions are found on exam. There is no evidence of cervical or axillary lymphadenopathy.

Thought Questions

- What is the differential diagnosis of this lesion?
- Which risk factors does this patient have?
- What are the key characteristics of this disease?
- What is the overall prognosis?

Basic Science Review and Discussion: Melanocytic Disorders

Benign Lesions vs. Malignant Melanoma   A **benign pigmented mole** is a small (less than 5 mm), well-circumscribed lesion with a well-defined border. It almost always has a single shade of pigment from beige to dark brown. An individual may have multiple moles, but they are generally similar to each other with respect to size, shape, and color. Benign moles are most often found on sun-exposed areas of skin such as the face, arms, and legs.

A **melanocytic dysplastic nevus** is a precursor lesion for malignant melanoma. Dysplastic nevi tend to be larger than benign common moles, and often have irregular contours and variegated coloring. In addition, dysplastic nevi may appear in non-sun-exposed areas as well as on sun-exposed body surfaces. Risk of transformation to melanoma increases with increased size of a nevus or increased number of dysplastic nevi on an individual.

Despite the benign-sounding name, all **melanomas** are by definition malignant invasive cancers. They are **aggressive tumors** that arise from melanocytic cells, which are normally located in the basal layers of the epidermis. There are four subtypes of melanoma: superficial spreading, nodular, acral lentiginous, and lentigo maligna. All four types exhibit the same general characteristics on physical exam, although they exhibit different rates of growth and carry different prognoses. Melanomas vary in shape from macules to nodules. These lesions exhibit wide pigmentation variabil-ity, covering the spectrum from black, brown, red, blue, purple, gray, and white. Melanomas have **asymmetric** and **ill-defined borders,** and are often larger than 6 mm. These findings can occur de novo or can be superimposed on a dysplastic nevus.

The most suspicious characteristic of a lesion is a **history of change** in color, shape, or size. Clinically, patients do not complain of the general constitutional symptoms that are associated with most cancers. Indeed, melanomas are usually asymptomatic, although they may exhibit itching or mild localized pain in the early stages. As the disease progresses, invasion through the dermis may cause ulceration or bleeding. Diagnosis is confirmed by histologic examination of a biopsy specimen. Definitive treatment involves surgical excision of the lesion, with chemoimmunotherapy reserved only for metastatic cases. Melanoma is curable before metastasis, but generally fatal after metastasis occurs.

Epidemiology of Melanoma   Melanoma is currently the seventh most common cancer in the United States, with the prediction that approximately 1 in 75 individuals will develop melanoma during their lifetimes. It affects adults in all age groups equally. The incidence of melanoma is increasing faster than any other cancer, with a trend toward a younger age incidence each year. The cause of this rising incidence is unknown. Melanoma is the leading cause of death from skin disease. However, increased awareness has led to earlier recognition at more curable stages, such that overall survival is now up to 90%.

Risk Factors for Melanoma   Multiple factors have been identified in association with the development of melanoma. **Excessive exposure to sunlight** is the most important environmental factor in the pathogenesis of melanoma. Light-haired, **fair-skinned** individuals, especially those with a tendency to burn rather than tan, also have a higher rate of melanoma. In addition, studies have linked blistering sunburns in childhood to increased rates of melanoma.

Dysplastic nevi are considered precursor lesions and confer an increased risk of melanoma. In addition, patients with many benign nevi or large congenital nevi are also at increased risk for the development of melanoma. Indeed, there are inheritable tendencies to develop hundreds of nevi (known as either the dysplastic nevus syndrome or the familial multiple mole and melanoma syndrome), which account for approximately 10% of all melanoma cases.

Melanoma Growth Patterns   It is important to note that melanomas exhibit two different patterns of growth: radial and vertical (Figure 35-1). **Radial growth** occurs in the initial phase, and consists of predominantly lateral growth within the epidermis. Because the cancerous cells do not leave the skin layer, melanoma in this stage demonstrates very little ability to metastasize. However, in later stages, **vertical growth** through the dermis predominates. This allows spread to lymphatics and blood vessels, and eventual formation of metastases. In contrast to patients with localized melanoma, patients with metastatic melanoma have a poor prognosis (median survival of 8 months). Due to the unique growth patterns of melanoma, tumor thickness (rough indicator of volume and depth of invasion) is the single most important prognostic factor for patients. Follow-up for life is important in the care of melanoma patients, as recur-

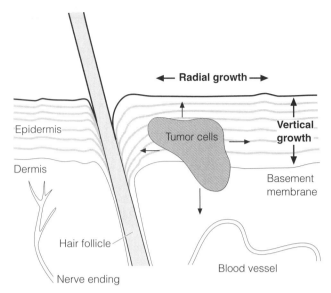

Figure 35-1 Melanoma growth patterns. Melanoma initially grows in the radial direction. Later stages of disease involve vertical growth with extension of tumor through the basement membrane.

rences can occur up to two decades after initial diagnosis and treatment.

Case Conclusion   DB underwent an excisional biopsy for diagnosis of his suspicious lesion. Microscopic sections showed asymmetric proliferation of melanocytes with large nuclei. There was extension of atypical melanocytic cells through the dermis to a thickness of 1.3 mm. The full lesion was surgically reexcised with 1-cm margins to establish local control. Because DB did not exhibit any clinical or radiographic signs of lymph node enlargement, regional node biopsy was deferred. Ten years after initial diagnosis, palpable axillary nodes were noted. CT scan also revealed liver lesions. Subsequent biopsies demonstrated metastatic melanoma. Treatment with chemoimmunotherapy was begun, but he passed away 1 year later.

Thumbnail: Melanoma

ABCDE of melanoma recognition:

Asymmetry

Border irregularities

Color Variegation

Diameter > 6 mm

Enlargement

Key Points

▶ Melanoma is an aggressive tumor that arises from melanocytes.

▶ Major risk factors include fair skin, excessive exposure to sunlight, precursor lesions (dysplastic nevi), and family history of melanoma.

▶ Melanoma exhibits radial (horizontal) and vertical growth patterns.

▶ Prognosis depends primarily on tumor thickness.

Questions

1. A 67-year-old man presents with a 10-year history of a slowly enlarging area of discoloration on the tip of his nose. The lesion is 4 × 5 mm, flat, dark brown, and has distinct borders. Which characteristic of this patient or his lesion is most worrisome for melanoma?

   A. Age of patient
   B. Gender of patient
   C. Color of lesion
   D. Size of lesion
   E. Enlargement of lesion

2. There are other skin lesions that may predispose toward the development of melanoma. Which of the following is a major risk factor for melanoma?

   A. Erythema multiforme
   B. Actinic keratosis
   C. Previous skin surgery
   D. Congenital nevus
   E. Psoriasiform dermatitis

3. In patients presenting with a diagnosis of melanoma, being able to counsel them as to their chances of cure is paramount. What is the most important prognostic indicator of outcome for patients with melanoma?

   A. Family history of melanoma
   B. Histologic grade
   C. Volume and depth of invasion
   D. Fair skin
   E. Positive margins at initial biopsy

HPI: KE is a 51-year-old man who presents to the ED after his wife saw him "have a seizure." After breakfast he collapsed to the ground for 4 to 5 minutes with outreached extremities experiencing jerky movements. He does not have a known seizure disorder. During the episode he was incontinent of urine and bit his tongue. He was disoriented to place and date for 20 to 30 minutes after the movements ceased. Past medical history is significant only for hypertension, for which he takes a low dose of hydrochlorothiazide. He does not smoke, and he drinks an occasional beer on holidays. His family history is significant for coronary artery disease, and both of his parents died in their 70s from MIs. On review of systems (ROS), it was noted that in the last 2 months he had been experiencing some new early morning headaches that were not relieved with over-the-counter analgesics. He said he generally felt more "clumsy" than usual.

PE: Overweight man sitting comfortably on gurney. Head and neck: pupils equally round and reactive to light and accommodation (PERRLA), extraocular movements intact (EOMI), conjunctiva clear. No lymphadenopathy. Neuro: CN II–XII intact. Motor: 4/5 on L upper/lower extremities; 5/5 on R; deep tendon reflexes (DTRs): decreased on the L bicep and knee jerk; negative Babinski test bilaterally. Sensory: intact to light touch. Gait: wide-based gait. Difficulty standing on heel/toe on L side. A head CT was ordered.

Thought Questions

- What are the most common types of brain tumors in adults? In children?

- Are "benign" brain tumors really benign?

- What is glioblastoma multiforme?

Basic Science Review and Discussion

It is estimated that 17,000 malignant tumors of the brain or spinal cord were diagnosed in 2002 in the United States. Approximately 13,100 will die from these malignant tumors. Cancer of the CNS accounts for approximately 1.4% of all human cancers and 2.4% of all cancer-related deaths, with men slightly more affected than women in a 3:2 ratio. CNS tumors are mostly intracranial; tumors of the spinal cord are much less frequent. Unlike other solid tumors in the body, primary malignant CNS tumors rarely metastasize.

In **adults,** the majority of intracranial tumors are **supratentorial** (occurring in the cerebral hemispheres). **Metastatic tumors are the most commonly occurring tumors of the brain,** followed by astrocytomas (including glioblastoma) and meningiomas. In **children,** the majority of intracranial tumors are **infratentorial** (occurring in the cerebellum/ brainstem), with **medulloblastoma** occurring most frequently. CNS tumors are about equal to acute lymphocytic leukemia as the most commonly occurring childhood cancer.

Brain tumors can be benign or malignant. Benign tumors have clear borders, do not invade adjacent brain tissue, and rarely reoccur after removal. Yet benign tumors can still result in devastating clinical consequences due to mass effect and compression of important brain structures.

Glioblastoma Multiforme Glioblastoma multiforme (GBM) is the most common and most malignant adult primary intracranial brain tumor. It is also known as the WHO grade IV astrocytoma. The peak incidence is age 45 to 70 years. The clinical history of patients with GBM is usually short (less than 3 months) and is consistent with the presence of a fast-growing diffuse brain lesion. Patients frequently present with headache, nausea, vomiting, and/or cognitive impairment. Patients can develop slowly progressing neurologic deficits such as motor weakness or visual changes. Seizures are not uncommon. It is widely accepted that several different genetic alterations may lead to the formation of glioblastoma. In approximately 40% of GBMs, the epidermal growth factor receptor (EGFR) is truncated, causing it to be continually turned on, leading to uncontrolled cell growth. Histologically, GBMs are composed of poorly differentiated, often pleomorphic astrocytic cells with marked nuclear atypia and brisk mitotic activity. Necrosis is an essential diagnostic feature, and prominent microvascular proliferation is common. A hallmark finding is a **pseudopalisade** arrangement of cells around an area of necrosis. Imaging studies are also essential to making the diagnosis of GBM. On CT, GMBs appear as irregularly shaped hypodense lesions with a peripheral ringlike zone of contrast enhancement and surrounding edema. MRI is also useful. Unfortunately, the prognosis for patients with glioblastoma multiforme is poor; survival is often less than 18 months after diagnosis. Treatment is primarily focused on palliation. Surgery is performed to debulk the tumor mass followed by radiation and/or chemotherapy to control remaining tumor cells.

Case Conclusion   The head CT revealed a large irregularly shaped intracranial mass spanning the right parietal region. A large area of edema surrounded the lesion and much of the parenchyma was compressed. A presumptive diagnosis of GBM was made. The patient was scheduled for surgery with the neurosurgeon, who removed a large portion of the mass. The pathology report commented on pseudopalisading glial cells around necrotic areas of tissue, confirming the diagnosis. The patient was scheduled to meet with both a medical and radiation oncologist for further follow-up.

Thumbnail: Nervous System Tumors

Tumor type	Who likely gets it	Significant features
Astrocytoma grade IV: glioblastoma multiforme	Age 45–70 Men > women	Most common adult primary intracranial tumor; neural tube origin; in cerebral hemispheres; hemorrhagic necrosis with pseudopalisading cells; highly malignant
Meningioma	Middle-aged women	Second most common adult primary intracranial tumor; originates in arachnoid cells; external to brain; neural crest origin; psammoma bodies on histology; benign, slow growing
Medulloblastoma	Children	Most common childhood intracranial tumor; in cerebellum; neural tube origin; highly malignant
Neuroblastoma	Children	Related to neuroblastoma of adrenals; in cerebral hemispheres; N-*myc* oncogene amplification; neural crest origin
Retinoblastoma	Young children	Retinal tumor; sporadic (unilateral) or familial forms (bilateral); linked to Rb (tumor suppressor gene) inactivation on both chromosome copies; neural tube origin
Schwannoma (acoustic neuroma)	Middle age to later life	Involves cranial nerve XIII; benign, often resectable; neural crest origin; presents with hearing loss, ataxic gait
Craniopharyngioma	Children	Most common supratentorial brain tumor in children; ectodermal origin (Rathke's pouch); enlarged sella turcica causing pituitary abnormalities, papilledema and bitemporal hemianopsia (tunnel vision)
Ependymoma	Children	Line ventricles, often 4th ventricle; obstructed CSF, hydrocephalus; rosette histology
Metastatic	Anyone	Most common brain tumor; usually from lung, breast, GI, melanoma, kidney, thyroid primaries

Key Points

▶ In adults, brain tumors are often supratentorial (cerebral hemispheres). Metastatic brain tumors are more common than astrocytomas (glioblastomas), which are more common than meningiomas.

▶ In children, brain tumors are often intratentorial (cerebellum); medulloblastoma is the most common type.

▶ Benign brain tumors can have devastating clinical consequences due to mass effect.

▶ Glioblastoma multiforme (grade IV astrocytoma) is the most common adult primary brain tumor; characterized by necrosis, pseudopalisading arrangement of cells and a poor prognosis.

Questions

1. A patient is found to have bilateral acoustic neuromas. What hereditary syndrome do you suspect?
   A. von Hippel–Lindau disease
   B. Neurofibromatosis type 1 (von Recklinghausen's disease)
   C. Neurofibromatosis type 2
   D. Li-Fraumeni syndrome
   E. Multiple endocrine neoplasia type I
   F. Multiple endocrine neoplasia type III

2. A 63-year-old man comes to your office after suffering from 2 months of new headaches, which do not resolve with over-the-counter analgesics. A CT of the brain shows multiple enhancing lesions in both cerebral hemispheres. What is your preliminary diagnosis?
   A. Glioblastoma multiforme
   B. Pilocytic astrocytoma
   C. Meningioma
   D. Medulloblastoma
   E. Metastasis

HPI: LS is a 37-year-old **hepatitis B virus (HBV)**-positive man who presents with **fatigue, weight loss,** and **increasing abdominal girth.** He originally comes from **Taiwan** and contracted HBV through vertical transmission from his mother. He had noticed increased difficulty with his work as a paramedic fire fighter for the last 5 months. In the last 3 months, he noticed having a hard time keeping on weight, even as he attempted to eat more and lift weights. In the last month, he has noticed a dull **sense of fullness** and **upper abdominal pain.** Over this time, he had also noticed his abdomen becoming more distended. He notes being a regular **alcohol** drinker, about two to five beers per day for 16 years.

PE: T 38.4°C HR 96 BP 125/70 RR 20 SaO$_2$ 98% at room air.
The patient is **thin,** pale, and ill-appearing. His exam is significant for a **distended abdomen** with a positive **fluid wave** and **migrating dullness to percussion.** He has diffuse **epigastric tenderness** and a **palpable liver edge.** He has no other stigmata for alcoholism including jaundice, palmar erythema, spider angiomata, or caput medusae.

Labs: WBC **17,500/μL** Hct **32%** AST **126** ALT **62.**
Abdominal ultrasound reveals marked **ascites** and a single **liver nodule.** An abdominal paracentesis is performed and **bloody ascitic fluid** is produced and quickly sent off for cytology. The α-**fetoprotein** levels are elevated. The patient is thus scheduled for a liver biopsy to further characterize the nature of the liver nodule.

Thought Questions

- How do viruses and other microbes promote the development of cancer?

- How does hepatitis virus promote the development of hepatocellular carcinoma?

- What are the clinical manifestations of hepatocellular carcinoma?

- How is hepatocellular carcinoma diagnosed and treated?

Basic Science Review and Discussion

Viruses and other microbes can promote carcinogenesis through (1) the **initiation** of a cell by genetic mutation, and then (2) the **propagation** of this mutation by cellular proliferation. Furthermore, the process of proliferation promotes the accumulation of additional mutations within a cell population steering it toward increased malignancy. Microorganisms that are well established in the pathogenesis of cancer include human papilloma virus (HPV), EBV, human T-cell leukemia virus type-1 (HTLV-1), *Helicobacter pylori,* and HBV.

The first step of initiation is commonly produced by the **integration of the microbial DNA into the infected cell's genome.** A classic example is **HPV** and its role in the carcinogenesis of cervical cancer. While HPV subtypes 1, 2, 4, and 7 produce **benign squamous papillomas** (or warts), **HPV types 16, 18, and 31** are strongly associated in the development of **invasive squamous cell carcinoma (SCC) of the cervix.** The initiating event occurs with integration of the HPV genome at its E1/E2 **o**pen **r**eading **f**rame (ORF, the regions of the

genome that are transcribed and translated into actual proteins). Integration at this site prevents the production of the E2 gene product, which normally represses the transcription of the downstream E6 and E7 proteins. E6 and E7 produce proteins that inhibit the tumor suppressor proteins *p53* and *pRb,* respectively. This disruption in two important cell cycle-regulating proteins establishes a cell's neoplastic potential. Some cofactors implicated in the development of cervical cancer include cigarette smoking and concurrent infections, both carcinogenic. Chronic cellular damage and regeneration with accumulation of genetic mutations promote the evolution toward greater malignancy.

The second step of carcinogenesis is the **propagation of a carcinogenic mutation by proliferation and selective survival of a malignant cell.** Often, this step is not preceded by a well-defined mechanism of genetic transformation as found in HPV. This is classically demonstrated by **EBV** and its role in the pathogenesis of Burkitt's lymphoma. EBV is a herpes virus that infects B-lymphocytes. **Burkitt's lymphoma** is a B-lymphocyte neoplasm common among children in Central Africa and New Guinea. EBV infects a B-cell and has the ability to immortalize that cell line by two mechanisms: (1) overexpression of *bcl-2,* an antiapoptotic gene, and (2) activation of growth usually triggered by T-cell cytokines. Among immunocompetent hosts, B-cell proliferation is usually controlled by T-cell-mediated suppression. In immunocompromised hosts, B-cell proliferation may continue unsuppressed. The transformation of B-cells toward unregulated proliferation increases the chance of developing a carcinogenic mutation like the t(8;14) translocation, which causes overexpression of the growth-promoting c-*myc* oncogene. Overall, EBV-mediated carcinogenesis highlights the important concept that an infection may not necessarily be directly oncogenic, but by promoting cellular proliferation, it predisposes an individual to developing the genetic mutation required to develop a malignant neoplasm.

HBV is similarly implicated in the pathogenesis of **hepatocellular carcinoma (HCC).** The HBV genome is integrated into the host genome. Although there is no well-defined site of integration, it appears to be a necessary initiating step in carcinogenesis. HBV promotes carcinogenesis by causing chronic hepatocyte injury and regenerative proliferation. As in Burkitt's lymphoma, the proliferation of a cell population increases the chance of acquiring more genetic mutations that can give rise to a malignant subpopulation. Also, HBV produces the HBx protein, which up-regulates expression of several growth-promoting genes like insulin-like growth factor I (IGF-I) receptor and IGF-II and interferes with the tumor-suppressor activity of *p53*. Hepatitis C virus is also strongly linked to HCC and may mediate tumorigenesis through similar mechanisms.

Paraneoplastic Syndromes　Some tumors produce disease as a function of the cellular products it secretes. For example, HCC produces IGF-II, a homologue of insulin. People with HCC may present with severe hypoglycemia as a result of IGF-II hypersecretion from this tumor. Often, well-differentiated tumors that retain the ability to produce hormones and peptides produce paraneoplastic syndromes. Less differentiated tumors are less likely to produce disease in this fashion and instead interrupt normal physiologic function through direct invasion of adjacent tissue.

Hepatocellular Carcinoma　HCC is the **most common organ tumor worldwide.** Although relatively rare in the Western world (U.S., Europe), it is quite common in Asia and Africa. Worldwide, HCC is strongly linked to HBV infection, which confers a 200-fold increased risk of developing the cancer. In the Western world, however, cirrhosis is the largest culprit in the pathogenesis of this disease. Other causes of HCC are **aflatoxin** exposure, **hemochromatosis,** and α_1-**antitrypsin deficiency.**

Case Conclusion　The liver biopsy reveals HCC in all specimens taken. The patient is referred to a surgeon, but his cancer is deemed too diffuse to resect. However, he was eligible for cryotherapy ablation of his tumors for the purpose of prolonging survival. Currently, he is stable and being followed to monitor the progression of his cancer.

Thumbnail: Summary of Hepatocellular Carcinoma

Epidemiology	Common in Asia and Africa, common among IV drug users (HBV/HCV+ risk), alcoholics with chronic liver cirrhosis; blacks > white; men > women; age 20 to 40 years
HPI	Weight loss, weakness, cachexia, epigastric abdominal pain, abdominal fullness
PMH	Exposure to aflatoxin, congenital α_1-antitrypsin deficiency, hemochromatosis
Family history	Congenital diseases that predispose one to chronic hepatic injury
Physical exam	Hepatomegaly, ascites, ±bruit or friction rub over liver
Lab findings	↑ α-fetoprotein, HBV/HCV+ serology, ↑ WBC, erythrocytosis (erythropoietin-producing tumor)
Diagnosis	Ultrasound, CT, or MRI, liver biopsy, abdominal paracentesis with cytology
Treatment	Liver resection or transplantation, tumor ablation (microwave, cryotherapy, radiation)

Key Points

▶ Viruses can cause genetic mutations that dysregulate tumor-suppression, activate proto-oncogenes, inhibit apoptosis, and promote proliferation via chronic cell damage and compensatory regenerative hyperplasia.

▶ Cellular proliferation propagates and makes permanent these cancer-promoting genetic mutations within a cell population.

▶ Although proliferation itself may not be directly oncogenic, it may increase the chance that a cell acquires a cancer-promoting genetic mutation.

Questions

1. LS reported a history of long-term alcohol consumption at moderate levels. What is the most likely mechanism through which this contributed to the pathogenesis of his hepatocellular carcinoma?

   A. His alcohol consumption led to the development of chronic liver cirrhosis, which predisposed him to developing hepatocellular carcinoma.

   B. He inherited a genetic predisposition from his mother, which predisposed him to developing HCC from moderate alcohol consumption.

   C. Alcohol suppressed his immune function enough to allow for HBV to proliferate in his liver, predisposing him to developing HCC.

   D. Alcohol potentiated the carcinogenic effects of chronic HBV infection by contributing to the continuous cycle of hepatocyte injury and regeneration.

   E. His level of alcohol consumption was unlikely to contribute to the development of HCC, and it is likely that his cancer arose solely from the influence of chronic HBV infection.

2. YR is a 30-year-old man with pulmonary emphysema with only a 10 pack-year smoking history who presents with abdominal fullness. He is HBV and HCV negative with only occasional alcohol consumption. His family history is significant for early-onset chronic obstructive pulmonary disease. His ultrasound of the liver reveals diffusely abnormal liver parenchyma with two liver nodules suggestive of some sort of neoplasm. Subsequent liver biopsy revealed hepatocellular carcinoma at both nodules. What is the most likely etiology of his cancer?

   A. Aflatoxin exposure

   B. Hepatitis B virus

   C. Hepatitis C virus

   D. Alcoholic cirrhosis

   E. α_1-antitrypsin deficiency

HPI: DC is a 55-year-old woman who presents with a **breast lump**. She had noted the lump 2 weeks ago in the shower and describes it as **painless**. She noted no bloody or green **discharge** from her nipples, no **nipple retractions, skin changes, breast dimpling** or **enlargement, axillary masses,** or **bone pain.** She has no **family history** of breast or ovarian cancer. She has no significant past medical history and no previous screening mammographies, and takes no medication. She has **never been pregnant.**

PE: The patient is a thin woman in no acute distress. She is afebrile with normal vital signs. She has no gross **breast asymmetry,** dimpling, skin changes, or retractions. She has a 2-cm **firm, nontender, and immobile breast nodule** at the **upper outer quadrant** of her left breast. She has no palpable **axillary lymph nodes** and no expressible nipple discharge.

Thought Questions

- How are tumors categorized histologically?

- What is the difference between benign and malignant tumors?

- What are the types of breast cancer? What risk factors are associated with this cancer?

- What is the basic diagnostic work-up of a breast lump and how is it treated?

Basic Science Review and Discussion

Each year, there are over 1 million people who are newly diagnosed with cancer, causing over 500,000 deaths in the year 2000. It is second only to cardiovascular disease as the leading cause of death in the United States. Yet there are often misunderstandings about the very definitions of "tumor" or "cancer," both words eliciting strong reactions from any person. Table 38-1 is a review of tumors, the terminology used, and the histologic and behavioral aspects of tumors that define them as benign or malignant.

Benign versus Malignant Tumors The basic difference between these two designations is that a malignant tumor is likely to grow in a way that would eventually cause enough disruption to a person's normal physiology to cause death, whereas with a benign tumor this is unlikely to happen. These are important designations because *a benign tumor is unlikely to become a malignant tumor.* Benign tumors are thought to be "benign" because they behave similarly to mature, well-differentiated cells and grow in a more controlled fashion, responding to regulatory signals like "normal" cells. They grow more slowly and compress (but do not invade) adjacent tissue. They do not spread to other parts of the body, and, if removed, will not recur. Malignant cells appear less differentiated, respond poorly to normal regulatory signals, invade surrounding tissue, and eventually metastasize to distant sites. Ultimately, these designations are mere *predictions* on the future behavior of

tissue. Along with tumor markers and patients' overall clinical pictures, these histologic characteristics can provide information on patients' prognoses and help them understand what is really meant when they are told they have a tumor.

Clinical Discussion: Breast Cancer Breast cancer is the second most common cancer and occurs in 1 of 8 American women, one third of whom succumb to the disease. Men represent less than 1% of those affected. The risk factors associated with breast cancer are those generally associated with *increased lifetime exposure to estrogen:*

1. **Increasing age:** majority of women are more than 50 years old
2. **Geographic/racial influence:** common in white women, rare in Asian women
3. **History breast cancer** in the contralateral breast or **endometrial cancer**
4. **Radiation exposure** and other mutagenic exposures
5. **Prolonged reproductive life:** early menarche and late menopause
6. **Nulliparity** or **late parity,** with first child at more than 30 years of age
7. **Obesity** causing increased estrogen synthesis in fat deposits, lower progesterone levels, greater number of anovulatory cycles
8. **Exogenous estrogen:** hormone replacement therapy (but not oral contraceptives)
9. **Family history of breast cancer** in mother, sister, daughter, especially if bilateral or before menopause
10. **Genetic predisposition:** germ line mutations in *BRCA-1, BRCA-2, p53, ATM* (ataxia-telangiectasia mutation), which are tumor suppressor and DNA repair genes

A woman may present with a palpable breast mass, nipple secretion, inflammatory skin lesions, or an abnormal mammogram during screening. A single, *nontender,* firm mass that is poorly circumscribed and fixed to skin or chest wall is

Table 38-1 The nomenclature of tumors

Terminology	Definition
Neoplasm	"New growth": abnormal tissue that undergoes uncontrolled or excessive growth
Tumor	"Swelling": includes the *parenchyma,* consisting of neoplastic cells, plus *supportive stroma,* including connective tissue and blood vessels
Nonneoplastic tumors	
Hamartoma	Tumor consisting of hyperplasia of normal differentiated cells located at its normal site
Hyperplasia	Tissue growth from cellular proliferation resulting in an *increased number* of cells
Hypertrophy	Tissue growth resulting from *increased size* of each cell, e.g., muscle growth
Metaplasia	The replacement of one type of fully differentiated cell by another type of fully differentiated cell, e.g., squamous metaplasia of Barrett's esophagus in chronic gastroesophageal reflux (GERD)
Benign tumors (-omas)	
Adenoma	Benign epithelial neoplasm that forms glandular patterns
Papilloma	Benign epithelial neoplasms forming finger-like or warty projections
Cystadenoma	Benign epithelial neoplasms forming large cystic masses
Malignant tumors/cancer	
Anaplasia	Very poorly differentiated cancers
Sarcomas	Malignant tumors arising from mesenchymal tissue (e.g., leiomyosarcoma)
Carcinoma	Malignant neoplasm of epithelial cell origin (any of three germ layers)
Adenocarcinoma	Carcinoma appearing in glandular growth pattern
Squamous cell carcinoma	Carcinoma with recognizable squamous cells
Teratoma	Mixed tumor consisting of tissue from two or three germ layers
Melanoma	Misnomer, *malignant* neoplasm of melanocytes

concerning for malignancy. Overall, 90% of women who present with a breast lump do not have cancer. But ultimately, *all such women must be evaluated to rule out the possibility of cancer.* This evaluation includes a thorough history and physical, mammogram, breast ultrasound, and biopsy, either fine- or large-needle aspiration or open excisional biopsy with subsequent histologic and cytologic examination (Table 38-2).

Staging and Histologic Subtypes of Breast Cancer Breast cancer, like many cancers, is staged according to a **TNM (tumor, node, metastasis) classification system.** Roughly speaking, T0, N0, and M0 mean no tumor, node, and metastasis. T*is* is carcinoma in situ, histologically malignant tissue that has not yet infiltrated the basement membrane. Tumor number increases with the tumor size. Node number also increases with progressive lymph node involvement. M1

Table 38-2 General clinical characteristic of benign and malignant breast lumps

	Benign breast lump	Malignant breast lump
History	< 50 years old, premenopausal, painful, esp. during premenstrual period, fluctuating size	Older (> 50 years old), white, family history of breast/ovarian cancer
Physical Exam	Breast mass *Fibroadenoma:* small, round, well-defined, mobile, rubbery, *tender* mass *Phylloides tumor:* large fibroadenoma *Fibrocystic disease:* multiple or bilateral tender masses Nipple discharge Bilateral discharge *Hyperprolactinemia:* milky discharge *Oral contraceptives:* clear serous, milky *Mastitis:* purulent discharge	Breast mass Single, nontender, firm mass, poorly circumscribed, fixed to skin or chest wall Nipple discharge Green or bloody discharge Appearance Breast enlargement or asymmetry Nipple or skin retractions Axillary lymphadenopathy Peau d'orange (edematous erythematous skin)

Table 38-3 Histologic subtypes of breast cancers

Breast cancer type	Percentage	Characteristics
Invasive carcinoma (70–85%)		
Ductal carcinoma	—	Carcinoma arising from the intermediate ducts
No special type	80%	Increased dense, fibrous tissue stroma → hard consistency Infiltrative attachment to surrounding structures with fixation causing skin dimpling and nipple retraction
Medullary	2%	Associated with *BRCA1* gene, better prognosis that NST cancer
Colloid	2%	Common in older women; slow-growing, well-differentiated, diploid tumor expressing hormone receptors → good prognosis
Tubular	6%	Younger women (late 40s); detected as spiculated (irregular) mass on mammography, often multifocal or bilateral; well-differentiated diploid tumors, expressing hormone receptors → good prognosis
Papillary	1%	Papillary architecture, similar to NST but better prognosis
Lobular carcinoma	10%	Often bilateral, multifocal, diffusely invasive, more likely to metastasize to CSF, ovary, uterus, and bone marrow
Inflammatory carcinoma	< 3%	Rapidly growing, painful mass that enlarges the breast with overlying skin erythema, edema, warmth; diffusely infiltrative
In situ carcinoma (15–30%)		
Ductal carcinoma in situ (DCIS)	80%	Malignant cells that do not infiltrate the basement membrane nor metastasize; often detected as mammographic calcifications
Paget's disease	1%	Form of DCIS that extends to nipple ducts, skin, and areola, causing a fissured, ulcerated, and oozing nipple lesion
Lobular carcinoma in situ	20%	Proliferation of terminal ducts (acini), often bilateral

denotes the presence of distant metastasis. Different combinations of the T, N, and M categorize a woman's breast cancer into a **stage,** which is useful for prognostication and deciding definitive therapy. Higher stages of disease yield poorer prognosis. **Tumor grade** is determined by microscopic evaluation of the biopsy's histologic subtype and degree of differentiation. The presence of normal cell markers like estrogen and progesterone receptors suggest more differentiated cells and better prognosis as well as eligibility for adjuvant therapy with tamoxifen. **Aneuploidy** (abnormal number of chromosomes), changed expression of oncogenes and tumor-suppressor genes (e.g., *Her2/neu, p53*), and evidence of accelerated proliferation and angiogenesis are poor prognostic markers (Table 38-3).

Case Conclusion Subsequent breast ultrasound reveals a 2-cm solid mass in the upper outer quadrant of the left breast. The mammogram shows a spiculated density with clusters of microcalcifications at this same location. The breast lump is biopsied by fine-needle aspiration, which reveals no pathology. The patient undergoes open excisional biopsy of the tumor and sentinel node. Histologic examination reveals ductal carcinoma no special type (NST) with no evidence of lymph node involvement. She is diagnosed with stage I disease and undergoes breast-conserving therapy. Five years later, she is healthy with no evidence of disease recurrence.

Thumbnail: Breast Cancer

Epidemiology	• > 50 year old women; white women > Asian women with breast lump	
History of present illness	• Breast lump painful or painless? • Lump size fluctuating with cycle?	• Nipple discharge? Color? • Skin changes? Dimpling?
Past medical history	• Prior breast cancer or other disease • Age of menarche and menopause	• Use of exogenous estrogens
Family history	• Breast or ovarian cancer in mother, sister, or daughter • Known *BRCA-1, BRCA-2,* or other breast cancer genes	
Physical exam (also self-breast exam)	• Appearance: breast dimples, asymmetry, skin changes • Palpate supraclavicular and axillary nodes • Palpate each breast superficial to deep; attempt to express discharge	
Diagnostic imaging	• Mammogram: calcifications, densities • Breast ultrasound to differentiate between solid and cystic masses	
Diagnostic procedures	• Fine needle/core needle biopsy • Open/excisional biopsy	• Axillary dissection • Sentinel node biopsy
Treatment	• Lumpectomy + axillary dissection or sentinel node biopsy + radiation • Rare modified radical mastectomy for more extensive disease • Hormonal therapy (tamoxifen) for estrogen receptor positive tumor • Chemotherapy	

Key Points

▶ A malignant tumor is likely to grow in a way that would eventually cause enough disruption to a person's normal physiology to cause death, whereas a benign tumor is unlikely to behave in such a way.

▶ Benign tumors are better differentiated and behave like normal cells, while malignant tumors are less differentiated and do not respond well to normal regulatory signals.

▶ Every woman should receive regular clinical breast exam and be taught to do monthly self-breast exam. All women with a breast lump must be evaluated to rule out the possibility of cancer.

Questions

1. A 23-year-old woman goes to her physician to ask about tender breast lump on her left breast. She has no family history of cancer and is taking low-dose oral contraceptives. On exam, she has a 2-cm, rubbery, round, mobile mass. An ultrasound is performed showing a solid mass. Core needle biopsy produces a sample with benign-looking morphology. What characteristic is seen on the sample?

   A. High nucleus to cytoplasm ration
   B. High fraction of cells with mitotic spindles
   C. Loss of glandular structure
   D. Cellular hyperplasia with glandular architecture
   E. Anaplastic cells

2. A 50-year-old woman presents with an abnormal mammogram showing clustered microcalcifications. She also notes recent spontaneous bloody discharge from her nipples. Her exam reveals no palpable breast, axillary, or supraclavicular masses. What is NOT a part of the appropriate diagnostic work-up for this patient?

   A. Excisional biopsy
   B. Fine-needle aspiration
   C. Sentinel node biopsy
   D. Cytology of expressed discharge
   E. Breast ultrasound

HPI: LS is a 78-year-old African American man who, during his annual checkup, is found to have a **palpable prostatic nodule** during digital rectal exam. In addition, he noted some **tenderness on his spine.** He also noted some difficulty in walking. He denied problems with urination, incontinence, numbness, weakness, or ataxia.

PE: The patient is afebrile with normal vital signs. His exam is significant for a 2-cm right-sided **prostatic nodule, spinal tenderness** at the L3 vertebra, and **mild inguinal lymphadenopathy.** He has a 4/5 left knee extensor **weakness,** and **numbness** on his left knee and inner thigh.

Labs: The patient has a markedly **elevated serum prostate serum antigen (PSA)** of 150. **Transrectal ultrasound (TRUS)** reveals a 3-cm **nodule** on the right **posterior region of the prostate** with extension into the prostatic capsule. Abdominal CT gave evidence of **lymph node involvement,** and pelvic lymphadenectomy was subsequently performed confirming malignant extension to these lymph nodes. In addition, **radionuclide bone scanning** revealed some radiopacity around the L3 vertebra. Subsequent **spinal MRI** showed impingement of the left L3 root as it exits the L3-L4 foramen.

Thought Questions

- How are tumors characterized histologically?

- What is the natural history of a tumor?

- How are tumors graded and staged?

- What is prostate cancer? What are its clinical manifestations?

- How is prostate cancer screened, diagnosed, and treated?

Basic Science Review and Discussion

Now that we have reviewed the behavioral differences between benign and malignant tumors (Case 38), *how does one determine when a tumor is cancer?* In large part, the histologic characteristics of a tumor biopsy are used to diagnose malignancy. The characteristics that suggest **anaplasia** (or poor differentiation) are included in Table 39-1.

A neoplastic tumor begins with a single transformed cell presenting at any stage of differentiation and behavior. This cell grows to form a distinguishable mass usually confined by some anatomic capsule or basement membrane.

Table 39-1 Characteristics of anaplasia

Cellular abnormalities	Architectural abnormalities
• Hyperchromatic DNA	• Disorganized growth
• ↑ Nuclear-to-cytoplasmic ratio	• Poor adherence to normal tissue architecture
• High mitotic rate; bizarre mitotic figures	• Scant vascular stroma with necrotic areas
• Giant cells: large with hyperchromatic nucleus	

Locally confined tumors are said to be in situ, which makes complete removal of all neoplastic tissue possible. However, if this membrane is breached, a neoplasm is said to have locally invaded adjacent tissue, which can be followed by metastasis via lymphatic or hematogenous spread.

Rate of tumor growth or **doubling time** depends on the fraction of cells in the replicative pool (**growth fraction**) and how much the rate of cell proliferation exceeds that of cell loss. The doubling time roughly correlates to the rate of clinical progression. Tumors with high growth fractions produce rapid clinical progression, if left untreated. But because such tumors have so many rapidly proliferating cells, chemotherapy quickly reduces or eliminates such tumors. On the other hand, tumors with smaller growth fractions and prolonged doubling times, while having a more indolent clinical course, are more resistant to chemotherapy.

As the tumor grows beyond 1 to 2 mm in diameter, the tumor requires neovascularization to supply the tissue with adequate oxygen and nutrients. Tumors cells stimulate **angiogenesis** by secreting angiogenic growth factors like **vascular endothelial growth factor (VEGF)** and **basic fibroblast growth factor (bFGF).** Newly formed endothelial cells reciprocally promote tumor growth by secreting **insulin-like growth factors,** PDGF, GM-CSF, and IL-1. **Neovascularization** supports not only tumor growth but also eventual metastasis.

Over time, a tumor may become more aggressive as a result of the dynamic evolution of the tumor cell population. Subpopulations may arise that divide more rapidly, are less responsive to hormonal therapy or chemotherapy, or are more prone to local invasion and metastasis. The underlying mechanisms of such shifts in behavior are thought to arise from genetic instability due to, for example, the loss of *p53,* which has a central role in DNA repair. If *p53* is lost, the rate of spontaneous genetic mutation accelerates. With rapid negative selection of nonadvantageous genotypes, a robust, rapidly proliferating subpopulation is bound to arise.

Eventually, a tumor cell gives rise to a subpopulation that has attained the ability to metastasize. These cells adhere and invade the basement membrane that contained the primary tumor, and attach to and degrade the local extracellular matrix (ECM). The cells pass through the ECM and **intravasate** into the local vasculature. Within the circulation, it may elicit immune attack and platelet aggregation, which causes the formation of a tumor cell embolus. This embolus can adhere to endothelium at a distant site, **extravasate,** and deposit itself within that tissue. Table 39-2 lists the routes through which metastasis occurs.

Eventually, such "selfish" growth and dissemination interferes with the normal function of cells around it. Thus, it is not the mere presence of neoplastic tissue that constitutes illness. It is the dysregulation of normal physiology by the proliferation of a neoplasm that ultimately produces the disease of cancer.

Clinical Discussion: Prostate Cancer   Prostate cancer is the most common form of cancer among men, with more than 300,000 new cases per year, resulting in 41,000 deaths. Risk factors include advanced age, increased fat consumption, and family history (a few susceptibility genes have been identified). Androgen levels are suspected to contribute, as evidenced by the tumor's response to antiandrogen therapy.

Most cancers arise in the posterior gland. The cancer grows until it abuts the glandular capsule. It first invades this capsule, and then infiltrates locally to the seminal vesicles and the bladder. After this, it spreads through lymphatic vessels to the deep pelvic nodes. Finally, it spreads hematogenously to the vertebral column and visceral organs.

Most men present asymptomatically during routine screening with a focal prostatic nodule found by **digital rectal exam (DRE)** or an **elevated PSA.** Relatively localized disease is unlikely to cause urinary symptoms, as prostate cancer is more likely to arise in the periphery within the subcapsular region away from the urethra. As the tumor grows, a patient may develop urinary problems. Back pain is an ominous sign, suggesting vertebral metastasis, and is virtually diagnostic of late-stage cancer with very poor prognosis.

Diagnosis

1. **DRE**

2. **Serum PSA** greater than 4 ng/mL (although the specificity is poor for prostate cancer); PSA may be also elevated in benign prostatic hypertrophy or prostatitis; adjusted for age and prostate size

3. **Transrectal ultrasound (TRUS)** for assessment of local spread

4. **Transperineal or transrectal biopsy** for histologic diagnosis of prostate cancer

5. **Radionuclide bone scan** for patients with symptoms suggestive of bony metastasis

6. **Fine-needle aspiration of pelvic lymph nodes** for those with lymphadenopathy

Pathology and Staging   For prostate cancer, the **Gleason system** is used to grade tumors on a five-point scale, based on *glandular pattern and degree of differentiation,* scored as 1 for well-differentiated tumors and 5 for the least differentiated. There are two grades assigned, with a combined score range of 2 to 10. Staging from A to D depends on the tumor size, focal or diffuse growth, glandular capsule invasion, and metastatic spread.

Grossly, prostate cancer appears gritty and firm, classically in the posterior location in the subcapsular region. Microscopically, a well-differentiated cancer appears glandular and crowded with "back-to-back" glands lined by a single layer of cuboidal cells. This tissue architecture deteriorates to a diffuse pattern with higher-grade lesions.

Table 39-2 Methods of metastatic spread

Route of spread	Metastatic destination	Example
Direct extension	Peritoneal cavity, pleural cavity	Ovarian cancer → intraperitoneal spread
Lymphatic spread	Draining lymph nodes	Breast cancer to axillary lymph nodes
Hematogenous spread Venous drainage		
Portal vein	Liver	Colon cancer metastasis to the liver
Inferior vena cava	Lungs	Renal cancer metastasis to the lungs
Paravertebral plexus	Brain or spinal column	Prostate cancer metastasis to spine or CNS
Arterial circulation*	Brain (depends on 1° tumor site)	Lung cancer spread via pulmonary vein → LV → aorta → internal carotid → CNS

*Metastasis through arterial drainage is less common, as the thick walls of arteries are more difficult to penetrate.

Treatment   For early-stage prostate cancer **transurethral radical prostatectomy (TURP)** and postoperative radiotherapy is performed. For those with advanced and metastatic cancer, **antiandrogen therapy** with such drugs as **finasteride** (an androgen receptor antagonist), **goserelin** [a gonadotropin-releasing hormone (GnRH) inhibitor], or **orchiectomy** (removal of testosterone-secreting testicular glands) suppresses tumor growth. However, such therapy does not induce remission, and testosterone-insensitive clones eventually arise. Such patients have a very poor prognosis.

Case Conclusion: Transrectal biopsy revealed a tumor with Gleason scores of 5 and 5. With such an advanced stage cancer, LS was thought to not be a candidate for surgical resection. Instead, he was treated with a combination of finasteride and goserelin. He also received IV dexamethasone and a 10-day course of radiation therapy to reduce the size of the spinal tumor with the hope of decreasing the spinal root compression. He is currently stable, receiving palliative therapy for end-stage prostate cancer.

Thumbnail: Prostate Cancer

Identification	• > 50 year old men	• Black > white >> Asian
History of present illness	• Asymptomatic • Dysuria • Frequency	• Hematuria • Difficulty starting/stopping stream • Bone or back pain
Family history	• First-degree relatives	• Early-age onset of prostate cancer
Physical exam	• Digital rectal exam • Glandular asymmetry • Palpable focal nodules	• Pelvic lymphadenopathy • Vertebral tenderness • Other bony tenderness
Diagnostic labs	• PSA > 4, age-, prostate-size adjusted	• Low free (unbound) PSA ratio
Diagnostic imaging	• Transrectal ultrasonography	• Radionuclide bone scan
Diagnostic procedures	• Transrectal/transurethral biopsy	• FNA of lymph nodes
Grading	• Gleason system: two points 1 to 5 (from most to least differentiated)	
Staging	• Stage A to D: tumor size, capsular invasion, nodal involvement, metastasis	
Treatment	• Transurethral radical prostatectomy (TURP)	• Hormonal therapy—finasteride • Orchiectomy

---

Key Points

▶ Malignancy is diagnosed histologically by the presence of cellular and tissue abnormalities including hyperchromatic DNA, high nuclear-to-cytoplasmic ratio, high mitotic rate, atypical or bizarre mitotic figures, and disorganized growth.

▶ Prostate cancer is the most common cancer among men, affecting older as well as African-American men.

▶ Early prostate cancer is usually asymptomatic and is picked up by DRE; late-stage prostate cancer may present with signs of local invasion and metastasis like dysuria and bone pain.

Questions

1. Of the following, which histologic characteristics would NOT be expected in LS's Gleason 5 and 5 tumor?

    A. Hyperplastic glands of cuboidal cells arranged back-to-back
    B. Frequent bizarre mitotic spindles
    C. High nucleus-to-cytoplasm ratio
    D. Hyperchromatic nucleus
    E. Areas of central necrosis

2. One year after starting finasteride, LS returned, complaining of increased dysuria and urinary hesitancy. DRE revealed a larger prostatic mass than what was felt several months before. His PSA was elevated severalfold higher than his previous level. What step in the pathogenesis of this new event is NOT likely to have occurred?

    A. Tumor growth was suppressed via androgen receptor antagonism by finasteride, as the relatively well-differentiated tumor cells require androgen stimulation for growth.
    B. Genetic instability led to the loss of *p53* function and normal DNA repair capacity causing acceleration in the rate of genetic mutation.
    C. A subpopulation of androgen-independent tumor cells arose against the selective pressure of finasteride therapy.
    D. A new primary prostatic tumor arose due to the selective pressure of finasteride.
    E. A subpopulation of highly proliferative tumor cells arose from spontaneous mutation yielding a high growth fraction and accelerated tumor growth.

HPI: FC is a 58-year-old woman who presents to her doctor concerned about a **palpable neck mass.** She first noticed it several months ago and has noticed it grow since. It is **painless,** and she reports having no difficulties with swallowing, hoarseness of voice, cough, or shortness of breath. She has no personal or family history of goiter or other thyroid disease. She did, however, work as an **x-ray technician** for 35 years.

PE: The patient is afebrile, with normal vital signs. Her exam is significant for a **left-sided, firm, nontender 1-cm nodule at the area of the thyroid gland** that moves along with the gland upon swallowing. She has no lymphadenopathy or bony tenderness.

Labs: Normal thyroid-stimulating hormone (TSH), triiodothyronine (T_3), and **free thyroxine (T_4) (FT_4) (thyroid hormone precursor); elevated thyroglobulin; elevated calcitonin** and **carcinoembryonic antigen (CEA).**
Ultrasound: Reveals a 0.8-cm, well-circumscribed solid nodule with no evidence of extension into the adjacent structures. This was followed by a fine needle aspiration biopsy (FNAB) of the nodule.

Thought Questions

- How do carcinogenic agents promote cancer development?

- What are the common carcinogens, and what cancers do they produce?

- What is thyroid cancer and in what forms does it occur?

- What are the clinical manifestations of thyroid cancer? How is it diagnosed and treated?

Basic Science Review and Discussion

There are many cancer-causing or **carcinogenic agents,** including environmental exposures like chemicals and radiation. **These agents are carcinogenic by virtue of their ability to cause genetic mutation.** Carcinogenic agents can either act directly to transform a cell or be metabolically processed by the host's cytochrome P-450 enzymes to produce such a chemical. Although not all mutagenic chemicals are carcinogenic, all carcinogenic chemicals are mutagenic. When specific genes called **proto-oncogenes, tumor-suppressor genes,** and **apoptosis-regulating genes** undergo mutation, normal cell function can become dysregulated in a way that furthers the survival and growth of that cell. The establishment of permanent DNA damage is termed the **initiation** of carcinogenesis, and is the first step of carcinogenesis. The agent that causes this damage is called an **initiator.** Without this initiator, a cell does not have the ability to give rise to cancer.

The second step of carcinogenesis is **promotion.** For a genetic mutation to remain within a cell population, this variant must be **promoted** by cellular proliferation and enhanced survival. Thus, it is not sufficient to simply have a genetic mutation. This mutation must promote its own reproduction and survival. Many things promote cell divi-

sion, the excess of which is termed **hyperplasia.** This includes growth-promoting hormones, viral infection, chronic cell damage and regeneration, and even "normal" physiologic replication. Also, a mutation may allow a cell to prolong its life span and resist cell death. This occurs when a cell resists its own programmed cell death, also called **apoptosis.** This arises from an imbalance between proapoptotic and antiapoptotic factors within the cell that causes it to lean toward survival. The prototypic antiapoptotic gene is *bcl-2* and its pro-apoptotic counterpart is *bax.* In fact, *p53,* the classic tumor-suppressor gene, promotes apoptosis by up-regulating *bax,* which counteracts the antiapoptotic influence of *bcl-2.* If *p53* is damaged, *bcl-2* will go unopposed, preventing apoptosis. An overabundance of *bcl-2* can give rise to a durable cell population that **promotes** itself by resisting death and prolonging its own life.

Common chemicals that *initiate* carcinogenesis include polycyclic aromatic hydrocarbons, direct-acting alkylating and acylating agents, aromatic amines and azo dyes, as well as natural plant and microbial products. **Polycyclic aromatic hydrocarbons,** carcinogens that are present in tobacco give rise to lung and bladder cancers. **Alkylating agents,** such as the cancer-chemotherapeutic agents **cyclophosphamide** and **busulfan,** have been known to produce leukemia and lymphomas. **Aromatic amines** and **azo dyes** are procarcinogens that are transformed into very powerful carcinogens by cytochrome P-450, some of which have been present in food coloring. Plant products including **aflatoxin B1,** a product of *Aspergillus flavus,* present in improperly stored peanuts and are associated with the development of hepatocellular carcinoma in Africa and the Far East. **Nitrosamines** are known to cause gastric cancer. **Asbestos** is implicated in the development of lung and gastrointestinal cancers, and **vinyl chloride** in hemangiosarcoma.

Radiation acts in a similar fashion to chemical carcinogens. **Ultraviolet radiation** (UV rays) from the sun is the established cause of squamous cell carcinoma, basal cell carcinoma, and possibly malignant melanoma of the skin. Although such damage can be repaired by DNA repair, such mechanisms can be overwhelmed by excessive sun exposure. This can lead to the persistence of unrepaired DNA, which can carry over into the next generation if the cell undergoes cell division without first correcting this "mistake." Other forms of **ionizing radiation** include *x-rays, γ-rays, α- and β-particles, protons,* and *neutrons,* many of which have been implicated in the increased incidence of cancer after major catastrophic nuclear fallouts, like the atomic bombings of Hiroshima and Nagasaki and the Chernobyl accident.

Clinical Discussion: Thyroid Cancer   **Thyroid cancer** is a common radiation-induced cancer. It can result from mere occupational or therapeutic exposure to ionizing radiation like **x-rays** and **radioactive iodine.** It is relatively rare, making up 1.5% of all cancers. It affects **women** more than men, especially in early and middle adulthood.

Patients usually present with a **single painless nodule** in the thyroid, perhaps with a history of **prior exposure to irradiation** to the head and neck. The tumor may spread through lymphatics to the lymph nodes and cause **cervical lymphadenopathy.** Patients may also have **dysphagia** or **hoarseness of voice,** suggesting infiltration of the tumor into cranial nerve X. In advanced cases, the tumor may infiltrate the trachea causing **cough** and **dyspnea.**

Fine needle asperation biopsy (FNAB) generally helps distinguish between benign and malignant lesions. An **ultrasound of the neck** helps distinguish benign cystic

nodules from more malignant solid lesions and may detect local spread. **Radioisotope studies** using ^{131}I **isotopes** that are not taken up well by poorly differentiated thyroid tumors help increase the level of suspicion for malignancy. These tumors are called "cold" nodules, in contrast to "hot" nodules that do take up isotope as well; however, some well-differentiated carcinomas can take up isotope. Some associated laboratory findings include **normal thyroid function tests (TSH, FT$_4$, T$_3$)** and **high serum thyroglobulin.**

There are four types of thyroid cancer (Table 40-1). Papillary and medullary carcinomas develop from radiation-induced mutation of the *RET* proto-oncogene. Mutation of this gene results in the overexpression of a constitutively active tyrosine kinase, which serves as a continuous growth signal for the cell. This promotes persistent cellular proliferation in thyroid cancer.

Treatment

- **Subtotal thyroidectomy,** leaving remnants of thyroid and parathyroid gland for continued hormone production.

- **Total resection and radiation** for poorly differentiated "cold nodule" tumors, like medullary and anaplastic carcinoma, with supplemental thyroid hormone therapy.

- **Radioisotope ^{131}I ablation** for patients with well-differentiated "hot" nodule tumors like papillary and follicular carcinoma.

- **External radiation therapy** for bony metastasis.

Table 40-1 Thyroid cancer subtypes

Cancer type	Frequency	Pathophysiology and pathology	Clinical characteristics
Papillary cancer	80%	• Well differentiated, least aggressive • Cuboidal epithelium, branching papillae • May transform into anaplastic cancer	• Ages 20s to 40s • Link to ionizing radiation exposure • 10-year survival 98%
Follicular cancer	15%	• Moderately well differentiated • Tumor from follicular epithelium • Widely invasive to bone, lungs, liver	• Women in 40s and 50s • Associated with multinodular goiter • 10-year survival 92%
Medullary cancer	5%	• Neuroendocrine neoplasm from parafollicular cells, or *C cells* • Secretes calcitonin, somatostatin, CEA, serotonin, vasoactive intestinal polypeptide (VIP), ACTH, corticotropin-releasing hormone (CRH) • Paraneoplastic syndrome from hormone secretion (e.g., serotonin syndrome)	• Often familial, ages 40s to 50s • Part of the multiple endocrine neoplasia (MEN)-IIA and -IIB syndrome • In MEN-IIB, it is aggressive with early hematogenous metastasis • 5-year survival 50%
Anaplastic cancer	1%	• Undifferentiated tumor of the follicular epithelium; aggressive, early metastasis • May arise from well-differentiated tumor that acquires loss of *p53*	• Older, 65 years old • Associated with multinodular goiter and prior history of papillary thyroid cancer • 5-year survival 5%; 100% mortality

Case Conclusion The FNAB of FC's thyroid nodule revealed a well-differentiated papillary thyroid carcinoma. FC underwent subtotal thyroidectomy. She was given levothyroxine postoperatively. Four months later, she returned for her first ^{131}I radionuclide body scan, which showed no evidence of recurrent cancer.

Thumbnail: Thyroid Cancer

History	Neck mass, hoarseness, dysphagia
Physical exam	Painless, firm nodule on thyroid, cervical lymphadenopathy, bony tenderness (metastases)
Labs	Normal thyroid function tests (TFTs), ↑ thyroglobulin, ↑ calcitonin, ↑ CEA, +*RET* proto-oncogene mutation
Diagnosis	FNA, ultrasound, chest x-ray or CT for metastases
Subtypes	Papillary, follicular, medullary, anaplastic
Treatment	Subtotal thyroidectomy, radioiodine ablation, radiation therapy, hormone replacement

Key Points

▶ Carcinogenic agents, including chemicals and ionizing radiation, can give rise to cancer by inducing genetic mutations of specific cancer-promoting genes.

▶ The establishment of permanent DNA damage to a cancer-promoting gene is termed the **initiation** of carcinogenesis. For a carcinogenic mutation to remain within a cell population, it must be **promoted** by cellular proliferation.

▶ Thyroid cancer is a common cancer that arises from exposure to ionizing radiation and subsequent mutation of a proto-oncogene; well-differentiated tumors may later transform into aggressive anaplastic carcinomas.

Questions

1. AP is a 72-year-old woman who presents with a new neck mass that had *quickly grown over the last 2 weeks*. On exam, she had a 2-cm firm and painless nodule in her left thyroid. She has a prior history of goiter. Currently, she has normal thyroid function tests as well as normal serum calcitonin and CEA levels. Given her clinical picture, what are the most likely diagnosis and prognosis?

   A. Follicular cancer—92% 5-year survival
   B. Anaplastic cancer—5% 5-year survival
   C. Papillary cancer—98% 10-year survival
   D. Medullary cancer—50% 5-year survival
   E. Multinodular goiter—100% 5-year survival

2. The following is a series of steps in the pathogenesis of FC's thyroid cancer. Which is least likely to be included?

   A. X-ray radiation induced mutation of the *RET* proto-oncogene that initiated the transformation of a single thyroid cell toward neoplastic growth.
   B. Chronic exposure to radiation likely promoted the accumulation of several carcinogenic mutations, increasing the likelihood of a single cell to become malignant.
   C. Normal physiologic proliferation of thyroid cells may have propagated a chance mutation into the following generations of cells, making that "mistake" permanent.
   D. Promotion of tumor growth occurred due to the acquisition of genetic mutations yielding more unregulated growth.
   E. Papillary carcinoma arose from excessive stimulation of normal thyroid cells by TSH.

HPI: MV is an 8-year-old girl who is brought in by her father after a month of markedly increasing "clumsiness." In the last month, he had noticed her frequently bumping into furniture and walls, although she denies blurry vision. She never had such symptoms before, and has no significant past medical history or any family history of any eye diseases.

PE: The patient is comfortable-appearing with normal vital signs. Her exam is significant for an **absent red reflex on the right eye,** normal visual acuity on the left eye, but **20/400 vision on the right eye.** She has a visual field consistent with **left monocular vision.** Her funduscopic exam revealed normal structures on the left eye and none in her right eye. She had no sensory or motor deficits, normal reflexes, negative Romberg's sign, but a slightly ataxic gait.

Thought Questions

- What are proto-oncogenes, tumor suppressor genes, apoptosis-regulating genes, and DNA repair genes, and how do these genes contribute to the development of malignancy?

- What is retinoblastoma and what are the underlying steps in its pathogenesis?

Basic Science Review and Discussion

Now that we have established the point that cancer arises from genetic mutations that promote unregulated cellular proliferation, we turn to the specific molecular events that mediate carcinogenesis. These molecular mechanisms fall under two main categories: (1) *those that promote growth,* and (2) those that *promote genetic mutation.* These two fundamental characteristics are mutually enhancing, that is, growth promotes mutation as mutation promotes growth. Under the categories of growth promotion, there are three contributing classes of genes: (1) **proto-oncogenes,** (2) **tumor-suppressor genes,** and (3) **apoptosis-regulating genes.** In the latter category, defective **DNA repair genes,** which normally act to maintain genomic integrity, increase the chance of developing a mutation in a growth-promoting gene and thus cause tumor growth indirectly. The following is a review of these main molecular mediators of neoplasia.

Proto-Oncogenes   Proto-oncogenes can be viewed as the "green-light" signal for the cell to undergo cell cycling. In a normal cell, the signal to divide is transiently released, and only after several molecular events occur. Such signals are normally tightly controlled by an elaborate system of growth-promoting and growth-inhibiting signals. But when a mutation compromises the regulation of a proto-oncogene, it can promote the uncontrolled growth of a cell (Table 41-1). The involved molecular mediators include (1) growth factors, (2) growth factor receptors, (3) signal transducers, (4) nuclear transcription proteins, and (5) cell-cycle regulating factors.

Growth factors are secreted proteins that bind a cell receptor and signal it to grow. Overexpression of growth factors due to a genetic mutation can promote cellular hyperplasia. **Growth factor receptors** receive the signal for growth and transmit that information to the intracellular compartment. Mutations in this class of proto-oncogenes can cause such a receptor to be *constitutively active* (e.g., it is always "on"), signaling a cell to undergo cell cycling, even in the absence of the growth factor. Alternatively, abnormal overexpression of the receptor on the cell surface may make a cell highly sensitive to even small amounts of growth factor and can also accelerate growth.

Signal-transducing proteins include any of the proteins within the cytoplasm that transmit the external signal for growth to the nucleus. Mutations in the **ras protein,** a tyrosine kinase involved in growth signaling, is one of the most common abnormalities found in tumors. It is activated by growth-factor receptors and ultimately promotes transcription and translation of *myc,* a cell-cycle regulator. There are many promoters, activators, and inactivators of the ras protein, and mutations that cause dysfunction of any of these regulators can cause constitutively active *ras* and thus uninhibited cell cycling. This is present in neurofibromatosis-1, wherein a defect in the *neurofibrin-1* gene prevents proper inhibition of the *ras* gene product. **Nuclear transcription proteins** are proteins that respond to the cytoplasmic growth-promoting signals and participate in intranuclear DNA binding that either up-regulates or down-regulates expression of specific genes. Important examples of such proto-oncogenes are *myc, max,* and *mad,* which interact to either promote or inhibit cellular replication. If *max* dimerizes with *myc,* proliferation and survival is promoted. If *max*

Table 41-1 Methods of mutagenesis and some examples

Point mutation	*ras* mutations in many cancers
Translocations	Burkitt's lymphoma: *c-myc* in front of immunoglobulin heavy chain gene Chronic myeloid leukemia: t(9,22) → *bcr-abl,* constitutively active tyrosine kinase
Gene amplification	*c-erb B2* amplification in breast cancer

dimerizes with *mad* (forming *mad-max*), cell growth is inhibited. Dysregulation of c-*myc* expression is present in Burkitt's lymphoma, breast, colon, and lung cancers.

Cell-cycle regulating proteins, or cyclins and cyclin-dependent kinases (CDKs) direct the orderly progression of the cell cycle during mitosis. CDK inhibitors inhibit cell-cycle progression. Overexpression of CDKs and hypo-functioning or insufficient expression of CDK inhibitors similarly promote tumor growth.

Tumor-Suppressor Genes   **Tumor-suppressor genes** act as the "brakes" of cellular proliferation in that they *inhibit the signals that promote cell cycling.* The ***Rb* gene** is the proto-typic tumor-suppressor gene found in patients with retinoblastoma. **pRb** (or the *Rb* gene product) binds a transcriptional activator, the E2F protein, and keeps it from binding DNA and promoting cell cycling. Normally, pRb is present throughout a cell's nonreplicating life. But as soon as a growth factor signals a cell to grow, pRB is inactivated by cyclin or CDK, thereby releasing E2F. This allows the cell to undergo cell division. Many things can interfere with pRb's ability to inhibit E2F. For instance, HPV produces a protein that binds *pRb.* This can result in the development of HPV-induced **cervical cancer.**

The other important tumor-suppressor gene is *p53,* also known as the "guardian of the genome" in that it acts through several mechanisms to protect the cell from genetic damage. *p53* senses DNA damage, promotes DNA repair, delays cell cycle progression (and thereby allows time for such repair), and induces apoptosis if the DNA is inadequately repaired. It repairs damage from UV light, irradiation, and other mutagenic substances. Loss of such important functions predisposes a cell to progressive accumulation of genetic mutations that may cause it to resist death or proliferate unregulated. *p53* is the most common mutation in human tumors and is present in over 50% of such cases.

Apoptosis-Regulating Genes   There are two classic regulators of programmed cell death, or **apoptosis.** *Bcl-2* inhibits apoptosis, while *bax* promotes it. Overexpression of *bcl-2* is implicated in the development in B-cell lymphoma.

DNA Repair Genes   Genetic mutations that cause defective DNA repair inherently predispose a cell to accumulating more cancer-promoting mutations. This mechanism of carcinogenesis is unique in that it does not directly promote tumor growth or survival but instead provides the condition within which a cell has an increased likelihood of acquiring a mutation in the genes that do so. This is present in **xeroderma pigmentosum,** where a congenital defect in DNA repair increases the risk of developing cancer due to DNA damage induced by UV light.

Two-Hit Hypothesis and Retinoblastoma   Retinoblastoma is a rare tumor of the eye, presenting in children from birth to 15 years of age. Among patients with retinoblastoma, it was noted that those with the familial form of retinoblastoma were heterozygotes for a mutant *Rb* gene, despite the fact that the disease is inherited in an autosomal-dominant fashion. From this, the **"two-hit" hypothesis of carcinogenesis** arose, wherein it is thought that the loss of two copies of a tumor-suppressor gene is required for malignant transformation. In those with familial retinoblastoma, a nonfunctioning *Rb* gene is inherited from a parent and is present in all somatic cells. Among those cells, particularly in the eye, one cell may acquire a genetic mutation that renders the remaining normal *Rb* gene non-functional. Only when this happens will one develop a retinoblastoma. Otherwise, in sporadic cases of retinoblastoma, the loss of two copies of the *Rb* gene occurs through two separate chance mutations, thus making it less likely an occurrence. This is an important concept and has been applied to many different tumors since it was first proposed for retinoblastoma.

Case Conclusion   An MRI of the head is performed, which reveals a tumor localized within the right orbit with no apparent extraorbital extension. MV is diagnosed with retinoblastoma and subsequently undergoes radiation therapy. She is currently stable 2 months after therapy.

Thumbnail: Genes and Proteins of Carcinogenesis

Gene or protein type	Subtype	Examples
Proto-oncogenes	Growth factors	FGF, bFGF, epidermal-derived growth factor (EDGF), transforming growth factor-α (TGF-α)
	Growth factor receptors	EDGF receptor
	Signal-transducing proteins	ras, abl
	Nuclear transcription factor	myc
	Cyclin and cyclin-dependent kinases (CDK)	Cyclin D, CDK4
Tumor-suppressor genes	—	p53, pRb
Apoptosis-regulating genes	Antiapoptotic	bcl-2
	Proapoptotic	bax
DNA repair genes	—	p53

Key Points

▶ Carcinogenesis is mediated by mutations in growth-regulating and DNA-repairing genes.

▶ Proto-oncogenes turn into oncogenes, which promote unregulated proliferation of cells.

▶ Tumor-suppressor genes inhibit factors that promote cell proliferation.

▶ Overexpression of antiapoptotic genes promotes cell survival and prevents the death of cells, even those normally destined for programmed cell death.

▶ DNA repair gene defects indirectly promote carcinogenesis by increasing the likelihood of developing mutations in the above genes.

▶ In the "two-hit" hypothesis, homozygote loss of tumor-suppressor gene function, like the *Rb* gene in retinoblastoma, is required for malignant transformation.

▶ Therefore those with familial retinoblastoma inherit one defective *Rb* gene in all somatic cells constituting the "first hit."

▶ A chance acquisition of a genetic mutation causing functional loss of the other *Rb* gene in just one of those cells constitutes the "second hit."

Questions

1. AG, a 32-year-old woman with known family history of hereditary nonpolyposis colon cancer (HNPCC) syndrome, is returning for her annual screening colonoscopy. One of the biopsy samples reveal changes concerning for malignancy. HNPCC results from defects in genes involved in DNA mismatch repair (i.e., repair of mismatched base pairs during replication, for example, C pairing to A). What step in the pathogenesis of this carcinoma is NOT likely to have occurred?

   A. AG inherited one defective DNA mismatch repair gene.

   B. One cell among all her colonic epithelial cells acquired a mutation that made the other copy of the repair gene nonfunctional.

   C. A chance error during replication led to a faulty pairing (e.g., G to T), which remained unrepaired.

   D. The defect in DNA mismatch repair transformed this cell into a malignant cell capable of unregulated proliferation.

   E. Accumulation of errors led to the dysfunction of several gene products involved in growth and cell-cycle regulation.

2. Burkitt's lymphoma is a B-cell lymphoma that results from the t(14;18)(q32;q21) translocation (32nd section of the long arm or "q" on chromosome 14 translocated upon q21 on chromosome 18). This translocation juxtaposes the site where immunoglobulin heavy-chain genes are found next to the *bcl-2* locus (on 18q21). What step in the pathogenesis of this cancer is NOT likely to occur?

   A. Chronic infection promotes B-cell differentiation into antibody-secreting plasma cells.

   B. A plasma cell with the t(14;18) translocation is stimulated to transcribe the immunoglobulin heavy-chain locus in the attempt to produce antibodies.

   C. *Bcl-2* is instead transcribed and translated to high levels of bcl-2 protein in the cytoplasm.

   D. The overabundance of *bcl-2* gene product promotes uncontrolled cellular proliferation of that transformed cell.

   E. The *bcl-2* gene product in excess forms *bcl-2* homodimers (bound pairs of bcl-2) producing an antiapoptotic signal that promotes cell survival.

HPI: JL is a 16-year-old boy who hurt his leg snowboarding 7 months ago. Since then, he has tried splinting, rest, elevation, and ice to alleviate the pain. It has waxed and waned, but has recently gotten worse. It responds partially to ibuprofen and acetaminophen. He now complains of an enlarging, firm, tender mass above the knee. PMH: no significant illnesses. PSHx: none. FamHx: both parents alive with no significant medical illness. Meds: ibuprofen, acetaminophen.

PE: T 36.9°C HR 64/min RR 14/min BP 114/63
General: alert, oriented teenager in no distress. Growth: Ht 70th %ile, Wt 60th %ile. Neck: supple, no masses. Chest: clear to auscultation with normal respiratory effort. GU: Tanner IV male, descended testes. Extremities: The right distal femur has a tender, palpable mass about 10 cm in diameter. All extremities are warm and well perfused.
Neuro: normal for age. Lymph: no enlarged lymph nodes.
An x-ray shows a lytic lesion with pronounced periosteal elevation.

Thought Questions

- What are the most common malignancies of bone?

- What imaging studies are needed?

- What additional studies are required for staging a malignant bone tumor?

- What are genetic features of bone tumors?

- What is the treatment and outcome?

Basic Science Review and Discussion

Metastatic bone disease and **multiple myeloma** are far more common than primary bone tumors. Bone sarcomas are extremely rare tumors that represent only 0.2% of new malignancies. The most frequent malignant tumors of bone are osteosarcoma, chondrosarcoma, and Ewing's sarcoma. The most frequent benign tumors are osteochondroma and giant cell tumor, which may be aggressive or transform into malignant tumors in certain familial syndromes.

Osteosarcoma Osteosarcoma accounts for over 20% of primary bone malignancies. It is common in adolescence and early adulthood, occurring almost exclusively during the pubertal growth spurt. It frequently arises in the diaphyses and metaphyses of long bones, particularly of the distal femur or proximal tibia (around the knee). Genetic factors implicated in the development of osteosarcoma include the loss of the tumor suppressor genes *p53* and *Rb*. Incidence is increased in **Li-Fraumeni syndrome** and congenital retinoblastoma. Radiation is a major risk factor for osteosarcoma, especially in genetically susceptible individu-

als. Under light microscopy, osteosarcoma consists of large, primitive cells producing disorganized osteoid. On x-ray imaging, the typical appearance is called the **"sunburst effect"** or **Codman's triangle**, which is created as the expanding tumor lifts the periosteum. Osteosarcoma metastasizes primarily to the lungs, via venous drainage. Therefore, lung imaging with x-ray and CT is critical for staging. Treatment is with intensive chemotherapy and surgery. Active agents are methotrexate, doxorubicin hydrochloride (Adriamycin), cisplatin, and, recently, ifosfamide. Osteosarcoma is resistant to radiation therapy.

Ewing's Sarcoma Ewing's sarcoma is the second most common primary malignant bone tumor of childhood. It can present as early as 3 years old. Like osteosarcoma, Ewing's can present in the long bones around the knee, but can also be found in pelvic bones, scapulae, and ribs. Ewing's sarcoma is characterized by a t(11;22) translocation that creates a fusion gene *EWS-FLI1*. This creates a chimeric transcription factor that leads to malignant transformation. Histologically, Ewing's sarcoma is composed of monotonous small round blue cells with little stroma. Similar to osteosarcoma, metastasis to the lungs is common.

Definitive resection with wide margins is essential to cure either of these tumors. This occurs after a period of induction chemotherapy to decrease the soft tissue component of the tumor. This commonly results in limb amputation; endoprostheses are in development. Radiation therapy may be used in place of surgery for Ewing's sarcoma. Prognosis depends on tumor stage. Overall, localized disease has a long-term survival rate of about 70%, but metastatic tumors only about 15%. Other risk factors for relapse include poor histologic response to chemotherapy, and large primary tumors.

Case Conclusion JL undergoes MRI of the leg, chest x-ray, and chest CT. These studies show four metastatic nodules in the chest. Bone biopsy reveals large malignant cells with immature osteoid, showing osteosarcoma. Immunohistochemistry for Her-2/neu is positive. No bone marrow biopsy is indicated. He is treated with high-dose methotrexate, cisplatin, Adriamycin, and ifosfamide. The primary lesion is resected with an above-the-knee amputation after 12 weeks of chemotherapy. The surgical specimen shows tumor necrosis of only 75%, indicating a poor response. Chemotherapy lasts 9 months, after which JL has no measurable disease and good function. However, he is likely to relapse within 5 years, and at that point will be a candidate for experimental therapy using anti-Her-2/neu therapeutics.

Thumbnail: Select Bone Tumors

Type	Location	Incidence	Description
Benign osteochondroma	Metaphyses: lower femur/upper tibia	Men under 25 years; most common benign bone tumor	Bony growth with cartilage cap projecting from bone surface; malignant transformation in *multiple familial osteochondromatosis*
Giant cell tumor	Epiphyses of long bones: lower femur, upper tibia	Women age 20–40 years	Multinucleated giant cells; "soap bubble" appearance on x-ray; aggressive regrowth
Malignant metastases	Variable	Variable; most common with kidney, thyroid, testes, lung, prostate, and breast primaries	Breast/prostate most common; breast: lytic and blastic; prostate: blastic; lung: lytic
Multiple myeloma	Skull, axial skeleton	Older adults	Punched out lytic lesions associated with hypercalcemia
Osteosarcoma	Metaphyses: lower femur/upper tibia	Boys age 10–20 years; most common primary malignant bone tumor; risk factors: Paget's disease, radiation, familial retinoblastoma	Bone-producing tumor; Codman's triangle on x-ray; ↑↑ alkaline phosphatase; early metastases to lung, liver, brain
Chondrosarcoma	Pelvis, spine, scapula, ribs, proximal humerus	Men age 30–60; ↑ in *multiple familial osteochondromatosis*	Cartilaginous tumor
Ewing's sarcoma	Long bones, pelvis, scapula, ribs	Boys under 15	Small cell tumor; 11;22 chromosomal translocation

Key Points

▶ Metastatic bone tumors and multiple myeloma are far more common than primary bone tumors.

▶ Osteosarcoma is the most common primary malignant bone tumor and it affects primarily children and adolescents. It is more common in boys.

▶ Ewing's sarcoma is the second most common primary malignant bone tumor in children.

Questions

1. An otherwise healthy 9-year-boy has a mass growing below his knee. At surgery, the mass is removed and sent to the pathology department. Sheets of hyperchromatic cells with small round blue nuclei are seen under the microscope. Cytogenic analysis reveals a t(11;22) translocation. What is the most likely diagnosis?

    A. Osteosarcoma
    B. Multiple myeloma
    C. Giant cell tumor
    D. Metastatic disease
    E. Ewing's sarcoma

2. Which bone tumor(s) frequently metastasize to the lungs?

    A. Osteosarcoma
    B. Ewing's sarcoma
    C. Giant cell tumor
    D. A and B
    E. B and C

HPI: DP is a 58-year-old man who presents with 2 months of progressively worsening **abdominal pain** with alternating bouts of **constipation and diarrhea.** He describes the pain as colicky, dull, and worsening before his bowel movements. He has noted a gradual **thinning of his stool caliber** with occasional **streaks of blood** on the stool. The consistency of his stool also alternates between firm and loose. He also notes worsening **fatigue and weakness.** He denies having fevers, chills, unexplained weight loss, urgency to defecate, or frank hematochezia. He has no significant past medical history. He has **one paternal uncle who died of colon cancer** at the age of 65.

PE: T 37.6°C HR 98 BP 115/85 RR 24, SaO2 96%
The patient is a thin, pale man in mild discomfort. His exam is significant for a soft, nondistended abdomen with moderate **diffuse tenderness to palpation** in the **hypogastric area** without peritoneal signs. There is a **palpable fullness in the left lower quadrant.** He has no hepatosplenomegaly. On rectal exam, there are no masses or frank blood in his rectal vault. His **stool** is brown but **positive for occult blood.**

Labs: **Hct 29%, MCV 79 fL,** normal liver function tests (AST, ALT, alkaline phosphatase, total and direct bilirubin), **CEA 32 ng/mL** (nl < 5.0 ng/mL).

Thought Questions

- What is the natural history of polyps and colorectal cancer?

- What molecular pathogenesis underlies the development of colorectal cancer?

- What are the clinical manifestations of colorectal cancer and how is it diagnosed and treated?

Basic Science Review and Discussion

Colorectal cancer is the second leading cause of death due to cancer. It is highly prevalent, affecting 6% of the U.S. population and is lethal if not detected early, killing 40% of those who have it. It not only is an important disease epidemiologically, but it also illustrates several fundamental concepts in oncology. For instance, colorectal cancer defies the age-old mantra that *benign tumors do not give rise to malignant tumors.* Colorectal cancer follows what is called the **adenoma-carcinoma sequence,** a process wherein progressive epithelial hyperplasia and dysplasia lead to the development of a carcinoma. Underlying this histologic tumorigenesis is a **multistep molecular carcinogenesis,** wherein sequential loss of critical DNA repair and cell-cycle regulating functions causes a polyp to progressively become more malignant. Familial syndromes provide examples of carcinogenesis governed by the **two-hit hypothesis** (see Case 41, Molecular Oncology). Lastly, tumor biology is revisited as the rate of tumor growth and the pattern of malignant spread have direct clinical importance in early detection, staging, treatment, and prognosis of colorectal cancer.

The Pathology of Colorectal Cancer Polyps are intraluminal protrusions of colonic mucosa. They include nonneoplastic tissue such as juvenile polyps (a hamartoma), hyperplastic polyps, and adenomatous polyps. **Adenomatous polyps** consist of proliferative mucosal epithelium in the colon. They grow and evolve over years, and a small percentage of them evolve into colorectal cancer. They have three architectural subtypes: (1) **tubular adenomas,** (2) **villous adenomas,** and (3) **tubulovillous adenomas** (Figure 43-1). Tubular adenomas are *pedunculated,* having long, slender fibrovascular stalks that tether the dysplastic epithelial glands to the intestinal wall. Villous adenomas are long, "finger-like" projections that are *sessile,* or without a well-defined stalk that separates the dysplastic glands from the colon wall. Thus these lesions invade earlier than tubular adenomas, and polypectomy is often not sufficient to remove all neoplastic tissue. Lastly, tubulovillous adenomas have properties intermediate to tubular and villous adenomas. Microscopically, the adenomas

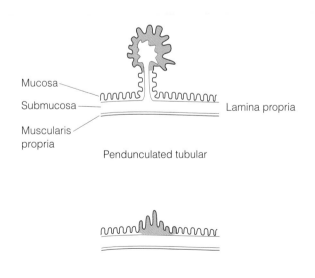

Figure 43-1 Morphology of adenomatous polyps.

consist of neoplastic glands lined with tall, hyperchromatic epithelium with varying degrees of disorganization depending of the level of dysplasia. Severe dysplasia confined to the mucosa is considered **carcinoma in situ,** a premalignant lesion. As soon as the dysplastic tissue invades the lamina propria, which separates mucosa from submucosa, the adenoma considered an **invasive carcinoma.** It is thought that over time, the population of cells within an adenomatous polyp can increase in malignancy, thus turning a benign hyperplasia into an adenocarcinoma. The slow rate of tumor growth makes early detection through screening highly effective at reducing rates of colorectal carcinoma

Multistep Molecular Carcinogenesis of Colorectal Cancer   The gradual transformation of a benign hyperplastic polyp to an invasive adenocarcinoma necessarily corresponds to a carcinogenic process occurring at the molecular level. Neoplastic transformation results from multiple stages of genetic mutation as a cell population increases in malignancy. Thus, no single defect can transform a normal polyp into a cancerous polyp. The gradual accumulation of mutations in cancer-related genes allows a cell population to evolve toward more rapid proliferation and spread. This is classically demonstrated by the molecular model proposed for the evolution of colorectal cancer (Figure 43-2).

Thus "malignancy" is not merely a designation based on the histologic presence of cells beyond an arbitrarily chosen boundary (e.g., the basement membrane). These cells demonstrate a clear deviation from normal behavior, which, by virtue of being "in the wrong place," strongly suggests a change in genetic information making such cells malignant.

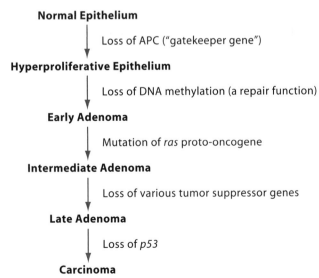

Figure 43-2 Multistep carcinogenesis of colorectal cancer. Progression of epithelial dysplasia is due to underlying genetic mutations that progressively increase the malignant behavior of the cell population.

Familial Syndromes   Familial adenomatous polyposis (FAP) is a classic familial polyposis syndrome. It has an autosomal-dominant pattern of inheritance and its **penetrance,** or the likelihood that the disease genotype will result in the disease phenotype, is 100% (i.e., all individuals with this condition will develop colorectal cancer within their lifetime). Whereas this disease is **genotypically** autosomal **recessive,** given that these individuals are born heterozygous for the mutation, it is **phenotypically** autosomal **dominant** in that all individuals are likely to become homozygous for the mutation and thus develop the disease. Those with FAP have inherited a germline mutation in one of the copies of their *APC* gene (adenomatous polyposis coli). This gene is considered the **"gatekeeper" gene** of colorectal cancer, as it is the necessary mutation required to initiate carcinogenesis in this disease. The APC protein works by binding and inactivating a transcription factor called β-catenin that normally initiates cell cycling. Without sufficient levels of the APC protein, β-catenin levels go unchecked and drive cellular proliferation. Those who acquire a mutation in the other copy of their APC gene acquire the homozygote genotype required for entry into multistep carcinogenesis. These individuals develop hundreds to thousands of adenomatous polyps in their colon, one of which will develop into adenocarcinoma within the individual's lifetime.

Hereditary nonpolyposis colorectal cancer (HNPCC) is a similar familial colorectal cancer syndrome that arises from a different genotype. This condition arises from a genetic defect in DNA mismatch repair genes, which confers genetic instability to a cell, which subsequently develops the homozygous genotype for the mutation. This malignancy is less likely associated with polyps, and multiple sites of cancer may be found within the colon.

Clinical Discussion   Colorectal cancer occurs mostly in older adults ages 60 to 79 years. Patients present with the signs and symptoms outlined in Table 43-1, depending on tumor location.

Laboratory findings may include iron deficiency **anemia** in those with chronic occult blood loss, **elevated liver function tests** for those with metastases to the liver, and elevated levels of **CEA,** a protein produced by the neoplasm, which can be used to monitor tumor progression after surgical resection. All patients over 45 years old with hematochezia, unexplained iron deficiency anemia, or occult blood in the stool with recent changes in bowel habits must be evaluated for cancer. Colonoscopy with biopsy is both the screening and diagnostic procedure of choice. Other diagnostic tools mentioned below are less sensitive. Other imaging modalities can be used to rule out metastatic spread. Definitive treatment is resection with or without chemotherapy or radiation therapy.

Table 43-1 Clinical presentation of colorectal cancer at different locations

Location	Clinical manifestations	Pathophysiologic explanation
Right-sided carcinoma	Fatigue Weakness Iron deficiency anemia	Exophytic mass projects into the lumen but rarely causes obstruction because of the right colon's large caliber; such lesions easily bleed from traction on the tumor causing chronic blood loss
Left-sided carcinoma	Occult bleeding, melena Diarrhea Constipation Crampy left-lower-quadrant discomfort	Tumor is often circumferential, causing significant obstruction of the smaller caliber left colon; this can cause symptoms of obstruction (e.g., constipation, crampy LLQ pain) with intermittent diarrhea as well as chronic blood loss
Sigmoidorectal carcinoma	Tenesmus Narrowed stool caliber Hematochezia	Obstruction due to severe narrowing of distal intestinal lumen causes narrowing of stool caliber; it can lead to painful spasms of the anal sphincter with an urgent desire to defecate; traction on the tumor caused by stool and straining can cause grossly visible rectal bleeding

Case Conclusion DP undergoes a colonoscopy and is found to have a 3-cm-long annular ("napkin ring") lesion constricting the distal bowel. He subsequently undergoes surgical resection of his distal bowel and lymph node dissection. Pathologic examination reveals extension of the neoplasm into the bowel wall with subserosal and serosal infiltration. Dissected lymph nodes reveal malignant infiltration. Full-body MRI reveals no evidence of metastatic spread. Thus DP is determined to have American Joint Committee on Classification (of colorectal cancer) (AJCC) stage III disease, giving him a 30% to 50% chance of survival at 5 years. He is started on adjuvant chemotherapy upon discharge. He is subsequently followed by an oncologist with regular clinical exams and labs every 3 months for the next 3 to 5 years.

Thumbnail: Colorectal Cancer

Etiology and pathogenesis	Adenoma → carcinoma in situ → invasive adenocarcinoma → metastatic disease Multistep carcinogenesis: mutations in DNA repair genes and tumor-suppressor genes		
Pathology	**Tubular adenoma**	**Villous adenomas**	**Tubulovillous adenomas**
Risk factors	Age ≥ 50 years old (peak ages 60–79); diets rich in fat/red meat and low in fiber, vitamins A, C, E deficiency		
History of present illness	R-sided proximal lesions • Fatigue and weakness • Iron deficiency anemia	L-sided distal lesions • Occult bleeding, melena • Diarrhea or constipation • Crampy LLQ pain	Sigmoidal/rectal lesions • Tenesmus • Urgency • Hematochezia
	Invasive/metastatic disease: low-grade fever, weakness, malaise, weight loss		
Past medical history	History of colorectal cancer, adenomatous polyps (esp. if multiple, > 1 cm, villous, or poorly differentiated); inflammatory bowel disease (ulcerative colitis, Crohn's disease)		
Family history	Familial adenomatous polyposis (FAP); hereditary nonpolyposis colorectal cancer (HNPCC)		
Physical exam	Usually normal unless disease is advanced (e.g., hepatomegaly with hepatic metastasis)		
Lab findings	Iron deficiency anemia, ↑ CEA, ↑ liver function tests		
Imaging	Barium enema; chest x-ray; abdominal CT for staging, pelvic MRI, endorectal ultrasonography		
Differential Dx	Inflammatory bowel disease, diverticular disease, ischemic colitis, infection, hemorrhoids, irritable bowel syndrome (IBS)		
Screening and diagnosis	• Colonoscopy (screening for those > 50 years old) • Flexible sigmoidoscopy (FS)	• Annual fecal occult blood testing (FOBT) • Barium enema	

Staging and prognosis	American Joint Committee on Classification		Dukes class	5-year survival
	Stage 0	Carcinoma in situ	—	—
	Stage I	Tumor invades submucosa or muscularis propria	Dukes A	80–100%
	Stage II	Tumor invades into subserosa, visceral peritoneum, or other organs and structures	Dukes B_1/B_2	50–75%
	Stage III	Bowel wall invasion with positive lymph node	Dukes C_1/C_2	30–50%
	Stage IV	Distant metastasis	Dukes D	5%

Key Points

▶ The adenoma-carcinoma sequence is a process of progressive epithelial hyperplasia and dysplasia leading to the development of a carcinoma.

▶ Tumorigenesis parallels a multistep molecular carcinogenesis as a tumor progressively becomes more malignant with the sequential loss of critical DNA repair and cell-cycle regulatory functions.

▶ The "two-hit" hypothesis governs the development of familial colon cancers.

▶ All patients over 45 years old with hematochezia, unexplained iron deficiency anemia, or occult blood in the stool with recent changes in bowel habits must be evaluated for cancer.

Questions

1. Which adenoma is most likely to be a stage III disease at the time of diagnosis?
   A. Tubular adenoma
   B. Carcinoma in situ
   C. Tubulovillous adenoma
   D. Villous adenoma
   E. Juvenile polyp

2. AG is a 25-year-old woman who presents complaining of fatigue and weakness and recent changes in bowel habits, including intermittent bouts of diarrhea and constipation. The following is a list of possible diagnoses that one must consider. Which is she least likely to have?
   A. Inflammatory bowel disease
   B. Chronic infectious gastroenteritis with intermittent dehydration
   C. Irritable bowel disease
   D. Sporadic colorectal cancer
   E. Familial colorectal cancer

3. TM is 76-year-old woman who presents with iron deficiency anemia, no changes in stool caliber or bowel habits, no hematochezia, no tenesmus or crampy abdominal pain. What would NOT be included in her diagnostic evaluation?
   A. Fecal occult blood test
   B. Colonoscopy with biopsy
   C. Barium enema
   D. Serum CEA levels
   E. Flexible sigmoidoscopy
   F. Complete CBC
   G. Liver function tests

HPI: PS, a 5-year-old boy, presents with 1 week of **low-grade fever,** sore throat, and persistent chest pain. The pain is localized to the sternum and is refractory to ibuprofen. The parents noted that he has not been as active during play, **bruised easily,** and had **frequent nosebleeds** in the past several months. They also noted constipation, with increased crying and distress associated with bowel movements in the last 2 days. **PMH:** Monthly episodes of upper respiratory infections including two hospitalizations for pneumonia in the last year.

PE: T 38.0°C HR 105 BP 100/63 RR 28 SaO$_2$ 97%
The patient is thin and pale. He has **multiple petechiae** in his oral mucosa with **pharyngeal erythema** and purulent exudate. **Sternal rub elicits tenderness.** The lungs are clear. Cardiac auscultation is normal. He has a **tender hepatosplenomegaly.** His extremities are cool with multiple **ecchymoses** on all extremities. Rectal exam reveals a small, tender perirectal mass compatible with an **abscess.** He is neurologically intact with no abnormalities on fundal exam.

Labs: **WBC 2200/μL,** Hg 6.5 g/dL, **Hct 20%,** platelets 75,000/μL, MCV 90 fL. The differential blood count shows 15% neutrophils, **74% lymphocytes,** 2% bands, 6% monocytes, and **3% blasts.** Na 139, **K 3.5,** Cl 100, HCO$_3$ 23, BUN 21, Cr 0.8. Throat cultures grow *Pseudomonas* sp. Given the **pancytopenia with predominance of lymphocytes,** a bone marrow aspirate and biopsy are performed showing **95% cellularity (normal 20–80%) with 75% blasts.**

Thought Questions

- What is the normal differentiation of hematopoietic cells?

- What is the genetic basis of acute leukemia? What is the etiology?

- What are the clinical manifestations of acute leukemia? What is in the differential diagnosis?

Basic Science Review and Discussion

All blood cells arise from a common pluripotent stem cell via hematopoietic differentiation. The first step in hematopoiesis is the differentiation into lymphoid and myeloid stem cells. These stem cells give rise to their respective blasts cells, the precursors to the final mature cells. Mature cells from the myeloid lineage include monocytes/macrophages, erythrocytes, megakaryocytes/platelets, neutrophils, eosinophils, and basophils. Mature lymphoid cells include T-lymphocytes, B-lymphocytes (which further differentiate into plasma cells), and possibly natural killer cells (Figure 44-1). As maturation progresses during normal hematopoiesis, there is a potential for a single cell to transform and divide unregulated by normal growth signals. In acute leukemia, malignant transformation of an immature "blast" cell with concurrent arrest of its maturation results in the rapid clonal proliferation of acute leukemia. In contrast, in chronic leukemia, the proliferating leukemic cells undergo full maturation, even though malignant transformation occurs at an earlier stage than it does in acute leukemia. The behavior of these more mature cells leads to a more indolent clinical course than that of acute leukemia. There are some conditions that

predispose one to developing acute leukemia, including Down syndrome, familial syndromes (e.g., Fanconi's anemia, ataxia telangiectasia), and previous exposures (e.g., cancer chemotherapy, radiation, benzene); however, most leukemias arise de novo.

Leukemia results from aberrant genetic rearrangements such as translocations, additions, or deletions at the chromosomal or genetic level in hematopoietic cells. Classically, leukemia is a consequence of a nonrandom, balanced chromosomal translocation that can result in the formation of a fusion gene, or **chimeric gene,** that causes, through varying mechanisms, the inappropriate expression of specific oncogenes. This can lead to the disruption of normal cell cycle regulation and thus lead to uncontrolled clonal proliferation. The ultimate phenotype of the leukemia is dependent on the specific genetic aberration and the subsequent behavior of the proliferating cells.

Acute lymphoblastic leukemia comprises 80% of acute leukemias of childhood. Acute myelogenous leukemia occurs mostly in adults, with a median age of onset of 50 years increasing with advanced age. Pathophysiologically, leukemic proliferation in the bone marrow leads to crowding out of normal hematopoietic cells, leading to bone marrow failure. Thus the clinical manifestations of acute leukemia are associated with the resulting **pancytopenia** (neutropenia, anemia, and thrombocytopenia), **leukocytosis,** bone marrow expansion, as well as the infiltration of leukemic cells into the bloodstream, major organs, and other tissues (Table 44-1).

The essential diagnostic feature of acute leukemia is a **hypercellular bone marrow with greater than 30% replacement by blast cells.** Other prominent features include **pancytopenia** and **blasts** in the peripheral blood smear.

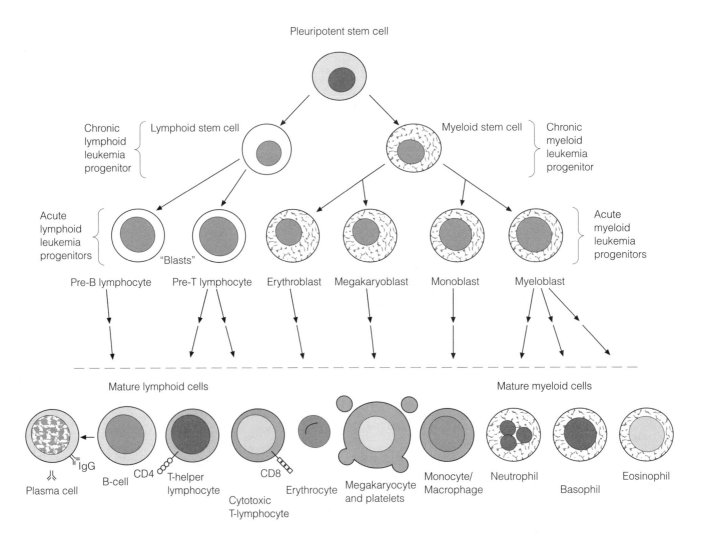

Figure 44-1 Hematopoietic cell differentiation.

Tests can also screen for evidence of soft tissue and bony infiltration as well other causes of pancytopenia or leukocytosis such as parvovirus B19 or infectious mononucleosis from EBV, respectively. Acute myelogenous leukemia (AML) is categorized by morphology and histochemistry from M0 to M7, roughly correlated to the least differentiated to the most differentiated leukemia. Acute lymphocytic leukemia

(ALL) is categorized by morphology into L1 (small uniform blasts of typical childhood ALL), L2 (larger, more variable size cells), and L3 (uniform cells with basophilic or vacuolated cytoplasm). ALL is further subdivided into B-cell and T-cell lineage by the immunohistologic identification of surface antigens, as listed on the next page. Cytogenetics provides significant prognostic information, as well (Box 44-1).

Table 44-1 Presentation of acute leukemias

Pathophysiology	Symptoms	Signs/lab abnormalities
Neutropenia	• Frequent infection, chronic fever • Anorexia • Sweats • Sore throat/oral sores • Rectal pain	• Fever, tachycardia • Weight loss/thin habitus • Diaphoresis • Pharyngitis/dental abscess/stomatitis • Rectal abscess
Anemia	• Fatigue • Dyspnea on exertion	• Pallor • Tachycardia, tachypnea, hypoxemia
Thrombocytopenia	• Excess bleeding • Easy bruising • Epistaxis • Menorrhagia	• Ecchymoses/petechiae • Retinal flame hemorrhages • Signs of chronic bleeding from hypocoagulability
Leukostasis	• Visual changes • Headache/altered mental status	• Leukocytosis with blasts > 100,000/μL • Hypoxemia
Bone marrow expansion	• Bone pain	• Local tenderness
Major organ infiltration esp. with monocytic leukemias	• Early satiety • Headache • Vision changes • Altered mental status	• Tender hepatosplenomegaly • Cranial nerve abnormalities • Papilledema/white retinal exudate • Spinal tenderness/leg weakness
Other soft tissue infiltration	• Skin nodules • Poor dentition • Neck or inguinal masses	• "Leukemia cutis" • Gingival hypertrophy • Lymphadenopathy
High cellular proliferation/death	• Muscle weakness, constipation • Gouty arthritis—joint pain • Vit. K deficiency → coagulopathy • Symptoms of DIC	• Hypokalemia • Hyperuricemia • ↑ PT, normal PTT • Low or falling fibrinogen

DIC, disseminated intravascular coagulopathy; PT, prothrombin time; PTT, partial thromboplastin time.

Box 44-1 Diagnosis of acute leukemia

Definition: **30% or more of bone marrow is replaced by blast cells**
(< 5% blasts is normal; 5–29% blasts is "pre-leukemia," usu. myelodysplasia)
Pearl: WBC > 60,000/μL is almost always some form of leukemia

Diagnostic marker	AML	ALL
Morphologic Cytoplasmic Auer rods	+	−
Histochemical Myeloperoxidase Nonspecific esterase	+ +	− −
Immunologic TdT	−	+

ALL subtype	Surface antigens
Early B-cell	CD10, CD19
T-cell	CD2, CD5, CD7

Differential diagnosis of abnormal blood count

Pancytopenia	Leukocytosis
Acute leukemia	Acute leukemia
Chronic leukemia	Chronic leukemia
EBV, HIV, CMV, parvovirus B19	Acute infection
Chronic infection in marrow	Infectious mononucleosis
Megaloblastic anemia	Corticosteroids
Aplastic anemia	Lithium carbonate intake
Bone marrow replacement	
Myelodysplasia	

Case Conclusion   PS was admitted, and further cytology was performed on the bone marrow biopsy. It was determined that the child had a hyperdiploid ALL. Induction chemotherapy was initiated over 7 days. He was supported with antibiotics and red blood cell and platelet transfusions. GM-CSF was started at the 4th week, and complete remission was achieved with a neutrophil count of 2000/μL, platelets 150,000/μL, and less than 5% bone marrow blasts. Several rounds of consolidation chemotherapy followed. At the age of 30, the patient is doing well, with no evidence of leukemia.

Thumbnail: Acute Leukemias

Pathophysiology	Genetic translocation, addition, deletion, or inversion → aberrant expression of oncogene → cell cycle dysregulation → lymphoid or myeloid blast cell proliferation
Epidemiology	ALL: peak ages 3–7 years old, 80% of childhood acute leukemias AML: more common in adults, 15–40 years old, 20% of childhood leukemias
Symptoms	Short-course of illness, fever, malaise, anorexia, weight loss, excessive bleeding, paleness, bone pain, sore throat, oral lesions, perirectal pain, neurologic deficits
Past medical history	Family history of AML (Fanconi, Bloom), Down syndrome Prior cancer (exposure to alkylating agents, radiation, topoisomerase II inhibitors) Occupational exposures (radiation, benzene, petroleum, smoking, paint, pesticides)
Physical findings	Fever, tachycardia, ecchymosis, papilledema, retinal hemorrhage/infiltrate, gingival hyperplasia, dental abscess, lymphadenopathy, sternal rub tenderness, hepatosplenomegaly, back tenderness, skin infiltration neurologic deficits
Laboratory findings	**Pancytopenia** (neutropenia, anemia, thrombocytopenia) or **leukocytosis** (esp. WBC > 60,000/μL), peripheral blast cells and abnormal PMNs/platelets; hypokalemia, hyperuricemia, ↑ PT, normal PTT, ↓ fibrinogen
Diagnosis	Bone marrow aspiration/biopsy: hypercellular bone marrow (normal 20–80%) **> 30% blasts** (normal < 5%) Differentiate between AML [Auer rods, myeloperoxidase (MPO), nonspecific esterase (NSE)] vs ALL [terminal deoxynucleotidyl transferase (TdT)]; further subtype leukemia according to morphology, surface antigen profile, and cytogenetics
Differential diagnosis	Acute or chronic leukemia, aplastic anemia, myelodysplasia, viral infection, megaloblastic anemia, mononucleosis, drug reaction, stress, infection, malignancy
Prognosis	**Favorable** / **Unfavorable**

Prognosis	**Favorable**	**Unfavorable**
	Younger	Older
	Hyperdiploidy	Complex cytogenetics
	Favorable cytogenetics	Unfavorable cytogenetics, e.g., t(9,22)
	Moderate leukocytosis	Severe leukocytosis
	De novo leukemia	Secondary leukemia
	< 4 wks to complete remission	> 4 wks to complete remission

Key Points

▶ Acute leukemia occurs from a malignant transformation and proliferation of a single leukocyte, giving rise to a monoclonal population of either myeloid or lymphoid cells.

▶ Malignant transformation in acute leukemia occurs at the "blast" stage, with arrest in cell maturation; while in chronic leukemia it occurs at an earlier stage, with no arrest in cell maturation, thus giving rise to a pleomorphic population of "mature" leukemic cells.

▶ The majority of the clinical manifestations arise from the pancytopenia and leukocytosis caused by the crowding out of normal bone marrow cells by proliferating leukemic cells.

▶ Diagnosis aims to identify the leukemia by morphology and histologic and cytogenetic markers, which direct treatment and provide information on prognosis.

Questions

1. A 7-year-old girl presents with a clinical picture suggestive of acute leukemia and a bone marrow biopsy performed showing greater than 30% blasts. Cytologic testing reveals Pre-B-cell ALL with L1 morphology. What diagnostic finding would not correlate with this diagnosis?

   A. TdT+ cells
   B. Small uniform blast cells
   C. CD7+ cells
   D. CD10+ cells
   E. CD22+ cells

2. A 53-year-old woman with a history of gouty arthritis presents with malaise, and bone and joint pain in the left femur and knee. She is slightly febrile and is found to have a WBC of 45,000/μL. What are the possible etiologies of her symptoms?

   A. Hyperuricemia from high cell turnover in acute leukemia, causing gouty arthritis
   B. Leukemic cell proliferation with bone marrow expansion
   C. Recent ingestion of contaminated meat, causing gastroenteritis
   D. Osteomyelitis from immunocompromise induced by steroid therapy
   E. All of the above

HPI: LA, a 42-year old, previously healthy man, presents with 2 months of **fatigue, night sweats,** and **low-grade fever.** He also noted increasingly **poor appetite** with **early satiety,** and 30-pound unexplained **weight loss** in the last 6 months. He has no other symptoms suggesting infection, and has had a recent negative PPD.

PE: T **38.5°C** HR 87 BP 125/85 RR 22 SaO$_2$ 98%
The patient is **thin-appearing.** His exam was remarkable for **sternal rub tenderness** and moderate nontender **splenomegaly,** with no hepatomegaly or lymphadenopathy.

Labs: WBC 150,000/μL, Hct 35%, platelets 515,000/μL. Manual differential on peripheral blood smear revealed **70% neutrophils, 6% bands,** 5% lymphocytes, **10% monocytes, 3% eosinophils, 2% basophils, 1% metamyelocytes, 1% myelocytes, 1% promyelocytes,** and **1% blasts.** A bone marrow biopsy revealed a **100% cellular bone marrow with myeloid and megakaryocytic predominance with less than 5% blasts.** Cytogenetic analysis was performed and the presence of t(9,22) translocation was confirmed.

Thought Questions

■ What are the chronic leukemias?

■ What are the fundamental molecular and cellular events that give rise to chronic leukemias?

■ What are the clinical manifestations of chronic leukemias? How is it diagnosed?

Basic Science Review and Discussion: Chronic Leukemias

Chronic leukemia is a major category of disease wherein mature-appearing blood cells proliferate in the bone marrow and appear in the peripheral circulation. Chronic leukemias consist of two major categories: myeloid and lymphoid lineage diseases (Figure 45-1). Myeloid disorders are

further categorized as myelodysplastic and myeloproliferative disorders. In myelodysplastic syndromes, damage to bone marrow tissue results in failed or insufficient hematopoiesis. In myeloproliferative disorders, damage results in the neoplastic proliferation of one or more hematopoietic cell lines. Lymphoid disorders are subdivided into B-cell and T-cell leukemias. The most common disorders are **chronic myeloid leukemia** (or chronic myelogenous leukemia) **(CML)** and **chronic lymphoid leukemia (CLL).**

CML originates from the nonrandom, balanced chromosomal translocation between chromosomes 9 and 22, or **t(9,22),** producing the *bcr-abl* **fusion gene,** also known as the **Philadelphia chromosome.** The *bcr-abl* gene product is a constitutively active tyrosine kinase enzyme, which continuously signals cell cycling, leading to unregulated cellular proliferation. This may occur in a single myeloid stem cell, causing **monoclonal proliferation** of that cell line, likely related to exposure to high-dose radiation.

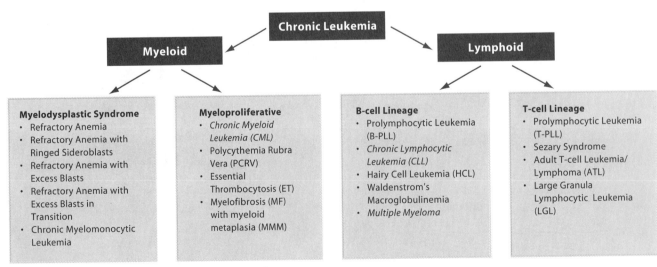

Figure 45-1 Chronic leukemias (common forms in *italics*).

The distinctive cytologic feature of chronic leukemia is the continuation of cellular maturation as the cell line proliferates, in contrast to that of acute leukemia where maturation is arrested. Clinically, this results in a more indolent course, wherein normal hematologic function is retained for many years before complete hematologic failure. Acute leukemia, on the other hand, follows a more fulminant course and is fatal without immediate treatment. In the chronic phase of chronic leukemia, leukemic proliferation continues while normal hematopoiesis is retained. But the malignant clone is chromosomally unstable, and it acquires additional genetic abnormalities. If left untreated, CML will progress to an accelerated phase, then eventually to a blast crisis, which is indistinguishable from acute leukemia.

CLL is a neoplastic proliferation of mostly B-lymphocytes. It is associated with several cytogenetic abnormalities, including those in chromosomes 13q and 14q, as well as trisomy 12. These abnormalities result in the accumulation of dysfunctional lymphocytes in the peripheral circulation, and thus manifest in **immunosuppression** from inadequate B-cell antibody production. Crowding out of normal hematopoietic cells in the bone marrow eventually leads to **bone marrow failure.** Leukemic cells infiltrate lymph nodes and other soft tissue as well. Unlike CML, CLL can also cause

autoimmune disease such as **autoimmune hemolytic anemia** and **immune thrombocytopenia,** from aberrant antibody production from neoplastic B-cells.

Clinical Discussion CML occurs in young and middle-aged adults, starting from age 30 and rising rapidly after the mid-forties. Most patients are diagnosed while asymptomatic during routine health screening. Table 45-1 outlines the pathophysiology of chronic leukemias and their clinical manifestations. Many patients present in the chronic phase with fatigue, night sweats, malaise, decreased appetite, and weight loss (also known as **B-symptoms**) from hypermetabolism due to white blood cell production and increased cytokine release. Early satiety or left upper quadrant pain or mass can result from **splenomegaly** secondary to **extramedullary hematopoiesis** (blood cell production outside of the bone marrow to compensate for insufficient hematopoiesis *in* the bone marrow). The patient remains in the *chronic phase* with stable blood counts for a median period of 3 years. With the accumulation of cytogenetic abnormalities, the disease progresses with changes in the hematologic profile and function. Patients may present with signs of **granulocyte or platelet dysfunction,** including frequent infection, thrombosis, or bleeding diathesis (tendency). Rarely, patients present with symptoms related to

Table 45-1 Pathophysiology of chronic leukemias and clinical manifestations

Pathophysiology	Symptoms	Signs/laboratory findings
Myeloproliferation with bone marrow expansion, hypermetabolism, increased cell turnover and cytokine release → B-symptoms	• Persistent low-grade fever • Night sweats • Weight loss • Malaise/fatigue/weakness • Symptoms of gout (joint pain) • Bone pain	• ↑ WBC > 100,000/μL • Normal Hct ± nucleated RBCs • Hypercellular bone marrow with left-shifted myelopoiesis • Elevated B_{12}/hyperuricemia • Sternal tenderness
Extramedullary hematopoiesis	• Early satiety • LUQ pain (splenic infarct) • Abdominal distension	• Splenomegaly (most common) • Hepatomegaly • Lymphadenopathy
Granulocyte dysfunction	• Frequent infections	• Mucocutaneous lesions/exudate
Lymphocyte dysfunction Immunocompromise autoimmune disease	• Frequent infections • Autoimmune hemolytic anemia • Immune thrombocytopenia	• Lymphocytosis • Direct Coombs' test—positive • Antiplatelet antibody test—positive
Anemia	• Palpitations • Fatigue	• Tachycardia, tachypnea, pallor • Low hematocrit/hemoglobin
Platelet dysfunction	• Thrombosis (DVT, PE, CVA, MI) • Bruising/bleeding/epistaxis	• Thrombocytosis, thrombocytopenia • Petechiae, ecchymoses, anemia
Basophilia → ↑ histamine release	• Pruritus, esp. with hot showers • Diarrhea • Flushing • Symptoms of peptic ulcer disease	• Excoriations • Signs of dehydration • Blanching erythema • Ulcer by endoscopy
Hyperviscosity	• Blurred vision • Priapism	• WBC > 500,000/μL • Or high hematocrit
Bone marrow failure	• Frequent infection • Bleeding diathesis	• Pancytopenia • Bone marrow fibrosis

Hct, hematocrit; RBC, red blood cell; LUQ, left-upper quadrant of abdomen; DVT, deep venous thrombosis; PE, pulmonary embolism; CVA, cerebrovascular accident (stroke); MI, myocardial infarction.

hyperviscosity due to leukostasis at WBC greater than 500,000/μL. As the patient enters the *accelerated phase,* the patient may present with worsening B-symptoms, increasing splenomegaly, **bone pain** from bone marrow expansion, and signs associated with **anemia** and **thrombocytopenia.** Blood and bone marrow blasts and basophils increase. **Basophilia** may result in symptoms of excess histamine production, namely pruritus, diarrhea, flushing, and even peptic ulcer disease from excess histamine-induced acid production. **Blast crisis** then ensues with blasts reaching **more than 30% of the bone marrow,** causing **bone marrow failure** manifested as increased bleeding and infection. Median survival at diagnosis of the blast crisis is 3 to 4 months.

CLL occurs mostly in those over 50 years old. Disease is often discovered incidentally while the patient is asymptomatic with a persistent isolated lymphocytosis on routine labs. **Lymphadenopathy** is a more common early sign, with progressive splenomegaly or hepatomegaly occurring later. Patients may also present with manifestations of anemia and thrombocytopenia from **autoimmune disease.** Other variants of CLL include **prolymphocytic leukemia,** which follows a more aggressive course, and **Richter's syndrome,** wherein an isolated lymph node becomes an aggressive large lymphoma. CLL can also evolve into ALL. The median survival is 10 years, and the major causes of death in CLL are infection, vital organ infiltration, and transformation into higher-grade neoplasm.

In chronic myelogenous leukemia, white blood count is typically greater than 100,000/μL with a myeloid predominance in the differential ("blood like bone marrow"). Other laboratory findings include elevated vitamin B_{12} and uric acid from high cell turnover. Peripheral blood smear reveals cells at several stages of differentiation, reflecting the continuation of maturation in these neoplastic cells (see Case 44, Acute Leukemia, Figure 44-1). The bone marrow is hypercellular, with myeloid and megakaryocytic predominance with normal to elevated blasts. **Definitive diagnosis of CML is established by the identification of the t(9,22), the Philadelphia chromosome,** which is found in 90% to 95% of patients with CML. Other diseases to rule out include reactive leukocytosis from infection where WBC is usually less than 50,000/μL and splenomegaly is absent.

CLL is diagnosed by the clinical picture and the persistent, unexplained presence of mature lymphocytosis greater than 5000/μL. The blood smear reveals a predominance of small, mature-appearing (but pathologic) lymphocytes with normal hematocrit and platelet count. If anemia and thrombocytopenia exist, **autoimmune disease** may be suspected and confirmed with the **direct Coombs' test** and **antiplatelet antibody test.** Bone marrow biopsy would reveal at least 30% lymphocytes. Further **immunostaining** of leukemic cells reveals **monoclonal** expression of typical **B-cell antigens,** few surface immunoglobulins, and an atypical expression of the T-cell antigen CD5. **Serum protein electrophoresis** may show low total IgG levels with a small IgG spike, reflecting the monoclonal nature of CLL.

Early chronic phase leukemias require no immediate therapy. Imatinib mesylate (Gleevec) has emerged as standard therapy for patients in the chronic phase of CML without a bone marrow donor. It inhibits *bcr-abl* tyrosine kinase activity, which interferes with cell cycling and promotes apoptosis of leukemic cells.

Other Myeloproliferative Diseases The other myeloproliferative diseases follow patterns of pathogenesis similar to those of chronic leukemia, but with differing consequences depending on the hematologic profile. These rare diseases underscore the direct relationship between the type of hematologic disturbance and the predominant clinical manifestations that result (Table 45-2).

Table 45-2 Summary of the clinical manifestations of other myeloproliferative diseases

Polycythemia rubra vera	**Erythrocytic leukemia:** high hematocrit, thrombocytosis, leukocytosis → *hyperviscosity*—headache, blurred vision, vascular occlusion (MI, CVA), massive splenomegaly; cyanosis
Essential thrombocytosis	**Megakaryocytic leukemia:** thrombotic, thromboembolic phenomena (MI, CVA)
Myelofibrosis with myeloid metaplasia	**Leukemic megakaryocytes with abnormal release of fibroblast-stimulating cytokines:** platelet-derived growth factor (PDGF) and transforming growth factor-β (TGF-β) promote fibroblasts collagen production and eventual bone marrow fibrosis and failure. Teardrop poikilocytosis on blood smear, hypercellular bone marrow with megakaryocytic predominance, hepatosplenomegaly, anemia, thrombocytopenia, bone marrow failure

Case Conclusion   LA is confirmed to have chronic myelogenous leukemia. Following this, his family is screened for ABO blood type and human leukocytic antigen (HLA) compatibility, but no one is found to be eligible to be a donor. He is started on imatinib mesylate, and his cancer enters remission after 3 months of therapy. Five years post-remission, he is doing well with no evidence of leukemic recurrence.

Thumbnail: Chronic Myeloid Leukemia vs. Chronic Lymphoid Leukemia

	Chronic myeloid leukemia	Chronic lymphoid leukemia
Pathophysiology	**t(9,22): Philadelphia chromosome** → *bcr-abl* tyrosine kinase → cell cycle dysregulation *Chronic phase:* myeloid proliferation and maturation in bone marrow in background of normal hematopoiesis, ± extramedullary hematopoiesis *Accelerated phase:* crowding out of normal hematopoietic cells → thrombocytopenia, anemia, basophilia, increasing leukemia *Blast crisis:* blast proliferation, bone marrow failure	Varied genetic abnormalities → clonal proliferation and maturation of lymphocytes → bone marrow lymphocyte infiltration, isolated lymphocytosis with aberrant cell function → immunosuppression, tissue infiltration, bone marrow failure
Clinical manifestations	*Chronic phase:* asymptomatic or B-symptoms, hepatosplenomegaly (HSM), lymphadenopathy (LAD) *Accelerated phase:* anemia, bleeding diathesis or thrombosis, basophilia, hyperviscosity syndrome *Blast crisis:* pancytopenia, infection, bleeding	*Early:* asymptomatic, or mild B-symptoms, LAD > HSM, isolated lymphocytosis *Later:* immunosuppression with frequent infections; tissue infiltration, autoimmune hemolytic anemia, immune thrombocytopenia *End stage:* pancytopenia, bone marrow failure; death usually from infection
Laboratory findings	WBC >100,000/μL with elevated mature myeloid cells, myeloid precursors in peripheral blood smear, thrombocytosis Hypercellular bone marrow with myeloid predominance, < 5% blasts Elevated B_{12}, uric acid	Persistent, unexplained lymphocytosis > 5000/μL (usu. 10,000–150,000/μL) with small, mature lymphocytes in blood smear Bone marrow > 30% mature lymphocytes Serum protein electrophoresis: low total Ig, monoclonal Ig spike
Diagnosis	Cytogenetic study: t(9,22) positive cells Molecular study: PCR detects *bcr-abl* messenger RNA (mRNA)	Monoclonal B-cells: positive for CD19, CD20, CD22, poor-IgG-staining, and **CD5**

MI, myocardial infarction; CVA, cerebrovascular accident or stroke; PUD, peptic ulcer disease.

Key Points

▶ Chronic leukemia arises from the neoplastic transformation of a hematopoietic stem cell that retains its ability to differentiate.

▶ Chronic leukemia follows an indolent clinical course as a result of the slow proliferation of these leukemic cells; unfortunately, this very quality makes it highly resistant to cytotoxic chemotherapy, as such drugs specifically target actively proliferating cells.

▶ The clinical manifestations of chronic leukemias arise from the myeloproliferation of leukemic cells and the subsequent interference of normal blood cell production.

▶ Imatinib mesylate, a *bcr-abl* ihibitor, has emerged as a highly effective therapy for CML.

Questions

1. A 52-year-old man presents with fever, night sweats, weight loss, and splenomegaly on routine exam. CBC reveals markedly elevated white blood cells at 200,000/μL and platelets at 455,000/μL. Which is NOT a possible cause of this blood count?

   A. Infection
   B. Chronic myeloid leukemia
   C. Chronic lymphoid leukemia
   D. Prolymphocytic leukemia
   E. Acute myeloid leukemia

2. A 65-year-old man with chronic myeloid leukemia is found to have markedly elevated platelets. What clinical consequence is NOT associated with thrombocytosis?

   A. Myocardial infarction
   B. Pulmonary embolism
   C. Perirectal abscess
   D. Deep vein thrombosis
   E. Stroke

3. A 63-year-old woman presents on routine exam with nontender lymphadenopathy with no hepatospleno-megaly. If she had some form of chronic leukemia, given her presentation, what is her most likely CBC with manual differential?

   A. WBC = 26,000/μL, 72% neutrophils, 6% bands, 12% lymphocytes, 7% monocytes, 3% eosinophils, Hct 32%, platelets 350,000/μL
   B. WBC = 325,000/μL, 65% neutrophils, 5% bands, 5% lymphocytes, 10% monocytes, 5% eosinophils, 5% basophils, 2% metamyelocytes, 1% myelocytes, 1% promyelocytes, and 1% blasts, Hct 37%, platelets 454,000/μL
   C. WBC = 60,000/μL, 25% neutrophils, 64% lympho-cytes, 7% monocytes, 3% eosinophils, 1% basophils, Hct 38%, platelets 350,000/μL
   D. WBC = 450/μL, 11% neutrophils, 3% monocytes, 2% eosinophils, 0% basophils, 75% blasts, Hct 25%, platelets 90,000/μL
   E. WBC = 8500/μL, 65% neutrophils, 27% lympho-cytes, 5% monocytes, 2% eosinophils, 1% basophils, Hct 35%, platelets 230,000/μL

Case 33

1. B
2. B
3. C

Case 34

1. B
2. C
3. A

Case 35

1. E
2. D
3. C

Case 36

1. C
2. E

Case 37

1. D
2. E

Case 38

1. D
2. B

Case 39

1. A
2. D

Case 40

1. B
2. E

Case 41

1. D
2. D

Case 42

1. E
2. D

Case 43

1. D
2. D
3. E

Case 44

1. C
2. E

Case 45

1. A
2. C
3. C

Answers

Case 1

1. D Increasing the activity of the Na$^+$/K$^+$ ATPase and the sodium channels in the collecting tubules. Aldosterone acts in the collecting tubules to increase the reabsorption of sodium and thus of water, increasing overall plasma volume. Loop diuretics (e.g., furosemide) act by blocking the Na$^+$/K$^+$/2Cl$^-$ channel (choice **A**). Antidiuretic hormone (ADH) is responsible for the insertion of aquaporins (choice **B**) in the collecting tubule cell, and parathyroid hormone (PTH) increases the reabsorption of calcium in the DCT (choice **C**). Carbonic anhydrase is an enzyme in the brush border of the PCT that is always active; aldosterone does not affect its activity.

2. B Dark staining with basal striations and debris in the lumen. The proximal convoluted tubule (PCT) is responsible for absorbing nearly all of the filtered glucose. When glucose transporters are overcome, this is usually indicative of diabetes mellitus, or in this case, gestational diabetes. The PCT is well designed for its role of absorbing 75% of the filtered load. It has a brush border of microvilli, which often become luminal debris during fixation. These basal microvilli are inhabited by many mitochondria, which stain darkly and thus form basal striations. **Pale staining with distinct borders between cells** describes the distal convoluted tubule. **Thin squamous epithelium lining a clear lumen** describes the thin descending limb of the loop of Henle. Choices **D** and **E** do not accurately describe any of the segments of the nephron.

3. D The loop of Henle. The osmotic gradient in the medulla is crucial for the concentration of urine in the collecting tubules. This gradient is established by countercurrent multiplication in the descending and ascending limbs of the **loop of Henle** (discussed in the sodium case). The **vasa recta** are the blood vessels that serve the renal parenchyma without disrupting the medullary gradient. The **peritubular capillaries** receive the reabsorbed solutes.

Case 2

1. A Median umbilical ligament. An urachal fistula is an abnormal connection between the bladder and the umbilicus. In normal development, the urachus is a canal that connects the allantois to the bladder in utero and over time becomes the fibrous **median umbilical ligament.** The **paramesonephric** (müllerian) and **wolffian** (mesonephric) ducts form the genital tracts and urinary collecting system, but are not involved in formation of the urinary bladder. The **vitelline duct** connects the yolk sac with the primitive gut in the embryo and is not involved in genitourinary development. The **medial umbilical ligaments** are the fibrosed umbilical arteries. There are two medial umbilical ligaments that lie lateral to the one median umbilical artery. A helpful way to remember this is that the media**L** ligaments lie **L**aterally while the o**N**e media**N** artery is centrally located.

2. D Bilateral agenesis of the ureteric buds. Lung hypoplasia and limb deformities occur when oligohydramnios (too little amniotic fluid) is present in utero. If the **ureteric buds** do not reach the metanephric tissue, they cannot induce the development of functional renal tissue, and bilateral renal agenesis (Potter's syndrome) results. Oligohydramnios is the consequence, as fetal urine is the primary source of amniotic fluid. **Unilateral renal agenesis** would not cause oligohydramnios since one kidney yields enough functional nephric tissue for adequate amniotic fluid. **Tracheoesophageal atresia** would lead to polyhydramnios (too much amniotic fluid), since the infant cannot swallow and infant swallowing is the main route of amniotic fluid reabsorption. **Duodenal atresia** causes polyhydramnios, intestinal obstruction with a double-bubble sign on ultrasound, and is associated with trisomy 21 (Down syndrome). **Congenital polycystic kidneys** result in renal insufficiency and death unless transplantation occurs.

Case 3

1. B 1000 mL/min. Recalling that the clearance of PAH is an estimate of renal plasma flow and using this equation:

$$RBF = ERPF/(1 - \text{hematocrit}) = 600 \text{ mL/min}/(1-0.40) = 1000$$

PAH clearance is a good marker for effective renal plasma flow as it is readily cleared by the kidney.

2. B 50 mL/min. Our patient has had a decline in his renal function. As his renal function is not normal (approximately 125 mL/min) or supranormal, choices C, D, and E are ruled out. To properly calculate creatinine clearance we use the following formula:

$$C_{Cr} = U_{Cr} * V/P_{Cr} = \text{mL/min}$$

$$U_{Cr} = \text{concentration of creatinine in urine} = 200 \text{ mg/dL} = 2 \text{ mg/mL}$$

$$V = \text{urine volume/flow} = 720 \text{ mL}/1440 \text{ min} = 0.5 \text{ mL/min}$$

$$P_{Cr} = \text{concentration of creatinine in the plasma} = 2 \text{ mg/dL} = 0.02 \text{ mg/mL}$$

$$C_{Cr} = 2 \text{ mg/mL} * 0.5 \text{ mL/min}/0.02 \text{ mg/mL} = 50 \text{ mL/min}$$

Serum creatinine is a good marker for renal function as it is endogenously produced at a constant rate, is filtered, not reabsorbed, and only slightly secreted. Serum levels are variable depending on age, muscle mass, and rigorous exercise. Inulin is a better measure of GFR but is used only in experimental settings.

3. C Glucose. The capillaries of the glomerulus allow the passage of small, neutral molecules through the endothelial wall. Larger and more negatively charged molecules such as dextran and albumin are effectively barred from passing into the filtrate by the negatively charged basement membrane. This patient most likely has a urinary tract infection, and her hematuria is most likely due to inflammation at the level of the bladder. The passage of albumin, protein, and red blood cells at the level of the kidney is indicative of damage to the glomerular membrane and is only seen in disease states. Slightly elevated levels of proteinuria may be seen after heavy exercise in healthy persons.

4. C 40 mL/min. The Cockroft-Gault equation is an estimate of creatinine clearance and thus of glomerular filtration rate. This is given by

$$C_{Cr} = \frac{(140 - age) * weight \text{ (in kg)}}{P_{Cr} \text{ (mg/dL)} * 72}$$

Thus,

$$C_{Cr} = \frac{(140 - 60) * 72}{2 * 72}$$

$$C_{Cr} = 80/2 = 40$$

One must consider the GFR when dosing medications in patients with renal insufficiency and advanced age. A number of medications, including antibiotics, diuretics, and digoxin, are eliminated by the kidney, and a decline in renal function can increase the serum drug concentration and contribute to drug toxicity.

Case 4

1. D 5000 mL. $C_1V_1 = C_2V_2 \cdot$ 500 mg/mL * 250 mL = 25 mg/mL * x. x = 5000 mL. Plasma volumes may be calculated under experimental conditions but are not used clinically.

2. A Intravenous 0.9% saline. Our patient is suffering from iso-osmotic volume contraction, and 0.9% saline is the replacement fluid of choice to rapidly replete the intravascular volume and restore his blood pressure. Over time, the water infused into the intravascular space also distributes to the interstitial space and more fluids may be needed. The 0.45% saline, a hypotonic fluid (as compared to plasma), more rapidly distributes from the vascular space to the interstitial space, making it a poor choice for fluid resuscitation. A 5% dextrose solution is the equivalent of giving water only, since dextrose readily diffuses into cells and is thus unable to exert any osmotic activity in the intravascular space. The 3% saline is used almost exclusively to correct life-threatening hyponatremia and is rarely used for volume contraction. Oral chicken soup with its high salt concentration is not a bad choice for fluid replacement in a volume-contracted patient. Oral replacement fluid is not appropriate in patients unable to tolerate oral intake or in patients with orthostatic hypotension. **Orthostatic hypotension,** also called postural hypotension, is an increase in pulse of 20 beats per minute and/or a drop in blood pressure of 20 mm Hg upon assuming an erect position. Our patient's complaint of dizziness stems from the drop in his blood pressure and decreased perfusion to his brain upon standing.

Case 5

1. B 336 mEq, 16 hours. The patient has had a rapid onset of hyponatremia and is symptomatic. Care must be taken not to "volume overload" the patient. The patient's sodium deficit can be calculated as follows:

Na+ deficit = (TBW) (Na+ desired − Na+ measured)

Na+ deficit = (0.60 * 70 kg) (130 mEq/L − 122 mEq/L) = (42 L * 8 mEq/L)

Na+ deficit = 336 mEq

The volume of 3% saline required to replace 336 mEq of sodium can be calculated as follows: Volume of 3% saline = 336 mEq/513 mEq/L = 0.650 L = 650 mL.

The rate of sodium correction is 0.5 mEq/L/h; 8 mEq/L should be replaced over 16 hours.

2. B Diabetes insipidus. Diabetes insipidus is the best choice given the clinical setting and the abrupt onset of polyuria, which is characteristic of central DI. The differential diagnosis for polyuria includes four of the five choices: DI, postobstructive diuresis, osmotic diuresis due to hyperglycemia, and inadvertent administration of diuretics. SIADH does not present with polyuria. Both DI and SIADH can occur, although not commonly, after subarachnoid hemorrhage.

3. E SIADH. SIADH presents with variable degrees of hyponatremia, and most patients are asymptomatic. A search for the cause of SIADH must be carried out. A mild weight gain is characteristic of mild water retention. Hyponatremia and weight gain could be characteristic of hypothyroidism, not hyperthyroidism, and must be ruled out as a cause of hyponatremia. Both advanced hyperglycemia and hyperlipidemia cause factitious hyponatremia, but there is no information to support those diagnoses. Surreptitious use of diuretics must be considered, but in light of a normal serum potassium, SIADH is the best answer.

Case 6

1. E All of the above. We treat hyperkalemia by antagonizing the effects of potassium, increasing the movement of potassium into cells and removing excess potassium. Our patient was given calcium chloride intravenously to antagonize the effects of potassium at the cardiac conduction system. Calcium is cardioprotective, but does not change the serum potassium concentration. Intravenous insulin preceded by intravenous glucose helps to shift potassium into the cells as does sodium bicarbonate. We also use β_2-agonists such as albuterol (a catecholamine agonist) to this effect. Sodium polystyrene sulfonate, not used in the urgent setting as it is slow acting, is an ion exchange resin that acts in the gastrointestinal lumen to absorb potassium in exchange for sodium, thereby removing potassium from the body. Dialysis is the proper treatment for this patient's severe hyperkalemia.

2. B Furosemide. Loop diuretics cause an increased flow of sodium and water to the distal nephron and cause potassium loss by disrupting the normal mechanisms for potassium balance. Increased sodium delivery to the distal tubules increases the action of the

Na^+/K^+ exchange pump there, increasing potassium loss in the urine. Aldosterone acts on the cortical collecting tubule to increase potassium secretion, and an excess, not a deficiency, of aldosterone would cause hypokalemia. Spironolactone is a potassium-sparing diuretic that can cause hyperkalemia. Metabolic alkalosis is associated with a shift of potassium into the cells and a lowered serum potassium. Hyperthyroidism does not affect serum potassium levels. Dietary deficiency is the most common cause for a decreased serum potassium. The ability of the kidney to conserve potassium is limited by the obligatory excretion of approximately 10 mEq/L in the urine even in the presence of hypokalemia.

3. E All of the above. All of the above ECG changes happen with hyperkalemia, and in general occur in the order listed. The final ECG in hyperkalemia looks like a sine wave. The increased serum potassium causes changes in the cardiac conduction system and can lead to supraventricular tachycardia, sinus arrest, AV dissociation, ventricular fibrillation, and cardiac arrest.

Case 7

1. C Renal insufficiency. Metabolic acidosis is one of the hallmarks of long-standing renal disease due to the accumulation of organic acids. This patient's renal disease is likely a result of hypertension and type 2 diabetes. He has a mild metabolic gap acidosis of 14. His elevated potassium is also likely caused by his renal insufficiency. **Hypertension** alone cannot cause decreased bicarbonate. **Diabetic ketoacidosis** is an emergent medical condition and often presents with a larger anion gap acidosis, obtundation, vomiting, and abdominal pain. **Diarrhea** causes a loss of bicarbonate and is a cause of a nongap or hyperchloremic acidosis. Chronic obstructive pulmonary disease causes a respiratory acidosis secondary to retained CO_2 and is usually accompanied by elevated serum bicarbonate as metabolic or renal compensation for a respiratory acidosis.

2. C Methanol. Hyperventilation is the appropriate response to a metabolic acidosis, allowing rapid diffusion of the volatile acid CO_2. Hyperventilation secondary to acidosis is often termed Kussmaul breathing, and is characterized by deep breaths. It is a prominent clinical sign of an acidemic patient. Severe acidosis may result in depression of cardiac contractility, hyperkalemia, and altered mental status. We can see from the blood gas that our patient is not **hypoxic**. **Diarrhea** causes a loss of bicarbonate and a hyperchloremic acidosis rather than an anion gap acidosis. **Vomiting** causes a metabolic alkalosis due to a loss of hydrochloric acid from the stomach. Chronic obstructive pulmonary disease results in retention of carbon dioxide and compensatory elevation of bicarbonate by the kidney.

3. C Hypocapnea and decreased bicarbonate. Acetylsalicylic acid, more commonly known as aspirin, causes a metabolic acidosis (decreased bicarbonate) due to ingestion of the acid and increased production or decreased removal of lactate by the liver. A concomitant respiratory alkalosis occurs due to direct stimulation of central respiratory centers, leading to hyperventilation and the "blowing off" of the volatile acid CO_2. Acute ingestion leads to nausea, vomiting, tachycardia, and tinnitus, and may result in coma, cardiovascular shock, and death.

4. D Vomiting. Vomiting results in a loss of potassium and hydrochloric acid from the stomach. Surreptitious diuretic use for weight loss can also deplete chloride; as a result, sodium must be reabsorbed with bicarbonate instead of chloride, causing alkalosis. The dehydrated alkalemic patient suffers from a (volume) "contraction" alkalosis. Consumption of antacids such as *calcium carbonate* with milk is a cause of milk alkali syndrome, but would not explain our patient's physical findings or hypokalemia. Milk alkali syndrome was seen more frequently when calcium-based antacids were used to treat peptic ulcer disease; alkalosis and hypercalcemia occurred in those patients with underlying renal insufficiency. *Renal failure* commonly causes acidosis, not alkalosis. **Polydipsia** can cause mild hyponatremia but would not cause alkalosis.

Case 8

1. C Hyperparathyroidism. Hyperparathyroidism is the most common cause of hypercalcemia due to an overgrowth of a single parathyroid gland, an adenoma. It is more common in women than in men. In addition to hypercalcemia, an important clue to an excess of PTH is the low serum phosphorus level due to the increased renal excretion of phosphorus. Long-standing renal insufficiency is more apt to cause hypocalcemia and hyperphosphatemia. Familial hypocalciuric hypercalcemia is a rare autosomal-dominant disease due to decreased urinary excretion of calcium. Diagnosis is confirmed by low levels of urinary calcium and corroborated with a family history of hypercalcemia. Pseudohypoparathyroidism is an inherited disorder of end-organ resistance to PTH, resulting in elevated levels of PTH, hypocalcemia, and hyperphosphatemia. It is a component of Albright's hereditary osteodystrophy, and patients usually have somatic features that include short stature, round face, short metacarpals and metatarsals, obesity, mental retardation, and basal ganglia calcifications. Excessive vitamin D results in elevated serum calcium and phosphorus due to increased absorption from the gut.

2. D Hypocalcemia and hyperphosphatemia. Chronic renal insufficiency that occurs with long-standing hypertension is characterized by small, scarred kidneys. With decreased nephron mass, less tissue is available for the hydroxylation of vitamin D and hypocalcemia results. A decreased glomerular filtration rate also occurs in long-standing renal disease, and as a result hyperphosphatemia is likely to be present. Other abnormalities such as hyperkalemia, acidosis, and anemia are also characteristic of kidney failure. Neither ACEIs nor beta-blockers have significant effects on renal excretion of phosphate or calcium.

3. B Hypocalcemia. This question is intended to remind us of what happens to serum ionized calcium levels in the presence of alkalemia. Our anxious medical student hyperventilated, inducing a respiratory alkalosis, leading to an increase of calcium bound to protein and ionized hypocalcemia. As discussed above, hypocalcemia may cause acral and perioral paresthesias. Both metabolic and respiratory alkalosis cause an increased binding of calcium to protein, and in the presence of low serum calcium may lower the threshold for tetany. Acidosis causes a decreased binding of calcium to protein and increased levels of ionized serum calcium.

Long-standing acidosis leeches calcium from bone and may contribute to renal osteodystrophy.

Case 9

1. E All of the above. Angiotensin-converting enzyme inhibitors (ACEIs) reversibly inhibit the conversion of angiotensin I to angiotensin II, a potent vasoconstrictor. Inhibiting systemic vasoconstriction results in vasodilatation and lowering of blood pressure. Reduced levels of aldosterone, causing less sodium and water reabsorption, also aid in reducing blood pressure. Angiotensin II aids in maintaining the glomerular filtration rate by causing vasoconstriction of the efferent arteriole. The loss of this mechanism may precipitate a usually reversible renal failure especially in those with impaired renal function at baseline. There is often a mild rise in serum creatinine upon institution of ACEIs, even in those with normal renal function. They may also result in hyperkalemia due to the decrease in aldosterone. Hyperkalemia occurs in approximately 5% of patients started on ACEIs, so serum levels of potassium must be monitored. There is a risk of hypotension with any antihypertensive medication. Angioedema is a common allergic reaction with any ACEI. A persistent dry cough is also a side effect of this class of drugs (the "captopril cough").

2. C Fibromuscular dysplasia. Causes of secondary hypertension are important to detect, as many are treatable. Our patient has many of the physical signs of long-standing hypertension, plus a carotid bruit indicative of fibromuscular dysplasia. Her young age, severe hypertension, and lack of family history should lead us to investigate causes of secondary hypertension. Hyperaldosteronism is usually due to an adrenal adenoma and leads to hypertension and hypokalemia. Cushing's syndrome is due to adrenal hyperplasia causing an excess of glucocorticoids and hormones that, like aldosterone, may have mineralocorticoid activity (aldosterone levels are usually normal). Findings associated with Cushing's syndrome include centripetal obesity, moon face and buffalo hump, peripheral muscle wasting, striae, and hypokalemia. Pheochromocytoma is usually an adrenal tumor but can be found extraadrenally and presents with episodic hypertension, palpitations, diaphoresis, and throbbing headaches. Atherosclerosis in a 29-year-old patient is unlikely. Drugs such as birth control pills, cocaine, and amphetamines may also cause hypertension.

3. E All of the above. Patients with inadequately controlled blood pressure are at risk for renal failure, retinopathy, left ventricular failure, and stroke. Long-standing hypertension increases the rate of decline in glomerular filtration rate. Eventually glomerular damage leads to proteinuria and microscopic hematuria. This process is retarded by ACEIs. Retinal changes can be seen early in hypertensive disease. On the fundal exam, one sees progressive narrowing of retinal arteries, retinal hemorrhages, and exudates, which can obscure vision, and nicking of the retinal veins by fibrotic retinal arteries that impede retinal venous flow. Increased systemic blood pressure increases afterload on the heart, leading to left ventricular hypertrophy and eventually ventricular dilation and congestive heart failure. Hypertension is the main risk factor predisposing to stroke. Elevations in systolic blood pressure correlate well with increased risk of stroke, and even small reductions in blood pressure can diminish that risk.

Case 10

1. E IgA nephropathy. IgA nephropathy (Berger's disease) is the most common form of acute GN worldwide, especially in Asia. It is most commonly seen in children, with boys outnumbering girls two to three times. It presents with gross hematuria 2 to 3 days after pharyngitis or a GI infection. Fifty percent progress to renal insufficiency. **Poststreptococcal GN** is also postinfectious, but presents 10 days to 2 weeks after streptococcal pharyngitis or skin infection, and is associated with elevated ASO titers and IgG deposition. **Henoch-Schönlein purpura** is indistinguishable from IgA nephropathy on microscopy and immunofluorescence, but is associated with palpable purpura, arthralgias, and abdominal pain. **Alport syndrome** is an X-linked mutation in the collagen IV gene that is associated with nerve deafness and eye problems. **Benign familial hematuria (thin basement membrane disease)** also results from hereditary defects in type IV collagen, but is asymptomatic, requires no treatment, and has no serious sequelae.

2. D This patient has **Goodpasture's syndrome,** in which circulating autoantibodies bind to the NC1 domain of the α3 chain of type IV collagen ("Goodpasture's antigen"), a normal component of the GBM. Since the GBM is a linear structure, the IgG autoantibodies form a linear pattern on IF. The lung endothelium also contains the same locus on type IV collagen. The binding of Ab to Ag starts the complement cascade leading to endothelial injury and hemoptysis and hematuria. **A** is not correct, as there are no circulating antigens in Goodpasture's. **B** is not correct because there is no mutation present. **C** is not correct because there are no exogenous antigens and antibodies tend not to be stationary. **E** is not correct because the pathophysiology is understood (at least in part).

3. B Churg-Strauss, like Wegener's granulomatosis, is a small-vessel vasculitis that often affects the renal vasculature. Both involve hematuria presenting in the context of systemic involvement. However, Churg-Strauss tends to occur in patients with a history of asthma or atopy (thus the connection with eosinophilic infiltration), whereas **Wegener's granulomatosis** is more commonly diagnosed in patients with upper respiratory (especially sinus) involvement. **Amyloidosis** also has systemic involvement but presents with nephrotic syndrome and Congo red staining of the mesangium due to light chains deposition. **Minimal change disease** and **thin basement membrane disease** also have no deposits seen on IF, but the former presents with nephrotic syndrome in *children* and the latter is a familial nephritic disease with no symptoms or sequelae.

4. B Alport's syndrome is classically described as an X-linked dominant mutation in components of type IV collagen (though there are other non-X-linked variants). It is associated with sensorineural hearing loss and abnormalities in the shape of the ocular lens. Hematuria can progress to serious nephritis and can cause renal failure in adolescence or young adulthood. None of the other syndromes are X-linked or associated with hearing or eye problems. **Goodpasture's syndrome** is also seen in young men, but is associated with hemoptysis. **Berger's syndrome (IgA nephropathy)** has IgA deposits in the mesangium. **Type IV lupus GN** is found more often in women and has IgG in a "wire loop" pattern on IF. **Type I**

membranoproliferative GN is also characterized by a split GBM on EM, giving the characteristic "train track" appearance, but it presents with nephrotic syndrome.

Case 11

1. B **Focal segmental glomerulosclerosis (FSGS). FSGS and minimal change disease** are both nephrotic syndromes characterized by normal findings on light microscopy and no immunoglobulin deposition on immunofluorescence. The only way to confirm these diagnoses is by visualizing effacement of foot processes on electron microscopy. As this requires an invasive renal biopsy, this is rarely done in practice. In this case, FSGS would be the more likely diagnosis for this older patient with multiple comorbidities, since minimal change disease is seen primarily in children 2 to 6 years old. **Membranous glomerulonephritis (GN)** demonstrates mesangial proliferation on light microscopy and significant immunofluorescence findings, and thus does not require electron microscopy (EM) for definitive diagnosis, though splitting of the GBM is seen on EM. **Lupus GN** and **diabetic nephropathy** also present with nephrotic syndrome, but are seen in the context of a systemic illness and have significant light microscopy and immunofluorescence findings (wire-loop and Kimmelstiel-Wilson nodules, respectively).

2. E **Amyloidosis.** Renal biopsy of a patient with **amyloidosis** will reveal deposits that stain Congo red under normal light microscopy and show apple green birefringence with polarized light microscopy. **Lesch-Nyhan syndrome** is a rare genetic syndrome characterized by spastic behavior, self-mutilation, and mental retardation. It results from a deficiency of the enzyme that catalyzes the central reaction in purine metabolism, resulting in hyperuricemia. This causes strongly birefringent uric acid crystals to precipitate, leading to uric acid kidney stones. **Diabetes mellitus** and **systemic lupus erythematosus** can lead to renal failure and nephrotic syndrome, but they have very different microscopic findings. **Diabetes insipidus** creates a water diuresis due to insensitivity to or inadequate production of antidiuretic hormone/vasopressin and does not lead to nephrotic syndrome.

Case 12

1. C *E. coli O1. E. coli O1* is one of the uropathic strains of *E. coli*. While it is not important to memorize which strains are uropathic vs. enterotoxic, it is important to recognize that a strain is NOT O157:H7. *E. coli* O157:H7 is enterohemorrhagic *E. coli*, responsible for inflammatory diarrhea plus hemolytic-uremic syndrome in children. Although it looks like other strains in most respects (green sheen on EMB agar), it can be distinguished by incubating it with sorbitol, since O157:H7 is the only *E. coli* strain that ferments sorbitol. *Staphylococcus saprophyticus* is a gram-positive cocci that causes 10% to 15% of UTIs in young sexually active women. *Serratia* and *Enterobacter* are coliforms found in hospitalized patients, many of whom have in-dwelling catheters.

2. D *Staphylococcus saprophyticus. S. saprophyticus* is a gram-positive cocci that causes 10% to 15% of UTIs in young sexually active women. *Staphylococcus aureus* is gram-positive but not

associated with UTIs, though it is associated with food poisoning, tampon-associated toxic shock syndrome, and various pyogenic infections (abscesses, osteomyelitis, endocarditis, etc.). *Chlamydia trachomatis* is a sexually transmitted bacteria that does not Gram stain well. Although it can cause urethritis and accompanying dysuria, this obligate intracellular bacteria rarely ascends as far as the bladder. It also causes mucopurulent cervicitis, pelvic inflammatory disease (PID), conjunctivitis, and arthritis. Its most common presentation, however, is asymptomatic infection. *Neisseria gonorrhoeae* is a sexually transmitted gram-negative diplococci that causes cervicitis, PID, and septic arthritis. *E. coli* is a gram-negative rod responsible for most community-acquired UTIs.

3. A **Struvite kidney stones.** Struvite stones are made of ammonium magnesium phosphate, which precipitates when urine becomes alkaline, as is the case with colonization with urease-producing bacteria. The urease converts ammonia to ammonium, absorbing excess hydrogen ions. These stones can become very large, filling the renal pelvis (a "staghorn"), and can harbor bacteria serving as a nidus for recurrent infections. These infections are often treatment refractory and require consultation with a urologist. An *imperforate hymen* can cause primary amenorrhea but not urinary tract infections; the hymen is the remnant of the joining of the müllerian/paramesonephric duct (the upper two thirds of the vagina) with the urogenital sinus (the lower one third of the vagina), and as such is located far from the urethral opening. *Calcium oxalate stones,* classic "kidney stones," are associated with hematuria and acute attacks of severe pain but not recurrent infections. *Systemic lupus erythematosus* is often diagnosed in young women and has multiple systemic effects, but is not particularly associated with UTIs. *Phimosis* is a nonretractable foreskin that causes urinary obstruction. As such, it is associated with recurrent UTIs in very young boys and is not a problem for women.

4. E **All of the above.** Cranberry juice is recommended for women with recurrent UTIs. Although initially thought to be helpful due to urine acidification, it is now thought that compounds in cranberry juice may inhibit *E. coli* adhesion to urinary tract epithelium. In addition, drinking lots of any fluid leads to increased urination, and good urine flow is the enemy of uropathic bacteria. Urinating after intercourse cleanses the urethral opening and distal urethra of bacteria. Condoms are not associated with increased incidence of UTIs, while *diaphragms* are. Diaphragms must be left in for several hours after intercourse to allow adequate sperm-killing. They compress the urethra, causing partial obstruction and stasis. Although recurrent UTIs warrant referral to a urologist, prophylactic antibiotics are considered in women who have more than three episodes of cystitis per year. Prophylactic antibiotics should never be used lightly, since the development of antibiotic-resistant bacteria poses a very real threat to public health.

Case 13

1. E **Struvite.** Struvite stones (magnesium ammonium phosphate stones) are strongly associated with infection by urease-producing bacteria like *Proteus* (most common), *Klebsiella,* and *Pseudomonas.* Urease metabolizes urea into CO_2 and ammonia, making the urine more alkaline (pH >7–7.5), which favors the precipitation of mag-

nesium ammonium phosphate salts. Struvite stones tend to be soft calculi that form a cast of the renal pelvis and calyces in a "staghorn" shape. This then serves as a nidus for future bacterial infections. It is more common to see this stone in women with recurrent treatment or refractory UTIs. They are radiopaque on x-ray and amenable to surgical treatment plus antibiotic sterilization of the urinary tract. Other types of stones can also be associated with urinary tract infection since they cause urinary stasis, a promoter of infection. However, this is a much less robust association than is found with struvite stones.

2. C Postrenal. Obstruction of any kind causes **postrenal** azotemia (increased BUN, a harbinger of kidney failure). This includes kidney stones (particularly the staghorn variety), benign prostatic hypertrophy, and phimosis (constriction of the foreskin which prevents retraction). Acute renal failure with anuria and severe azotemia result only with *bilateral* obstruction of the ureters, unilateral obstruction of one functioning kidney, or obstruction of the urethra.

3. E All of the above. Recurrent UTIs and **pyelonephritis** are associated with struvite stones. **Hydronephrosis** is associated with large stones that completely obstruct a ureter, leading to increased back-pressure, which causes dilation of calyces and resulting kidney damage, which can be permanent. **Acute renal failure** results from postrenal obstruction (see question 2).

4. B Cystine. **Cystine** stones are pathognomonic of cystinuria, an uncommon (1/7000) inherited defect of an amino acid transporter in the PCT. This transporter is responsible for transporting **c**ystine, **o**rnithine, **l**ysine, and **a**rginine **("cola"),** the dibasic amino acids. Cystine stones are uncommon in adults but are the most common stone observed in children.

Case 14

1. E When taking a family history, be certain to ask about these related complications. ADPKD has varied presentations. **Berry aneurysms in the circle of Willis** can rupture, causing subarachnoid hemorrhage, often leading to death or permanent neurologic impairment. **Mitral valve prolapse** is seen in 20% to 25% of ADPKD patients. It is usually asymptomatic and can be heard on a careful cardiac exam as a late systolic murmur and faint systolic click best heard at the apex or left lower sternal border. The same process that encourages cyst formation in the kidney leads to diverticula in the colon, making **colonic diverticular disease** a very common extrarenal finding in ADPKD. **Nephrolithiasis** is found in 20% of patients, with calcium and uric acid stones predominating.

2. E Renal infections are more common in patients with ADPKD. Cysts can become infected and turn into abscesses requiring parenteral antibiotics. An increased incidence of kidney stones can lead to urinary obstruction and stasis, increasing the likelihood of UTI. Consequences of repeated infections can be dire in ADPKD, since the resolution of infection often results in the scarring and fibrosis of an already compromised kidney. **Abdominal pain** results from infection, bleeding into cysts, and nephrolithiasis. Cyst

drainage may be necessary to alleviate chronic pain. **Chronic renal failure** is a common complication of ADPKD, with 50% of patients progressing to ESRD by age 60. **Hypertension** is present in 75% of adults with ADPKD, and increases with age. Cyst-induced renal ischemia is thought to activate the renin-angiotensin system with resulting hypertension. Aggressive treatment of hypertension and cyst decompression can decrease blood pressure and slow the progression to ESRD. Because of increased blood pressure and atherosclerosis, heart disease is a common development and 40% of ADPKD patients ultimately die of hypertensive heart disease.

Case 15

1. D 1%, of limited use in this nonoliguric patient. Although the correct answer is <1%, FE_{Na+} is useful only in oliguric patients. The calculation is as follows:

$$FE_{Na+}\ [\%] = \frac{U_{Na+}/P_{Na+} \times 100}{U_{Cr}/P_{Cr}}$$

$$= \frac{5/140 \times 100}{25/3.5}$$

$$= 0.5\%$$

2. C Benign prostatic hypertrophy (BPH) → postrenal failure. This patient's age and sex makes BPH likely, and BPH leads to postrenal obstructive failure. **Kidney stones** do cause postrenal failure; however, they are usually very painful, and one might expect an elevated blood pressure or tachycardia. In patients with both kidneys, stones cause ARF only if they are lodged in the urethra or the bladder-urethral junction, not in one of two ureters. **Diabetes mellitus** is common in this age group, but most often leads to chronic renal insufficiency rather than ARF. **Sepsis** is a common cause of prerenal ARF in elderly men, but this patient has no other signs or symptoms of systemic illness. **Goodpasture's syndrome** is a vasculitis that can cause glomerulonephritis and intrinsic ARF, but occurs in young men with hemoptysis.

Case 16

1. E All of the above. Hyperkalemia occurs when GFR falls below 10 mL/min, though there is increased incidence in patients with diabetes mellitus. **Osteitis fibrosa cystica** is one of the disorders of mineral metabolism that occur as part of renal osteodystrophy. Normocytic, normochromic **anemia** results from decreased erythropoietin production. Uremic toxins irritate the pericardium, causing a fibrinous pericardial effusion and the pericardial friction rub characteristic of **pericarditis.**

2. C Furosemide is the most appropriate choice. Many patients with chronic renal failure receive this diuretic. It is a potassium-wasting diuretic that is useful in severe CRF where hyperkalemia is a common and life-threatening complication. The diuretic **triamterene,** like amiloride, blocks the Na^+/K^+ ATPase in the collecting duct, diminishing the Na^+ gradient used to reabsorb Na^+ and water, and resulting in diuresis. However, it is one of the potassium-sparing diuretics remembered with the mnemonic "K+ **STA**ys around" for **s**pironolactone, **t**riamterene, **a**miloride. **Spironolactone** blocks the aldosterone receptor, blocking aldosterone's effects in the collecting tubules. Aldosterone normally up-regulates the Na+/K+ ATPase and increases the activity of the Na+ reabsorption pump to increase the amount of Na+ and water retention. Blocking these effects is not a bad idea in CRF, but again, it is a potassium-sparing diuretic and can lead to dangerous hyperkalemia. **Acetazolamide** inhibits carbonic anhydrase causing increased concentrations of luminal HCO_3^- creating an osmotic diuresis. However, this also depletes body stores of the important base bicarbonate, not a good idea in patients already prone to developing metabolic acidosis. **Mannitol,** neither secreted nor reabsorbed, also creates an osmotic diuresis, with increased excretion of free water far and above the excretion of sodium. It would not be a good choice for CRF, because it can cause pulmonary edema and hypernatremia, dangerous in a volume-overloaded patient with electrolyte disturbances. It can be used in **acute** renal failure to maintain urine flow or to decrease intravascular volume emergently in cases of increased intracranial pressure. It is parenterally administered.

Case 17

1. A Wilms' tumor and neuroblastoma. If our patient was 3 rather than 63, the differential diagnosis for RUQ abdominal mass, fever, and weight loss, would be neuroblastoma vs. Wilms' tumor. Neuroblastoma, a malignancy of the neural crest cells, is a common tumor of childhood. Thirty percent of neuroblastomas arise in the adrenal medulla, which lies on top of the kidney. Therefore, neuroblastoma is clinically difficult to distinguish from a Wilms' tumor. Wilms' tumor is a malignant mixed kidney tumor, composed of embryonal elements such as blastemic, stromal, and epithelial cell types. As is true for all cancers, the less differentiated the mixture of cell types, the more aggressive the tumor. Gross specimens reveal large, tan masses that tend to appear in the lower kidney poles. They are usually solitary, well circumscribed, and unilateral, though 10% are bilateral. **Renal cell carcinoma** and **polycystic kidneys** are found in adults.

2. C Prader-Willi syndrome. The important point to this question is that the syndromes that cause Wilms' tumor are unified by chromosome 11 mutations, all within or near the *WT*-1 gene (11p13). The product of the *WT-1* gene is a transcription factor that seems to be necessary for kidney formation. Transgenic mice lacking both copies have complete renal agenesis. **WAGR syndrome** is characterized by an increased incidence of **W**ilms' tumor (33% chance), **a**niridia (absence of the iris), **g**enital anomalies, and mental **r**etardation. It results from a sporadic deletion of genetic material at chromosome 11p13. **Denys-Drash syndrome** is characterized by male pseudohermaphroditism, nephropathy, and Wilms' tumor in most patients. There is a missense mutation at chromosome 11p13 that affects the ability of *WT-1* to bind DNA. **Beckwith-Wiedemann** syndrome is characterized by enlarged organs, renal medullary cysts, adrenal hypertrophy, and an increased incidence of Wilms' and other malignant tumors. The implicated gene is on chromosome 11p15.5, just distal to *WT-1*. This locus has been dubbed "WT-2" but its function is unknown. **Prader-Willi syndrome** is characterized by obesity, hypogonadism,

short stature, and mental retardation but has no effects on the kidney. It is an imprinting disorder caused by a deletion of 15q12 in the paternal gene and inactivation of the maternal gene.

Case 18

1. C Blood loss is the most common cause of iron deficiency anemia. The GI tract is the most common source of blood loss for men and postmenopausal women. Malignancy, ulcers, gastritis, hemorrhoids, and vascular abnormalities are all potential causes. You certainly don't want to miss a colon cancer! (A digital rectal exam and guaiac stool test would be a good thing to do in the office.) If this work up is negative, then you would give iron supplementation and follow up the Hct in 6 weeks.

2. D Plummer-Vinson syndrome is characterized by the classic findings of iron deficiency (anemia, glossitis, koilonychia) and upper esophageal webs. It is most prevalent in women; typical age range at diagnosis is 40 to 70 years. This syndrome is associated with a higher incidence of squamous cell carcinoma of the esophagus. **Fanconi anemia** is an inherited disease leading to bone marrow failure (aplastic anemia). Patients are usually diagnosed by age 12 and often die of acute myelogenous anemia (AML) by adulthood. **Lead poisoning** directly inhibits heme synthesis and is characterized by gingival lines, GI colic, and renal lesions. **Porphyria** is associated with abdominal pain, neuropsychiatric complaints, and sometimes photosensitivity. It is caused by buildup of toxic intermediates in the heme synthesis pathway, caused by various enzyme deficiencies.

Case 19

1. D The question stem correctly describes part 1 of the Shilling test. A low urinary excretion of vitamin B_{12} suggests malabsorption in a broad sense, but calls for part 2. Here the test is repeated and intrinsic factor is given. If excretion improves (therefore absorption has improved) the patient must be deficient in intrinsic factor (pernicious anemia). If excretion (hence, absorption) does not improve with the administration of IF, then malabsorption is due to problem with the bowel (e.g., resection, Crohn's disease, sprue, bacterial overgrowth, etc.).

2. C Vitamin B_{12} levels should be checked in every patient with a suspected macrocytic anemia, even if folate levels are low. It is important **not** to give folate to a patient with vitamin B_{12} deficiency. This may improve the anemia, but may actually worsen the neurologic problems. The early diagnosis of vitamin B_{12} deficiency is extremely important, as chronic neurologic deficits (e.g., >1 year) are often irreversible despite treatment. It would be wise to check iron studies, as many patients have a combination of deficiencies.

Case 20

1. D This boy has sickle cell disease. Ceftriaxone, a third-generation cephalosporin, is the treatment of choice for probable salmonella osteomyelitis, which is associated with sickle cell. Salmonella is a gram-negative organism and would not be covered by penicillin G or vancomycin. Azithromycin covers primarily gram positive and atypical organisms (*Mycoplasm, Legionella, Chlamydia, Neisseria*). Isoniazid is an antituberculosis drug that is only used alone for prophylaxis against TB infection.

2. A Target cells are sometimes seen in sickle cell patients because the RBC membranes become too large for the sickling cells. (Howell-Jolly bodies can also be seen if the person is physically or functionally without a spleen.) Hypersegmented neutrophils are seen in vitamin B_{12} and folate deficiency. Auer rods are diagnostic for acute myeloid leukemia. Spherocytes are classic findings in hereditary spherocytosis and autoimmune hemolytic anemias. Schistocytes are seen in microangiopathic hemolytic anemias.

Case 21

1. C Silent carriers 50%; also note that 25% will have α-trait genotype and 25% will be normal (Table A-21). It is useful to draw out the Punnet square for these types of questions.

Table A-21 Punnet square of two silent carriers of α-thalassemia

	$-\alpha$	$\alpha\,\alpha$
α	$-\alpha/-\alpha$ (α trait)	$-\alpha/\alpha\,\alpha$ (silent)
$\alpha\,\alpha$	$\alpha\,\alpha/-\alpha$ (silent)	$\alpha\,\alpha/\alpha\,\alpha$ (normal)

2. D β-Thalassemia major is an autosomal-recessive disease. Using the **Hardy-Weinberg equation:** $p^2 + 2pq + q^2$; p^2 (normal genotype, β/β), q^2 (homozygous disease genotype, $\beta°/\beta°$), and $2pq$ (heterozygous genotype $\beta/\beta°$). Therefore, $q^2 = 1/1600$, $q = 1/40$ (or 0.025). Using the fact that $p + q = 1$; $p = 0.975$. The probability for heterozygosity is $2pq$ or $2\,(0.975)\,(0.025) \approx 1/20$.

Case 22

1. D During an osmotic fragility test, a patient's RBCs are mixed with salt solutions of varying concentration. As the salt concentration decreases, the solution becomes more hypotonic, and water seeks to move into the cell, causing it to burst. Normal RBCs lyse at about 50% NaCl. Fragile cells tolerate less water influx, causing them to burst at higher concentrations of salt.

2. C Plasma haptoglobin would be decreased because more of it is complexed to free Hb (released during hemolysis). The Hb-haptoglobin complex is taken up by liver cells, leaving less in the plasma.

Case 23

1. F This is a normocytic anemia that makes iron deficiency and thalassemia (microcytic) and vitamin B_{12} deficiency (macrocytic) less likely. There is no evidence of a hemolytic anemia (the bilirubin is normal and the patient is not jaundiced). Hereditary spherocytosis would show spherocytes on the peripheral blood smear. There is no evidence that this patient is bleeding acutely.

Given the progressive renal failure, it is likely that this patient's kidneys are unable to produce normal amounts of erythropoietin to stimulate RBC production, resulting in this clinical picture.

2. A Polycythemia vera (PV) is characterized by erythrocytosis, leukocytosis, thrombocytosis, splenomegaly, and decreased erythropoietin. In PV, red cells are produced independently of erythropoietin. Secondary causes of polycythemia (hypoxia, tumors) are associated with increased erythropoietin.

Case 24

1. C This correctly describes the direct Coombs' test. Choice A describes the indirect Coombs' test, which is the procedure used for blood "type and screening" before a transfusion.

2. A RhoGAM is given to all Rh-negative pregnant women at 28 weeks' gestation and when they undergo any procedures where fetal cells may be introduced into maternal circulation (e.g., amniocentesis). It is given again postpartum to any Rh-negative women who have delivered an Rh-positive baby. RhoGAM prevents the formation of anti-D (Rh) IgG antibodies, which could potentially cross the placenta during a subsequent pregnancy, and which might otherwise cause hemolytic anemia of a Rh-positive fetus. IgM antibodies do not cross the placenta. Because RhoGAM (IgG anti-D antibodies) is given in a small quantity, it does not cause hemolytic disease of the newborn. Rh-positive women do not need RhoGAM because they will not mount an antibody response to the anti-D antigen.

Case 25

1. B FXII deficiency is unique in its ability to increase a patient's PTT yet not lead to clinical bleeding episodes. The current recommendation with FXII deficiency is to proceed with any planned surgeries and inform the family that it is unlikely the patient will ever express a bleeding disorder. It is important to inform the patient in case the lab work is repeated later in life.

2. E The transmission of HIV and other infectious organisms to hemophiliacs is a highly sensitive issue that has involved the medical, legal, and government arenas. Severe hemophiliacs have received purified blood products for over a decade, and new technology has produced recombinant FVIII, which involves in some cases little, and in others no, human blood derivatives. Many parents and patients who lived through the 1980s will be concerned about their own or their child's safety on replacement therapy. This issue should be discussed when patients with severe hemophilia start a prophylactic treatment program.

3. A Patients with mild hemophilia A rarely present with bleeding unless it is due to trauma or surgery. Following significant trauma, bleeding is a concern for any patient with factor levels less than 30%, and in very severe cases—less than 50%. Labs on this patient indicate a FVIII activity of 14%, a prolonged PTT, and a normal PT. Recombinant FVIII replacement therapy was provided to a 100% correction due to the possibility of brain trauma and hemorrhage.

4. E Briefly following birth, some children experience decreased vitamin K levels and thus slightly elevated PT and PTT values. In this case description, the repeated times are normal following this dip, indicating no suspected coagulopathy. The presentation of repeated bruising with rib fractures that have continued over time is highly suspect of child abuse. While domestic abuse, by law, does not require reporting to protective services, in abuse of children and the elderly reporting is required, and it is an offense if it is not done within strict time guidelines. It is important to know the state's and specific hospital's policies on reporting suspected child/elder abuse.

Case 26

1. C von Willebrand's disease is the most common inherited bleeding disorder. Deficiencies in vWF occur in 1% of the population and are equal between genders, ethnicities, and ages. Von Willebrand's disease follows an autosomal-dominant inheritance pattern. Knowledge of their family history allows patients to be tested and provide treatment in the case of excessive menorrhagia, surgery, or trauma.

2. B Following activation of platelets and during plug formation, the contents of their granules are released, furthering the clotting process. Within α-platelet granules are fibrinogen, FV, vWF, thrombospondin, and platelet factor 4. Within δ-platelet granules are ADP, serotonin, calcium, and lysosomal enzymes. Deficiencies of these proteins result in storage pool disease and abnormal platelet function. VWF is unique in its ability to act as a carrier protein for FVIII. Cueing the release of vWF also increases circulating FVIII levels.

3. E Only type 3 vWD includes a clinical presentation of hemarthroses in addition to a quantitative decrease in vWF. Quantitative reductions occur in types 1 and 3. Type 2 vWD is a functional deficiency with no quantitative loss. Type 2A is a decrease in high molecular weight multimers, type 2M vWF contains a mutated GPIb binding site, and type 2N vWF lacks affinity for FVIII.

4. B The type of bleeding rules out either form of hemophilia from the differential. Due to the inheritance pattern described, von Willebrand's disease is unlikely. Differentiating between Glanzmann's thrombasthenia and Bernard-Soulier disease is possible based on the aggregation studies. In this case, poor aggregation is seen with both ristocetin and thrombin. This allows the diagnosis of Bernard-Soulier disease to be made.

Case 27

1. C Congenital leukocyte adhesion deficiencies (LAD) cause defects in tight adhesion of leukocytes and can lead to deficits in recruitment of neutrophils toward a site of tissue damage and infection and can cause poor wound healing. Release of chemokines from the site of injury will occur normally and induce proliferation and release of neutrophils from the bone marrow, causing a leukocytosis and neutrophilia. However, neutrophils will not properly bind

to endothelial cells and subsequent diapedesis and migration toward the site of injury will be impaired leading to poor wound healing in such patients. Answers D to F are incorrect because WBC and absolute neutrophil count would both normally increase in response to cytokines released by tissue damage. Answers A and B are incorrect as LAD is associated with poor wound healing with paradoxical neutrophilia.

2. B The triad of rheumatoid arthritis, neutropenia, and splenomegaly suggests Felty's syndrome. While congenital causes of neutropenia usually present in early childhood, it is feasible for a patient to present later in his or her teenage years. Large granular his or her lymphocytosis (LGL), a disorder of clonal proliferation of neutrophil-killing NK-cells or T-cells, is also associated with autoimmune disease like rheumatoid arthritis, and may present with neutropenia and splenomegaly. However, SR's CBC reveals a low WBC count with an isolated neutropenia, while LGL should cause a lymphocytosis from the clonal proliferation of the abnormal lymphocyte; thus C is incorrect. Answers A and D are incorrect, as these diseases are expected to produce either highly elevated WBC counts with abnormal blasts (in acute leukemia) or myeloid precursors (in chronic myeloid leukemia) on blood smear. Lastly, E is incorrect, as myelofibrosis with myeloid metaplasia is associated with a pancytopenia in late stages of the disease, and teardrop-shaped red blood cells, immature myeloid cells, and giant platelets on the peripheral blood smear.

Case 28

1. D Fanconi's anemia is unlikely the cause of AA's aplastic anemia as defined by his peripheral pancytopenia with hypocellular bone marrow. Such congenital anomalies are more likely to present earlier in life rather than at the advanced age of 68 years. Other clues in the history make possible several etiologies of aplastic anemia. His recent viral infection after visiting his granddaughter who had been ill with a fever and rash suggests parvovirus B19 infection as a possible cause. Children with this infection may present with fever and the "slapped cheek" rash, while adults may present with nonspecific pharyngitis, abdominal discomfort, and arthralgias from immune complex deposition. His history of hepatitis with negative serologies in fact may be from the as-yet-unidentified hepatitis virus thought to precede many cases of aplastic anemia. The mechanism of this disease is thought to arise from a cross-reactivity of the immune response to the virus causing autoimmunity to hematopoietic precursors. Benzene exposure (from working in a petroleum plant) is also related to aplastic anemias. Lastly, even subclinical deficiencies in hematopoiesis, as in sickle cell trait, can predispose one to fulminant aplastic anemia if newly infected with a hematopoietic cell-tropic virus, such as CMV or EBV.

2. C Parvovirus B19 is the most unlikely cause of her pancytopenia as this is usually accompanied by a significant but transient hypocellular bone marrow. Poor nutrition is a common cause of pancytopenia among elderly, especially those with comorbid conditions and poor social structure. Such patients are susceptible to vitamin B_{12} and folate deficiency from poor food intake. Otherwise, older patients can develop an autoimmune condition that targets **intrinsic factor,** a protein that binds to vitamin B$_{12}$ and aids its absorption in the terminal ileum. Loss of this protein's function can cause pernicious anemia, a condition where normal hematopoiesis is inhibited by the absence of a necessary substrate for nucleic acid synthesis, vitamin B$_{12}$. Lastly, both drugs and alcohol cause pancytopenia by ill-defined mechanisms. The diseases mentioned above are often associated with a cellular bone marrow.

Case 29

1. C The clinical presentation indicates in the first sentence the likely finding of generalized stem cell deficiency. Pallor and fatigue are mentioned to illustrate the presentation of anemia. Infection is likely due to a neutropenic state. The petechiae and ecchymoses are due to the patient's thrombocytopenia. As mentioned previously, the most likely cause of this state is generalized bone marrow failure, i.e., stem cell depletion. Stem cell depletion presents microscopically, as described in answer C. Lab values expected would include thrombocytopenia, neutropenia, and anemia.

2. D Obstetric complications are by far the most common cause of DIC. DIC is a highly significant concern not only in premature births but also throughout pregnancy. Complications such as amniotic fluid embolism, premature separation of the placenta, eclampsia, retained placenta, and septic abortions may lead to DIC. If the fetus is near term, C-section may be required to save both the mother and baby.

3, 4. E, B Pertinent negatives described in the clinical presentation allow the proper diagnosis to be made. Based on the patient's labs, aplastic anemia is ruled out. Mention of prior infection or symptoms such as diarrhea would be necessary to suspect hemolytic uremic syndrome. Systemic lupus erythematosus presents with systemic findings and connective tissue symptoms. The lack of neurologic findings decreases the likelihood of thrombotic thrombocytopenic purpura. Her thrombocytopenia is therefore a result of idiopathic thrombocytopenic purpura. The molecular basis of ITP is the formation of an autoantibody that cross-reacts with glycoprotein IIb/IIIa or glycoprotein Ib complex.

Case 30

1. A Factor V Leiden mutation is the most common inherited thrombophilia yet discovered. Until 1994 the link of 40% of hereditary thrombophilia to this mutation was unknown.

2. A The half-lives of the clotting factors inhibited by warfarin (Coumadin) are important to know since they determine the length of double therapy required with another anticoagulant. Factor VII has a half-life of less than 24 hours. Thrombin's half-life is just under 5 days. Only after this amount of time is it safe to switch a patient to single therapy of warfarin.

3. B Coumadin prevents the normal activity of vitamin K in the γ-carboxylation of the glutamic acid residues within serine proteases (factors II, VII, IX, and X). A prolonged PT and PTT result from Coumadin therapy or intoxication due to FVII's role in the extrinsic pathway and FIX's role within the intrinsic pathway. Platelet counts are not affected by Coumadin therapy.

4. D Patients presenting with recurrent thrombotic events and multiple miscarriages have a high likelihood of an antiphospholipid antibody syndrome. In this case, the specific antibody is thought to be related to the patient's comorbid SLE. Unique to this thrombophilia, an elevated PTT is observed due to the lupus anticoagulant. This presentation without the elevated PTT is possible in women on hormone therapy or with other autoimmune diseases.

Case 31

1. D Enoxaparin (low molecular weight heparin) has many benefits over standard heparin, which includes reduced rates of HIT and osteoporosis. However, for patients who have already developed HIT from standard heparin, a significant degree of cross-reactivity exists. In most cases, a direct thrombin inhibitor is preferred such as hirudin, lepirudin, or argatroban.

2. C Warfarin antidote is a combination of vitamin K and fresh frozen plasma. Protamine is an antidote for heparin overdose. Aminocaproic acid is the recommended treatment for tPA or streptokinase overdose. Flumazenil provides the antidote for benzodiazepine overdose.

3. E Treatment of cerebral strokes may include urokinase, streptokinase, or tPA. However, the imaging studies reveal a possible cerebral hemorrhage, which in the majority of cases rules out fibrinolytic therapy. If fibrinolytic therapy were necessary, tPA would be recommended over urokinase or streptokinase due to its localization to thrombi. This is achieved by tPA's selectively increased affinity to fibrin.

Case 32

1. E This African American male fits the demographic for G6PD deficiency. The antimalarial quinine drug has precipitated a bout of hemolysis by causing an increase in free radicals. You would also expect to see Heinz bodies within RBCs on the peripheral smear. Answer A describes warm-reacting antibody hemolysis, and answers B and D describe cold-reacting antibody hemolysis. Answer C is the mechanism for microangiopathic hemolytic anemia.

2. B This woman has the classic symptoms of thrombotic thrombocytopenic purpura (TTP): fever, anemia, thrombocytopenia, and renal and neurologic abnormalities. TTP is one of the causes of microangiopathic hemolytic anemia, which is characterized by schistocytes on the blood smear (fragmentation due to damage over microthrombi in small vessels). Bite cells are seen in G6PD deficiency; target cells in thalassemias; spherocytes in autoimmune hemolytic anemias and hereditary spherocytosis; hypersegmented PMNs in folate and vitamin B$_{12}$ deficiencies.

Case 33

1. B Anemia, bone pain, and blurry vision are most likely due to multiple myeloma. Anemia is almost universal in multiple myeloma. Bone pain occurs from bone marrow replacement with neoplastic plasmacytic cells. Blurry vision is associated with blood hyperviscosity due to elevated paraprotein (or IgM produced by the malignancy). Waldenstrom's macroglobulinemia is not usually associated with bone pain. The other lymphomas listed primarily involve lymph nodes and lymphoid tissue and only later spread to bone marrow. They would least likely present with bone pain and anemia. Therefore, answers A, C, D, and E are incorrect.

2. B The identification of Reed-Sternberg (RS) cells first classifies the lymphoma as Hodgkin's disease. Staging is then the next most important predictor of prognosis. Single-node involvement is classified as stage 1, multiple nodes on the same side of the diaphragm as stage 2, nodal involvement traversing the diaphragm as stage 3, and diffuse involvement as stage 4. The patient also does not have fever, night sweats, or weight loss and thus is considered category A. Overall, she is expected to have a good outcome, with high likelihood of cure. Thus, she does not have stage IIA or IB HD. Also, given the fact that RS cells were identified, she does not have non-Hodgkin's lymphoma (NHL), such as follicular lymphoma or large diffuse B-cell lymphoma.

3. C The lymphomas associated with HIV are Hodgkin's disease, diffuse large B-cell lymphoma, and Burkitt's lymphoma. Anergy due to T-cell dysfunction can be due to advanced HIV or Hodgkin's disease. Impaired T-cell function can predispose one to fungal and mycobacterial disease and may cause the recrudescence of previous mycobacterial infection. B-symptoms can result from the lymphoma or mycobacterial infection. Multiple myeloma is the least possible etiology of this clinical presentation, as it is a B-cell disorder and less likely associated with T-cell dysfunction and more so with anemia, bone pain, and hyperviscosity; therefore, C is the least likely to explain her symptoms.

Case 34

1. B Actinic keratosis is only a precursor lesion for squamous cell carcinoma. Excessive sunlight exposure and chronic inflammatory skin conditions predispose to both squamous cell and basal cell carcinomas. Tanning salons use equipment that emit ultraviolet A and B radiation, which are just as damaging to the skin as sunlight, and increase the risk of both squamous cell and basal cell malignancies. Dysplastic nevi are precursors of melanoma.

2. C Keratin pearls (circular whorls of keratinization) are the histologic hallmark of squamous cell cancer. Acanthosis is abnormal epidermal thickening often seen in chronic inflammatory conditions. Basal cell carcinoma cells are "basaloid" in appearance with palisading nuclei. Basal cell carcinoma is histologically most similar to follicular cells.

3. A The vast majority of basal cell carcinomas arise on the structures of the head and neck, most prominently the nose and ears.

However, remember that there are no hard-and-fast rules; any location may potentially give rise to skin malignancy, so be sure to biopsy all suspicious lesions!

Case 35

1. E The most worrisome characteristic of any lesion is a history of change in color, shape, or size. In this case, although the lesion is not technically enlarged (it is < 6 mm diameter), a history of enlargement of the mole is concerning for melanoma. The presence of multiple colors suggesting a "mottled appearance" would be more worrisome than a single shade of dark brown. Neither advanced age nor gender are associated with increased rates of melanoma, although men have worse survival rates once the disease is diagnosed.

2. D Large congenital nevi greatly increase the risk of developing melanoma. Erythema multiforme is a rash that is triggered by the herpes virus. Actinic keratoses are skin lesions composed of atypical keratinocytes, and are considered precursor lesions for squamous cell carcinoma of the skin. Psoriasiform dermatitis (psoriasis) is an inflammatory dermatitis characterized by a chronic scaly rash. History of previous skin surgery is not a risk factor for melanoma.

3. C Overall prognosis is most closely associated with tumor thickness, which is a rough indicator of volume and depth of invasion. As such, tumor thickness is a predictor of the ability of the melanoma to metastasize. Remember that melanoma is curable before metastasis, but generally fatal after metastasis occurs. Histologic grade is not as strongly associated with prognosis. Family history of melanoma and fair skin are both risk factors for the development of melanoma, but are not predictors of outcome. Positive margins at initial biopsy would be followed up with surgical reexcision, which should adequately establish control over the cancer.

Case 36

1. C Neurofibromatosis type 2 (NF2) is a multisystem genetic disorder associated with bilateral vestibular schwannomas, spinal cord schwannomas, meningiomas, gliomas, and juvenile cataracts. The manifestations of NF2 result from mutations in (or rarely deletion of) the *NF2* tumor suppressor gene located on the long arm of chromosome 22. Half of affected individuals have NF2 as a result of a new (de novo) gene mutation. Neurofibromatosis type 1 (NF1) is a multisystem genetic disorder that commonly is associated with cutaneous (café-au-lait spots), neurologic (optic nerve gliomas), and orthopedic (arthroses or dysplasias) manifestations. Li-Fraumeni syndrome (LFS) is a cancer predisposition syndrome associated with soft tissue sarcoma, breast cancer, leukemia, osteosarcoma, melanoma, and cancer of the colon, pancreas, adrenal cortex, and brain (medulloblastoma, gliomas). The combination of parathyroid tumors, pancreatic islet cell tumors, and pituitary hyperplasia or tumor formation is called MEN-I. MEN-III (or IIB) includes pheochromocytoma, medullary carcinoma and multiple mucocutaneous neuromas.

2. E The multiple lesions spanning both cerebral hemispheres is a tipoff for metastatic disease. Statistically, this answer is your best bet because metastatic brain tumors account for over 50% of all intracranial tumors. Pilocytic astrocytomas are often well-circumscribed, localized lesions. Meningiomas are external to the brain and most frequently occur in the convexities of the cerebral hemispheres. Medulloblastomas are found in the cerebellum and are found mostly in children.

Case 37

1. D Alcohol potentiates the carcinogenic effects of chronic HBV infection by adding to the cycle of hepatocyte injury and regeneration. The more the cells in a tumor divide, the more likely a tumorigenic genetic mutation will occur within that cell population. Thus alcohol consumption, even at moderate levels, can accelerate one's development of HCC; thus, E is incorrect. The patient's level of alcohol consumption is unlikely to have produced alcoholic cirrhosis; thus, A is incorrect. He probably did not inherit a genetic predisposition toward development of HCC. Instead, he "inherited" an infection by vertical transmission of HBV from his mother, which predisposed him to developing HCC; thus, B is incorrect. Chronic alcoholism can cause immunosuppression, but usually only in severe alcoholics with poor nutrition; LS does not fit this picture; thus, C is incorrect.

2. E α_1-Antitrypsin deficiency is an autosomal-recessive disorder caused by a deficiency in an antiprotease, a major inhibitor of the tissue-damaging enzyme neutrophilic elastase. This leads to a syndrome that arises from increased susceptibility to tissue degradation. Among the clinical manifestations of this disease is early-onset emphysema in individuals who have even minimal histories of cigarette smoking. This arises from unopposed activity of the neutrophilic elastase, causing destruction of the elastin in alveolar walls of the lung. Another manifestation is chronic hepatic injury. Chronic cirrhosis from this disease can predispose someone to developing hepatocellular carcinoma. Aflatoxin exposure is a possibility but is unlikely in the U.S. Aflatoxin is a product of *Aspergillus flavus* present on improperly stored peanuts, common in Africa and the Far East, and is strongly associated with the development of hepatocellular carcinoma; thus, A is incorrect. Given his negative serology for HBV and HCV, his HCC is unlikely from infectious etiologies; thus, B and C are incorrect. His level of alcohol consumption is unlikely to be sufficient for developing alcoholic cirrhosis as a precursor to HCC; thus, D is incorrect.

Case 38

1. D Benign tumors are expected to have normal cellular morphology as well as good adherence to normal tissue architecture. High nucleus-to-cytoplasm ratio, frequent mitotic spindles, loss of glandular structure, and anaplasia suggest poorly differentiated malignant cells. Thus, answers A, B, C, and E are incorrect.

2. B It would be inappropriate to do a fine-needle aspiration for this woman given the fact that she has no palpable breast mass. Normally, one would use radiographically guided needle biopsy directed toward the clustering of microcalcification. For the most part, microcalcifications are highly specific for ductal carcinoma, which warrants open biopsy with sentinel node dissection. The sentinel node is the draining lymph node of the breast tissue suspected to be involved and would be detected using dye or radioisotope injected into the tumor site preoperatively, which is subsequently detected intraoperatively and then removed. Prior to these invasive diagnostic procedures, it would also be appropriate to perform a breast ultrasound to look for masses.

Case 39

1. A Hyperplastic glands arranged back to back are histologic patterns expected in well-differentiated tumors. PC has a high-grade, poorly differentiated tumor. Frequent bizarre mitotic spindles suggest cytogenetic instability that may arise from *as well as* lead to genetic rearrangements that give rise to greater anaplasia. High nucleus-to-cytoplasm ratio and hyperchromatic nucleus also appear in high-grade tumors. Lastly, as the tumor proliferates rapidly, outgrowing its vascular supply, unless adequate neovascularization occurs to keep up with the rate of tumor growth, there may be central areas of necrosis, representing tumor cells that have died due to lack of oxygen and nutrients.

2. D The development of a second primary prostatic tumor is a highly unlikely event, especially under the pressure of anti-androgen therapy. Tumor cells that normally respond to the growth-stimulating signal of endogenous testosterone are deprived of this stimulus via antiandrogen therapy. A random mutation may give rise to an androgen-independent clone. Such a cell will necessarily outgrow those cells that require androgen stimulation. Eventually, these finasteride-resistant cells will make up the majority of tumor, and the tumor will grow despite this therapy. Thus, A and C are incorrect answers. The likelihood of this random mutation occurring may have increased secondary to the loss of the DNA repair function of *p53*. Thus, B is incorrect. Lastly, any genetic mutation can give a cell and its progenitors a selective advantage over other cells. Such phenotypes include any phenotype yielding rapid, perhaps uncontrolled, cell proliferation. Thus, E is incorrect.

Case 40

1. B An older patient with a rapidly growing thyroid nodule should lead one to suspect anaplastic thyroid carcinoma, although this requires biopsy and histologic characterization to diagnose. Anaplastic carcinoma can arise de novo, from chronic inflammatory or hyperplastic thyroid diseases, or from undetected well-differentiated thyroid cancers, like papillary carcinoma. The cancer may arise in a rapidly proliferating thyroid gland that has lost the important cancer-suppressing function of *p53*, leading to rapid progression toward malignant transformation. Thus this cancer is the least differentiated and most aggressive thyroid cancer and carries with it a very poor prognosis. All the other cancers are possible but unlikely; however, they can only be ruled out with fine-needle biopsy. Thus, A, C, and D are incorrect. Anaplastic carcinoma may arise from multinodular goiter, as chronic thyroid cell hyperplasia may increase the chance of developing cancer-promoting genetic mutations. But given the patient's solitary nodule, she is unlikely to have *multinodular* goiter. Also, her normal thyroid function tests are more concerning for malignancy than they would be if they were abnormal. Thus, E is incorrect.

2. E Proliferation of normal thyroid cells through TSH stimulation is insufficient for the development of a neoplastic thyroid nodule. Carcinogenesis requires the acquisition of a cancer-promoting genetic mutation for *initiation* of neoplastic growth. Without this step, the development of cancer is impossible. In fact, there are many forms of physiologic cellular proliferation that the body must be able to do in order to carry out its normal functions, including glandular proliferation of breast tissue for breast milk production and endometrial proliferation during a woman's reproductive cycle. All these processes can proceed without necessarily giving rise to cancer. It is the tight regulation of genetic integrity by DNA pair mechanisms that keep this from happening. However, papillary thyroid carcinoma can arise from radiation-induced mutation of the *RET* proto-oncogene, giving rise to a constitutively active tyrosine kinase signaling continuous cell growth. Thus, A is incorrect. Chronic exposure to mutagenic irradiation may increase the likelihood of developing the *RET* proto-oncogene mutation, either directly or through the development of defective DNA repair. Thus, B is incorrect. Normal physiologic cellular proliferation may also propagate a genetic mutation if a faulty genetic sequence is read by the cell's replicative machinery before it has been repaired. This mutated sequence is carried on to the next generation as a chemically "normal" entity and is thus no longer detectable by the cell's DNA repair mechanisms. Thus, C is incorrect. Tumor growth subsequently results from rapid proliferation of cells that have acquired crucial cancer-promoting genetic mutations, usually yielding the phenotype of unregulated growth. This is a fundamental characteristic of a neoplasm. Thus, D is incorrect.

Case 41

1. D A defect in a DNA repair gene does not directly transform a cell toward unregulated proliferation. Instead, these defects increase the likelihood that cell will develop such genetic mutations. In the case of the familial disease of HNPCC, family members must undergo routine screening for colon cancer, as they have inherited one defective DNA mismatch repair gene in all their somatic cells (the first "hit") in a way that puts all their colonic epithelial cells at risk for developing into a cell homozygous for the defect. Loss of both genes will lead to a cell that is impaired in its abilities to maintain the integrity of the genome. This increases the likelihood of developing errors in many growth- and cell cycle-regulating genes that can subsequently transform the cell into a rapidly proliferating cell. Answers A, B, C, and E are included in the pathogenesis of HNPCC, and these are incorrect answers.

2. D Overabundance of *bcl-2* expression does NOT lead to uncontrolled cellular proliferation. Instead, *bcl-2* provides an *antiapoptotic signal,* which promotes *cell survival* rather than cell division. This is a very important distinction. This illustrates that even the persistence of a cell beyond its programmed life span is also a cancer-promoting event, as it defies the normal cycle of cell death and regeneration. It can be overexpressed in the case of Burkitt's lymphoma wherein the *bcl-2* open reading frame is translocated to a sort of "pro-

moter" region of the immunoglobulin heavy chain, which, if stimulated to produce heavy chain, will produce *bcl-2* transcripts instead. Thus, A, B, and C are incorrect. The abundance of *bcl-2,* which eventually forms *bcl-2* homodimers, mediates signaling that favors cell survival. Thus, E is incorrect. There are many more steps in the development of Burkitt's lymphoma. However, for the purpose of the board exam, it is important to understand the concept of apoptosis regulation as a step in the pathogenesis of cancer.

Case 42

1. E Ewing's sarcoma is characterized by small round blue-staining cells. This patient fits the demographic of patients affected by the disease. Multiple myeloma is a plasma cell disorder that causes lytic lesions in the bones, but is extremely rare in children. Giant cell tumors are characterized by multinucleated giant cells and most commonly affects young to middle-aged women. Metastatic bone disease is rare in children. Osteosarcoma consists of spindle cells and osteoid formation.

2. D Lung metastases are common in both osteosarcoma and Ewing's sarcoma. Giant cell tumors have aggressive growth, but are considered benign; they do not spread outside of the bone.

Case 43

1. D The villous adenoma is the most likely to be a stage III colorectal cancer, or a carcinoma that invades the entirety of the bowel wall and spreads earlier to the lymph nodes than all the other tumor types. Tubular adenomas and tubulovillous adenomas are more pedunculated than villous adenomas, and thus are less likely to have invaded beyond the mucosal layer because of this extra margin of tissue separating the anatomic locations; thus, A and C are incorrect. Carcinoma in situ, by definition, is a tumor that has not invaded beyond the lamina propria and remains within the mucosal layer; thus, B is incorrect. A juvenile polyp is hamartoma and is inherently benign, and very rarely goes beyond the mucosal layer; thus, is incorrect.

2. D This 25-year-old woman is least likely to have the sporadic form of colorectal cancer, given her age (it is possible, but very unlikely). Sporadic forms of colorectal cancer are thought to develop from the acquisition of two mutations, nonfunctional cancer-related genes (e.g., tumor-suppressor or proto-oncogene). That requires developing a mutation in a single gene, then developing it *again* in the same gene on the other chromosome in the same cell line of the original cell that first acquired the mutation, a highly unlikely event. This is thought to be possible, however, over many decades of gradually accumulating random mutations in colonic epithelial cells (probably due to chronic exposure to unknown carcinogens in our diets). Thus the acquired form of colorectal cancer tends to develop later in life. Those with *familial* forms of colorectal cancer have already acquired a mutated, poorly functioning or nonfunctioning gene in *all* their somatic cells. All they need is the acquisition of a mutation in the normal functioning gene copy in just *one* cell out of millions of somatic cells to set off the process of carcinogenesis; thus, E is included in the differential and therefore is an incorrect answer. Bowel changes can occur with infectious gastroenteritis causing diarrhea. Dehydration from diarrhea can also cause constipation, fatigue, and weakness; therefore, B is an incorrect answer. Alternating bouts of constipation and diarrhea can occur with both inflammatory bowel disease (IBD) and irritable bowel syndrome (IBS). While IBD is associated with distinct pathologic findings, IBS is thought to be a *functional* disease, not correlated with any gross or histologic pathology; thus, A and C are incorrect answers.

3. E All the above diagnostic tests are reasonable tests to order, with the exception of the flexible sigmoidoscopy. The presence of iron deficiency anemia without symptoms suggestive of obstruction suggests a right-sided or proximal lesion. Flexible sigmoidoscopy would be inadequate in evaluating a proximal lesion, as it does not reach far enough into the colon to evaluate the proximal colon. Colonoscopy would be the only useful endoscopic diagnostic test; thus, B would be included and is an incorrect answer. All the other diagnostic tests are included in the standard diagnostic work-up for this patient.

Case 44

1. C Most childhood ALL is of the L1 subtype, which morphologically consists of small uniform blast cells. Initial cytologic screening would reveal TdT+ blast cells but no Auer rods, myeloperoxidase, or nonspecific esterase activity. Once lymphoid lineage is determined, it is further subtyped to B- vs. T-cell leukemias. The primitive B-cell leukemia is common, staining with surface antigens CD10, CD19, CD20, CD21, CD22. CD7 falls under the category of T-cell leukemias whose surface antigens consist of CD2, 3, 5, and 7, (Hint: CD-prime numbers under 10) as well as CD4 and CD8 in more mature T-cells.

2. E All of the above are possible explanations for different aspects of the clinical case. Hyperuricemia occurs from the rapid lysis of a large cell load as found in acute leukemia as a breakdown product of nucleic acids. This can induce an acute exacerbation of gouty arthritis, which is caused by the deposition

of uric acid crystals in joints, causing inflammation and pain. Bone pain can be caused by the rapid expansion of leukemic cells in the bone marrow. The femur is a common site of bone pain from leukemia. Recent ingestion of meat can also cause exacerbation of gouty arthritis by introducing a large nucleic acid load into the body, thereby causing hyperuricemia. If the meat were contaminated, this may explain her fever and leukocytosis. Lastly, people taking corticosteroids chronically are immunocompromised and are susceptible to serious infections like osteomyelitis, an infection of the joint, which can be fatal if untreated. This would explain her knee pain, fever, and leukocytosis as well.

Case 45

1. A The most important point of this question is that a markedly elevated WBC, especially $> 100{,}000/\mu L$ should prompt immediate work-up for malignancy. Answers B to D are leukemias that can produce such high leukocytosis. This level of leukocytosis is rarely caused by infection.

2. C Perirectal abscesses are usually caused by granulocyte dysfunction rather than thrombocytosis. Thrombocytosis is associated with thrombotic and thromboembolic phenomenon from activation of high concentrations of platelets, leading to vasoocclusive diseases such as myocardial infarction, stroke, deep venous thrombosis, and pulmonary embolism. Thus, A, B, D, and E are incorrect.

3. C Isolated lymphadenopathy without hepatosplenomegaly is usually associated with a lymphoid-origin leukemia, the most common being CLL. Therefore, the WBC would be elevated usually in the range of 10,000 to $150{,}000/\mu L$ with normal hematocrit and platelet count. Answer A reflects a CBC and differential of reactive lymphocytosis due to infection, as reflected by the neutrophilia and bandemia. Answer B reflects the profile for CML with marked leukocytosis and myeloid precursors present in peripheral circulation. Answer D reflects the profile for acute leukemia as reflected by pancytopenia (neutropenia, anemia, and thrombocytopenia) accompanied by the presence of blast cells in peripheral circulation. Finally, answer E reflects a normal CBC.

Index

Index note: page references with *f, b,* or *t* indicate a figure, box or table.